Metacognition, Metahumanities, and Medical Education

This persuasive volume develops a novel approach to medical education and medical humanities, making a case for the integration of the two to explore the ways in which 'warm' humanism and 'cold' technologies can come together to design humane posthumanist futures in medicine.

There are many problems with conventional medical education. It can be overly technocratic, dehumanising, and empathy-eroding, introducing artefacts that lead to harm and reproduce inequality and injustice. Use of the arts, humanities, and qualitative social sciences has been pursued as an antidote or balance to these problems. Arguing against the purely instrumentalist use of medical humanities in this way, this book addresses the importance of a genuine and open-ended engagement with humanities approaches in medicine. It discusses the impact of artificial intelligence and emerging theoretical frameworks and posthumanist perspectives, such as object-oriented ontology, on meaning making in medicine. It demonstrates how the key to such a transition is the recovery of the intrinsic art and humanity of metaphor-heavy biomedical science, in turn framed by models of dynamic complexity rather than static linearity.

This book is an important contribution to debates around the medical humanities and its role in medical education. It is an essential read for scholars with an interest in these areas, as well as those working in science and technology studies and the sociology of health and illness.

Alan Bleakley is Emeritus Professor of Medical Education and Medical Humanities at Plymouth University Peninsula School of Medicine, UK. He is Past President of the Association for Medical Humanities.

Rachel Ellaway is Professor in the Department of Community Health Sciences and Director of the Office of Health and Medical Education Scholarship at the Cumming School of Medicine, University of Calgary, Alberta, Canada. She is also Editor in Chief of the journal *Advances in Health Sciences Education.*

Quentin Eichbaum is Professor of Pathology, Immunology and Microbiology at Vanderbilt University Medical Centre, where he co-directs the Transfusion Medicine Service, and Professor of Medical Education and Administration at Vanderbilt University School of Medicine where he was Assistant Dean and developed and directed the College Colloquium medical humanities programme.

Routledge Advances in the Medical Humanities

Rethinking Pain in Person-Centred Health Care
Around Recovery
Stephen Buetow

Medical Education, Politics and Social Justice
The Contradiction Cure
Alan Bleakley

Poetry in the Clinic
Towards a Lyrical Medicine
Alan Bleakley and Shane Neilson

Critical Humanities and Ageing
Forging Interdisciplinary Dialogues
Edited by Marlene Goldman, Kate de Medeiros and Thomas Cole

Palliative Care Nursing as Mindfulness
Embodying a Relational Ethic through Strong Emotion, Uncertainty and Death
Lacie White

From Loneliness to Solitude in Person-centred Health Care
Stephen Buetow

Ageism and Person-Centred Care
Rehabilitating Bias for Age-Friendly Practice
Stephen Buetow

Metacognition, Metahumanities, and Medical Education
Thinking Without the Box
Alan Bleakley, Rachel Ellaway and Quentin Eichbaum

For more information about this series visit: www.routledge.com/Routledge-Advances-in-the-Medical-Humanities/book-series/RAMH

Metacognition, Metahumanities, and Medical Education

Thinking Without the Box

Alan Bleakley, Rachel Ellaway, and Quentin Eichbaum

Routledge
Taylor & Francis Group
LONDON AND NEW YORK

First published 2025
by Routledge
4 Park Square, Milton Park, Abingdon, Oxon OX14 4RN

and by Routledge
605 Third Avenue, New York, NY 10158

Routledge is an imprint of the Taylor & Francis Group, an informa business

British Library Cataloguing-in-Publication Data
A catalogue record for this book is available from the British Library

Library of Congress Cataloging-in-Publication Data
Names: Bleakley, Alan (Alan Douglas), author. | Eichbaum, Quentin G., author. | Ellaway, Rachel, author.
Title: Metacognition, metahumanities, and medical education : thinking without the box / Dr Alan Bleakley, Dr Rachel Ellaway and Dr Quentin Eichbaum.
Description: Abingdon, Oxon ; New York, NY : Routledge, 2025. | Includes bibliographical references and index.
Identifiers: LCCN 2024026180 (print) | LCCN 2024026181 (ebook) | ISBN 9781032687322 (hardback) | ISBN 9781032696898 (paperback) | ISBN 9781032687339 (ebook)
Subjects: LCSH: Medical education. | Medical education--Philosophy. | Medical education--Social aspects. | Metacognition.
Classification: LCC R737 .B57 2025 (print) | LCC R737 (ebook) | DDC 610.71/1--dc23/eng/20240708
LC record available at https://lccn.loc.gov/2024026180
LC ebook record available at https://lccn.loc.gov/2024026181

ISBN: 978-1-032-68732-2 (hbk)
ISBN: 978-1-032-69689-8 (pbk)
ISBN: 978-1-032-68733-9 (ebk)

DOI: 10.4324/9781032687339

Typeset in Times New Roman
by SPi Technologies India Pvt Ltd (Straive)

Contents

Illustrations

Figures

Tables

Authors

Dr Alan Bleakley is Emeritus Professor of Medical Education and Medical Humanities at Plymouth University Peninsula School of Medicine, UK. He is Past President of the Association for Medical Humanities.

Dr Rachel Ellaway is Professor in the Department of Community Health Sciences and Director of the Office of Health and Medical Education Scholarship at the Cumming School of Medicine, University of Calgary, Alberta, Canada. She is also Editor in Chief of the journal *Advances in Health Sciences Education.*

Dr Quentin Eichbaum is Professor of Pathology, Immunology and Microbiology at Vanderbilt University Medical Centre, where he co-directs the Transfusion Medicine Service, and Professor of Medical Education and Administration at Vanderbilt University School of Medicine where he was Assistant Dean and developed and directed the College Colloquium medical humanities programme.

Preface

In this book, we set out to 'make strange' or 'defamiliarise' taken-for-granted processes of thinking and feeling as these apply to medical education, through advancing the concepts and practices of metacognition (embracing meta-affect) and metahumanities. Clearly, medicine has both cognitive and affective elements at its core, reflected for instance in clinical reasoning and face-to-face patient encounters. To 'make strange' (or defamiliarise) was devised by early 20th-century Russian Formalists such as Victor Shklovsky and Roman Jakobson as 'close reading' of texts in the context of literary studies. We adapt the praxis (a fusion of concept and practice) to apply it to how we might think differently about processes of thinking and feeling (and sensing and intuiting) in clinical contexts and to provide a commentary on the pedagogical challenges that conceptual thinking about thinking (metacognition) may bring.

Thinking about thinking (or critical reflexivity) and thinking about feeling (or insight after catharsis) transform medical humanities into 'metahumanities', a plural, holistic, complex, transdisciplinary/circumdisciplinary position that is a product of perspectives from the biomedical sciences and the complex of arts/humanities/qualitative social sciences. By transcending outdated and unproductive oppositions between science and art (and between other aspects of human experience and knowledge), we shift focus rather to the quality, intensity, and innovative potential of synthesising perspectives from the biomedical sciences and the arts/humanities to transcend reductive instrumentality. In doing so, we embrace a wider spectrum of values: ethical, aesthetic, and political ways of knowing and being.

'Making strange' has been re-invented in pedagogy as forms of 'reflective practice' (Schön 1983, Bleakley 1999). These describe the human capability to reflect after an event ('what have I just done?') or during an event as a way of monitoring one's behaviour, thoughts, and feelings. Donald Schön (1983) calls the former 'reflection-on-action' and the latter 'reflection-in-action'. Reflection therefore becomes an 'event-within-an-event'.

In the contexts of both pedagogy and psychotherapeutic education, Alan Bleakley (1999) has progressed Schon's model to note that we have the capacity to set up a trail of reflections-on-reflections, as 'reflexivity'. Moreover, such reflections-on-reflections can take on a critical nature, where we adapt behaviours, thoughts, or feelings according to the ways in which we reflect on and build meanings around them. Bleakley (ibid.) calls this 'critical reflexivity'. Such chains of reflection are metonymic – linking words and actions through logical conceptual association to form chains of ideas at one level described by coherent sentences at another. Through enacted practices, governed by semiotics (signs and symbols), such metonymic chains describe how actions and activities unfold with a sense of sequential logic. Such logic itself can be interrupted or re-invented through critical reflexivity.

These ongoing chains of reflection-upon-reflection are typically conducted in social contexts where ideas and thoughts can be shared with the aid of artefacts (such as computers). These socially situated and artefactually enhanced reflections are forms of 'refractive practice' where each person's individual reflections or considerations – either in the event or after the event – are refracted through the whole of the social–artefactual context. As an example, consider the shared thinking-on-one's-feet necessary in a 'crash' scenario or running a code, or the shared post-activity reflections that constitute debriefing in clinical team contexts. Collaborative self-regulation characterises democratic teamwork and invites the use of subjunctives ('it might', 'we could') rather than indicative moods and imperatives ('it is', 'we will'). Democratic healthcare teams with flattened hierarchies are of necessity well-practised in critical reflexivity and refractive practices, and as a result tend to have better patient outcomes, better patient safety records, and higher worker satisfaction than teams who work hierarchically and rely largely on indicative or directive exchanges (Bleakley 2021). Indeed, impeding or limiting shared reflection raises resentment amongst those lower on the hierarchy, so that their reflective work is in danger of being skewed away from attention to the patient towards self-absorption through emotional states of resentment. It is therefore imperative that healthcare education cultivates refractive practices as democratic habits.

Reflexive and refractive practices are now more commonly framed as forms of metacognition and meta-affect – individuals thinking-about-thinking and feeling-about-feeling brought up a gear to engage specific social contexts as shared and negotiated thinking-about-thinking and feeling-about-feeling. Such extended and situated cognition and affect embraces the use of artefacts and languages/semiotics (sign and symbol systems such as mathematics, chemical formulae, and standardised uses of languages such as English for Medical Purposes).

In the healthcare education literature, nursing studies have been more proactive than medical pedagogy in promoting ideas of metacognition and reflexivities in practice. For example, Ruth Anne Kuiper and Daniel J Pesut (2004) described 'Promoting cognitive and metacognitive reflective reasoning skills in nursing practice: self-regulated learning theory' some two decades ago. However, their analysis is confounded by a reductive instrumental language, where, for example, 'Reflective clinical reasoning in nursing practice depends on the development of both cognitive and metacognitive skill acquisition' (ibid), revealing an instrumental bias. Neither cognition nor metacognition can be meaningfully reduced to linear 'skills' to be performed as needed; they are complex capabilities that rely on reflection, metacognition, and meta-affect. Moreover, the article focuses on intra-personal rather than inter-personal reasoning and fails to account for extended cognition as a product of the extension of cognition through use of artefacts and situated cognition as specific tailored strategies used for specific contexts.

Kuiper and Pesut's (2004) review is cited in a recent integrated review by Jerusalem Merkebu and colleagues (2024) – 'The Case for Metacognitive Reflection: A Theory Integrative Review with Implications for Medical Education' – where the authors note that 'The concepts of metacognitive reflection, reflection, and metacognition are distinct but have undergone shifts in meaning as they migrated into medical education' and call for 'conceptual clarity'. Their review set out to understand 'what metacognitive reflection is'. Only 87 articles met their inclusion criteria, demonstrating a lack of conceptual clarification in the field over the past two decades. The authors note a difference between 'root metacognitive reflection' and more advanced 'cycles of reflection', and that further sophistication shows in models that describe 'affective component, transformational nature, and contextual factors' in metacognition, 'to develop a richer conceptualization'.

However, Merkebu and colleagues conclude that 'a theory of how metacognitive reflection works is elusive'. Of course, it is a fool's errand to search for a single, unifying theory, and we must accept that a topic as broad, complex, and dynamic as 'metacognition', when interfaced with meta-affect, is necessarily going to provide multiple and even conflicting models that show dynamic change. The authors themselves note a lack of conceptual clarity and agreement across articles relating to key concepts. This is because metacognition and meta-affect are not linear, closed, mechanical processes, but dynamic, open, complex, adaptive, nonlinear systems moving to maximum complexity at the edge of chaos, sometims falling into chaos or crystallising and collapsing, and often reformulating spontaneously at higher levels of complexity.

Merkebu and colleagues (2024) then say,

> Metacognitive reflection involves heightened internal observation, awareness, monitoring, and regulation of our own knowledge, experiences, and emotions by questioning and examining cognition and emotional processes to continually refine and enhance our perspectives and decisions while thoughtfully accounting for context. We argue that metacognitive reflection brings a shift in perspective and can support valuable reconceptualization for lifelong learning.

We cannot disagree with the concluding line, and we applaud reference to affect as well as thinking, but we differ on the nature of the route map towards that conclusion. Merkebu and colleagues' conclusion is prone to the personalistic and individualistic fallacy that haunts psychological models of metacognition such as the Ur-text of Pina Tarricone (2011), whose taxis is to the interior cognitive maze of the human mind, ultimately grounded in 'memory'. In other words, the metacognitive gaze is seen to have an introspective taxis.

We prefer the direction of travel that the philosopher of cognition Andy Clark (2023) takes in a series of texts since the 1990s, where cognition is extended to embrace social and material worlds spatially; and, in a remarkable temporal move, Clark suggests that thinking does not inhabit current time, but is 'predictive' or 'inhabits' split-second future time. Based on such 'predictive processing', our bodies adjust to what our minds expect. But Clark, we think, also falls short in not attending fully to the role of emotional or affective life in his model of cognition. Thinking humans are shot through with affect whatever the occasion – and this relationship between cognition and feeling, as neuropsychology has long informed us, is a paradoxical one. Affect expression is inhibited (or suppressed if you are a Freudian) in social contexts as much as it is expressed (as such expression is shaped according to social norms and etiquette). For example, medical students are often taught to keep affect in control in the face of alarming sets of stimuli, such as sudden exposure to suffering and death. To do so is to hold to professional integrity but it cannot be done without a personal cost that should not remain unacknowledged or unexamined. As Freud noted, continuous repression or suppression of affect can cause such emotions to return in a distorted form – for example as anxiety, burnout, and suicide ideation.

In this book, we pay attention to both metacognition and meta-affect, and we resist attempting a unifying theory or overarching position. While adopting a range of critical positions, we survey the fields of metacognition and meta-affect as they relate to contemporary medical education practices. Our starting point, therefore, is one of pedagogy rather than biology and is focused on the structures and cultures of medical education rather than the intricacies and varieties of clinical practice. This does not mean that we shy away from comment on clinical work or clinicians' related experiences. Our aim is to inform and improve medical education through better understanding of systems of metacognition and meta-affect.

We are advocates of face-to-face 'warm' humanist pedagogies, placing learners at the centre of the experience of medical education. Our learners are primarily medical students, and we want them to place patients at the centre of their work, and to work democratically with clinical and non-clinical colleagues to achieve this. However, we are also advocates of artefacts such as information technologies to support and expand human consciousness. Our challenge in this book is then to set out an agenda for bringing together 'warm' humanism and 'cold' technologies to work towards humane posthumanism futures in medical education and clinical work. We consider differing routes to such a metahumanist perspective, and we present these ideas at the verge of simultaneously exciting and terrifying developments in posthumanism, transhumanism, and AI. This book takes a bold perspective on these complex topics and seeks to outline a challenging new vision.

In the process, we present a critical overhaul of established medical education and medical humanities paradigms. We propose a complex 'deep', plural medical humanities – as metahumanities – embracing extensions and augmentations of the human condition that engage aesthetic, ethical, political, and transcendental (meaning) values beyond the instrumental. We are passionate about productive engagement between sciences and the arts, supporting the preservation and recovery of the intrinsic art and humanity of biomedical science that is in turn framed by models of dynamic complexity rather than static linearity.

References

Bleakley, A. 1999. From reflective practice to holistic reflexivity. *Studies in Higher Education*. 1999; 24: 315–30.

Bleakley, A. 2021. *Medical Education, Politics, and Social Justice: The Contradiction Cure*. Abingdon: Routledge.

Clark, A. 2023. *The Experience Machine: How Our Minds Predict and Shape Reality*. London: Allen Lane.

Kuiper, R.A., Pesut, D.J. Promoting cognitive and metacognitive reflective reasoning skills in nursing practice: self-regulated learning theory. *J Adv Nurs*. 2004; 45: 381–91.

Merkebu, J., Veen, M., Hosseini, S., Varpio, L. The case for metacognitive reflection: A theory integrative review with implications for medical education. *Adv Health Sci Educ Theory Pract*. 2024. doi: 10.1007/s10459-023-10310-2

Schön, D. 1983. *The Reflective Practitioner: How Professionals Think in Action*. New York, NY: Basic Books.

Introduction

Alan Bleakley, Quentin Eichbaum, and Rachel Ellaway

Stepping out from under the cloud of AI

The exponential growth of artificial intelligence (AI) has impacted both academic and lay communities, not least through fears that 'rogue' AIs will one day displace their human parents and come to either control or destroy humanity as a contemporary analogue of Frankenstein's monster. Although many AI applications are playing a positive role in fields such as medicine (e.g., in clinical imaging diagnostics), there remain many concerns, particularly related to the value of human thought and experience. Indeed, technological change is proving an existential threat, most notably through the evolving planetary climate crisis.

Considering these developments, we ask in this book: have we exhausted the coffers of our flesh-and-blood human potential? Our cognition is not bound by our skulls but extends across social activities as these are augmented by 'soft' and 'hard' artefacts including languages and tools, all of which are central to medical education. How we construct curricula, learn, and teach are intimately bound up with individual and collective cognition extended by an ever-growing repertoire of technologies and systems.

And yet, the heart of clinical encounters is still about flesh-and-blood exchanges between doctors and patients, and between doctors and other health professionals working with and around their patients. At the heart of this clinical work, often carried out under conditions of ambiguity and uncertainty, is the necessary expression, exchange, and regulation of emotions and feelings guided by the senses, and the exercise of the most mysterious of human qualities: intuition and imagination (typically expressed as forms of creativity).

Despite the exponential growth of sophisticated technologies such as AI, we are still puzzling over how to best *educate* and *cultivate* such human qualities generally and specifically in the field of medical education. It is this challenge of pedagogy – how to cultivate more sophisticated ways of thinking, feeling, sensing, and intuiting – that this book frames as *aspiring to the 'meta'* (or 'greater than'). This embraces metacognition (thinking-about-thinking, or sophisticated forms of reflection) and meta-affect (gaining insight into feeling states), and it seeks to unite them through the concept of 'metahumanities' as this also embraces complex and artistic biomedical science.

DOI: 10.4324/9781032687339-1

We propose 'medical metahumanities' as a critical extension of a tradition of medical humanities encompassing the shift in values from the linear instrumental to the complex of ethical, aesthetic, political, and transcendental (encompassing meaning) (Bleakley 2023, 2024). We are close here to the work of del Val (n.d.-a, b, last accessed 2024), who defines metahumanism as challenging and transcending perceived faults of traditional humanism that casts 'the human as [a] distinct and superior species, distinguished by rationality, autonomy, individual subjectivity and free will'; this has become 'associated to [a] hegemonic subject that is predominantly European, white, male, high-class, neurotypical, [and] heteropatriarchal' and engages in 'a colonial project of domination of nature, other humans, other species and the planet and to an all-encompassing thrust to rationalisation'.

Metahumanism (del Val n.d.-a, b, 1,2, Tuncel 2023), as a critically reflexive set of stances on humanism, both critiques and offers alternatives to areas of traditional humanism that may be perceived as potentially oppressive. There is emphasis upon not losing the body and qualities of embodiment to abstractions; the importance of a relational ethics set within a philosophy of Nietzschean transvaluation of values that does not strive for utopianism; and, importantly, a political dimension embracing resistance and activism in the face of perceived oppression (Tuncel 2023). Sand (2013) notes that del Val embraces a transhumanism that supports a critical and selective approach to technological enhancement, but also seeks humane ways of challenging inequities and inequalities to provide quality of life for all, echoing the 'capabilities' approach championed by Amartya Sen and refined by Martha Nussbaum (see Chapter 9).

We follow this approach and embrace technological enhancements and expansions of the person, including AI, where AI is regulated from within the purview of the expansion of human qualities rather than the 'doom' scenario of replacement of such qualities in a shift from a carbon-based to a silicon-based life web. Medicine has benefitted enormously from AI, particularly radiology diagnostics, and medical education benefits particularly in learning through simulation.

Our focus then is one of realising potential in flesh-and-blood persons – specifically medical students and junior doctors – through new horizons in studies of cognition and affect. These horizons include forms of attention and perception; sense-making and the making of meaning; quality of linguistic registers embracing production of metaphors; forms of intuition; tacit dimensions to knowing; the socially and artefactually extended mind; using heuristics or short-cut solutions to complex problems; thinking in patterns and other forms of augmentation; educating for complex capability rather than linear competence; tolerating uncertainty and 'wicked problems' that cannot be solved but must be faced; appreciating the differences between linear problem-solving and problematising in complex situations; and relating to others at a deeper level of identification (compathy rather than empathy).

As we develop these accounts of human potential that can inform pedagogical strategies for learning medicine, we recognise that we are also developing a new form of the medical humanities. Traditionally seen as the introduction of arts and humanities into a medicine curriculum to compensate for an overload of reductive biomedicine, we sophisticate this view of the role of the medical humanities. Metahumanities are introduced as trans-disciplinary (or circum-disciplinary) forms of translational pedagogies. Such pedagogies are characterised by raising quality, intensity, and complexity of education through movement from a baseline, reductive instrumentalism to embrace other human values and experiences to include embodied ethical, aesthetic, political, and transcendental ways of knowing and being. In this model, biomedical sciences and medical humanities are not seen as antagonistic; and neither are medical humanities treated as a cure for the symptoms of an ailing biomedical scientific system of education. Rather, where both arts/humanities and biomedical science can be instrumental and reductive, they can both be expressive and complex. Welcome to the flesh-and-blood world of metacognition, meta-affect, and metahumanities as these expand medical pedagogies.

'Meta' has an origin myth

In some Greek mythology accounts, Aegeus was the founder and first King of Athens. His first wife was Meta – meaning 'beyond', or better, 'untouchable' – who did not bear him a child, and so Aegeus re-married (to Chalciope). This marriage also failed to result in a child. During the marriage, Aegeus was made drunk by Pittheus, the King of the Peloponnesian province Troezen, and under the influence he slept with Pittheus' daughter Aethra. She bore the child Theseus, who, according to most Greek mythological accounts, founded the city of Athens. Theseus also famously slayed the Minotaur in a labyrinth in Crete, helped by Ariadne who provided the thread that allowed Theseus to find his way out of the maze after killing the monster.

At this point, only a few pages into this book, you may also be feeling lost in the labyrinth or mired in the maze. So, let us re-state two threads for the sake of clarity. First, the account above, like many re-tellings of Greek myths, is biased towards the patriarchy. Thus, Meta and Chalciope 'fail' to provide offspring for Aegeus. Aethra, while the mother of Theseus, is cast in the role of seductress defined only in terms of those she can seduce. This might be rectified in many ways: perhaps Meta might choose not to bear Aegeus a child because she thinks he may be a poor father. Perhaps, living up to her name, she has insight beyond the norm, a meta-perception, and remains – for Aegeus – untouchable, a person in her own right.

Today, we are familiar with 'Meta', perhaps from the re-branding by Mark Zuckerberg of 'Facebook, Inc.' as 'Meta Platforms, Inc.', including Instagram, Threads, and WhatsApp. But, of course, 'meta' is a common preposition and prefix, meaning 'more than' or 'greater than' (such as metaphysics, metatarsal, and metastasis). The Greek derivation can mean 'after', 'beyond', and 'behind' – spatial terms that shift whatever is our focus of attention away from the centre or the norm. The 'metaverse' then implies conversations beyond the everyday to grasp the beyond, the future, the hidden. Indeed, in current slang, 'meta' has taken on an adjectival persona: 'that's so meta!'

But 'meta' – as the Greek root – also means 'along with' and 'among'. Meta can imply raising the stakes or quality of a phenomenon from within its own being or constituent parts, rather than some abstract or mythical state signifying something out of the ordinary. It is within the ordinary that meta explodes as the flowering of the extraordinary through deliberate development rather than serendipity.

It is within the known and achievable that new visions can emerge as metacognitions, a thinking-about-thinking. Thinking happens and then thinking-about-thinking happens, not only as reflection after the event, but also as reflection within the event (reflection-in-action). And then something remarkable occurs. Such thinking-about-thinking is subject to another (or several) layers of reflection as a critical 'holistic reflexivity' (Bleakley 1999). These include ethical considerations, aesthetic shaping, political awareness, and transcendental (meaning) formations. Thinking for yourself becomes thinking about others (relational empathy or compathy) in considered ways. Such ways are critical (questioning habits), reflexive (thinking things through), and humane (caring for others). These are the values that can drive a medical education to go beyond the technical or instrumental bottom-line of biomedical knowledge and application.

Thinking without the box

The title of this book is comprised of two descriptive terms – metacognition and metahumanities – both of which we define later in relation to medical education. First, let us deal with the book's subtitle, one that is, we admit, intentionally ambiguous. 'Thinking without the box' may mean that we have abandoned the box altogether. 'Without' does not just mean bereft of something, but also 'outside' or nearby (a less used term nowadays). So, let us imagine that we have abandoned the box in the sense of abandoning a raft that keeps capsising but is still nearby so that we still have one hand on the raft. Thus, it is with metacognition and metahumanities – they are beyond the ordinary, but they are nevertheless within reach. As the book progresses, we will add 'meta-affect' to metacognition and metahumanities and explicitly foreground this in some chapters. For the moment, let us imagine that metacognition is used as a catch-all to include both cognition and emotion. We will unpack differences between metacognition and meta-affect later.

Back to the box. Thinking within the box means strictly following protocols and rules while anchoring in the territory of the known. The educationalist Yrjö Engeström (2008, 2016) calls this a 'stabilization knowledge' (as opposed to a 'possibility knowledge') and a 'will-to-stability' (as opposed to 'spearheads of innovation'). Thinking without the box can mean abandoning the box altogether (dangerous – you may drown) or thinking outside the box with one hand still on the capsized raft. The latter is a better learning strategy, commonly known as 'scaffolding', where learners are encouraged to take leaps into the unknown ('possibility learning') on the basis that they have a safety harness, or one foot in the known (provided by their expert facilitator). The unknown territory into which the learners leap ('without' the box as outside norms and protocols) has been described by Engeström (2008, 2016, 2018) as 'learning for change', comprised again of 'spearheads of innovation' – strategies that upend previous thinking in the field (while maintaining a tangible tether). Engeström has long called this 'learning what is not yet there' or 'expansive learning'.

Let us give an illustrative example. In 2022, a 34-year-old male patient (a heavy smoker) was admitted to the emergency department of a hospital in Evanston, Illinois, after reporting acute shortness of breath. He was diagnosed with influenza A and prescribed a course of antibiotics. He rapidly developed a lung infection that proved resistant to the antibiotics. His condition deteriorated rapidly, and he was admitted to intensive care where he continued to decline so badly that a double lung transplant remained his only option for survival. He was transferred to a specialist unit – the Northwestern Medicine Canning Thoracic Institute, under the care of Dr Ankit Bharat, head of the unit. Faced with the urgency and complexity of the case, Bharat could not retreat to the known but had to think without the box. He devised a spearhead of innovation, combining two temporary breast implants to hold the heart in place, and an artificial lung, until a donor lung was available. Both infected lungs were removed, the chest cavity debrided to clear the infection, and double D breast implants were used as support for the heart. Heidi Splete (2023), who reports this case in 'Medscape' says: 'it was time for outside-the-box thinking … with the lungs taken out, we needed something to support the heart. Breast implants came to mind, and double Ds were the largest available'. A crash course in management of the breast implants was given to the surgical team by plastic surgeons. Serendipity stepped in – while the lung team imagined that their innovation would be required for weeks, the patient improved rapidly once the infected lung tissue was removed, and a donor was found within 24 hours. As a secondary innovation, the surgeons also created an artificial lung system devised of conduits to keep the blood pumping in the temporary absence of lungs.

The patient was discharged to rehabilitation therapy after several months in intensive care. Again, serendipity may follow spearheads of innovation as calculated risk-taking. The chief surgeon Bharat said: 'a lot of stars aligned … we were surprised how quickly he recovered once we removed the infected lungs … [and yet] this was uncharted territory'. Returning to our metaphor of 'without the box', or one hand on the raft and the body already in the water, Bharat's surgical team drew on established procedures as well as innovating. For example, removal of both lungs had already been shown to prevent cross-contamination in lung cancer patients.

After the procedure, and blessed with hindsight, the patient said in a press conference: 'you should not inhale anything into your lungs except oxygen'. We suggest that when thoughts are oxygenated in creative experts, innovation naturally follows. This case study is a good example of a mix of linear and complex systems at work. The human body is an open, nonlinear, complex, adaptive system, but aspects of it, such as anatomy and physiology, are stable attractors within that complex system working in a more-or-less linear fashion. The body is subject to entropy (we are sure to die), such that medicine can be understood to involve the impossible art of cheating entropy, while medical education provides the instrumental, ethical, aesthetic, and political values webs that cradle such an essentially hubristic activity. We would argue that metacognition is perhaps the most sophisticated way that we have of cheating death.

The case study is also a good example of the interplay between what the philosopher Nassim Taleb (2012) calls 'fragility and antifragility' as the potential interplay of disorder and order, noting 'things that gain from disorder' (of which the lung transplant above is a shining example). Just as complex systems working at maximum complexity at the edge of chaos can either fall into chaos or re-order at a higher level of complexity, so Taleb invents a parallel notion of 'fragility' – as opposed to stability or 'antifragility'. Some things are clearly fragile – when stressed, they break, such as a porcelain plate. The human body too is fragile, but has great flexibility or has a range of antifragility. We can exercise and eat well to gain strength for example. We can recover from addictions. The patient's smoking in the example above was a lifestyle event leading to lung fragility.

Medicine (and surgery), Taleb reminds us, has been a culture of fragility, where until relatively recently medicine did more harm than good to bodies. Now, that effect has been reversed. Medicine has become a culture of antifragility that treats the fragile. Taleb (ibid.) suggests that, paradoxically, 'the comfortable is what fragilizes'. Many conditions of ill-health in high-income countries are products of chosen or forced lifestyle: polluted air, fatty foods, alcohol and tobacco consumption, lack of exercise, work-related stress and anxiety, depression, and so forth. While medicine is now a culture of antifragility ('resilience' is the buzzword), it is also permeated by fear of failure and of medical error (leading to death, harm, and professional and legal penalties). While medicine typically adopts a 'tough-minded' attitude, it also follows Engeström's 'will-to-stability' and 'stabilization knowledge' that resist risk as innovation in case of error. This gives medicine an aura of fragility (fear of taking risks) just as it develops an 'antifragility' culture embodying intolerance of ambiguity. 'Antifragility' does not literally mean 'toughen up' – although metaphorically this may be the case. Rather, it means extending cognition and affect to adapt to challenging contexts, something medicine strives to do and medical education hopes to teach. Again, encouragement to think without the box. We are back to the necessity of the 'meta'.

Originary sources on metacognition: Pina Tarricone and Andy Clark

The educational psychologist Pina Tarricone (2011) can be credited with writing the first exhaustive text on metacognition. Tarricone's model differs from what might be seen as the cutting edge of metacognition modelling developed by the cognitive philosopher Andy Clark (1997, 2010, 2016, 2023).

Where Tarricone is interested in the retrospective, she ties thinking and reflection (thinking-about-thinking) to the anchor of memory. In contrast, Clark ties reflection to prediction, drawing up the anchor. This can be partly explained by differing discipline interests: Tarricone comes from traditional experimental cognitive psychology while Clark comes from future-focused and speculative information processing and AI.

Where Tarricone loops reflexive awareness back to a memory base and is interested particularly in the regulation of memory (as metamemory), Clark privileges a looping forward, from memory through reflexive consciousness to a future-facing cognition. Here cognition, as prospective not retrospective, extends beyond the bounds of the skull to give primacy to the way that the environmental context for thinking affords cues that shape thought (see Chapters 2 and 5). Tarricone, in contrast, remains within the confines of the skull in 'self-knowledge' created through reflexive awareness of what has been done (memory) and how things may be improved for the individual.

For Tarricone, such improvement rests with a 'metamemory' – both knowledge and regulation of memory. In this, Tarricone echoes the interests of psychoanalysis in memory, but where psychoanalysis looks at memory content as largely actively repressed matter, Tarricone is interested more in the organisational framework of memory as a process – how memory actively shapes strategies for cognition such as planning, monitoring, and controlling consciousness. She does not draw on Michael Polanyi's (1966) account of tacit knowing, or models of a 'cognitive unconscious', such as Arthur Reber's (Reber and Allen 2022) account of 'implicit learning' and 'tacit knowing', where we learn more than we can say, and we cannot consciously recover the rules by which cognition operates, such as language use. Tarricone's interests rest rather with the conscious than the unconscious aspects of memory.

Our concern here is not with the details of differences between models of metacognition, but what makes for a leap from cognition (thinking) to metacognition (thinking-about-thinking). Is it primarily the past that shapes metacognition (e.g., a doctor relying on stored facts and information to make a clinical judgement) or does future-focus stimulate innovation (e.g., a doctor makes a leap-of-faith diagnosis based on a hunch)? Or do both play a role depending on context? Tarricone would say that metamemory is not about recovering experiences and knowledge as uncontaminated facts. Rather, following Aristotle, she sees memory as a process of associations that weave a credible picture through recollection. A memory that invents, rather than simply recovers, is already a metamemory; and an account of that meta-memorising of course adds another layer of reflection. Memories are then not directly recalled experiences, but translations of those experiences. This is close to William Wordsworth's famous definition of poetry as emotions recalled in tranquillity.

It is telling that where Tarricone's system provides a hierarchical taxonomy of regulatory factors in metacognition and her analysis is then a closed system describing metacognition as a closed system, Clark in contrast offers the analogy of 'surfing' for his model, as keeping just ahead of the breaking part of the wave to avoid a 'wipeout', a precarious adventure in an open, complex system. Returning to Yrjö Engeström's work on expansive learning, Andy Clark's model of cognition can be seen as embracing 'possibility knowledge' and 'learning for change' through 'spearheads of innovation' to embrace 'learning what is not yet there'.

The originary source on meta-affect: John Heron

What then are the key differences between metacognition (thinking-about-thinking) and meta-affect (feeling about feeling)? The latter draws affect and cognition together, for John Heron's (1977, 1989, 1992, 1998, 1999, 2001) view on catharsis, or the release of emotion (feeling states) sees catharsis as empty without subsequent insight after the cathartic event. Here, cognition develops in the wake of catharsis, as if the emotional event clears the way for clarity of thought. From a modernist perspective, we can think of catharsis as being deeply personal, but there is another view. Ancient Greek culture coined the word *katharsis* to refer to a public, collective 'cleansing' of feeling states through theatre. Tragic dramas played out tangled emotional scenes, where the audience undergoes catharsis through identification with the players and the chorus – a group of singers who comment on the unfolding storyline of the play. David Brooks (2023) suggests that such collective catharsis was developed as a 'tragic sensibility' as strife, hardship, and war are every day. 'The tragic sensibility', suggests Brooks, 'prepares you for the rigors of life in concrete ways', teaching you humility, a prudent approach to life, caution, and suspicion towards one's own rage to develop rather an outrage at injustice. This includes contempt for hubris and anything that dehumanises. Finally, collective catharsis can translate into empathy and compathy (see Chapter 12).

During the late 1970s, the psychologist John Heron developed a collaborative research project at the University of Surrey, Guildford, UK, on the place of 'catharsis in human development'. By catharsis, Heron meant release of emotion or affect that might otherwise create symptom. Aristotle had initiated study on catharsis referring to identification with tragedy (common to Greek theatre) as noted above. This was identified as the paradox of 'tragic pleasure' – again, the audience engaged in a common catharsis through identification with actors and chorus playing out the tragedy.

The practice of catharsis became the mainstay of psychoanalysis from Breuer and Freud onwards, where patients were encouraged to engage with often painful repressed memories and, in their unearthing, would, through emotional release, gain post-cathartic insight into the dynamics and meaning of these memories. Heron followed this psychoanalytic line, placing emphasis upon the gaining of insight during the cathartic episode itself. This mirrored Donald Schön's (1983, 1990) account of *ad hoc* 'reflection-in-action', rather than post hoc 'reflection-on-action'. As noted in the Preface, Alan Bleakley (1999) progressed Schön's model to consider a 'critical reflexivity' ('reflection-as-action') that occurs in activity, but as an intensive source of insight shaping and guiding action, common to 'expert practice' (Kneebone 2020). Such critical reflexivity engages both metacognition and meta-affect simultaneously.

Heron recognised that, particularly in a cultural context of suspicion about displaying emotions (such as stereotypical 'English reserve'), potentially cathartic episodes would often be rationalised away or become stilted. Arguing that blocked and frustrated catharsis is the basis to psychological distress (a key tenet of psychoanalysis), Heron argued for general education into the field of affect (and emotional lability) and specific therapeutic work as individuals in releasing chronic cathartic blocks as personal distress. He termed this 'human development', progressing Harvey Jackins' praxis of 'co-counselling' or 're-evaluation counselling' first developed in the USA in the 1950s as a democratic model for therapeutic engagement, with the main aims being insights that could accompany cathartic episodes along with bodily re-alignments such as posture, breath, and quality of proxemics (non-verbal signals in social settings). Once taught the basics, those with interest and ability can act as both therapist and client, swapping the roles within an agreed protocol.

Jackins' and Heron's key contribution was to raise counselling and psychotherapy from an instrumental activity to one laced with ethical, aesthetic, and political concerns. For example, cathartic episodes in a traditional psychoanalytic or psychotherapeutic context are typically tied up with the politics (power structures) of the occasion, where the therapist's power is reflected in either passive observance (positive transference from client to therapist) or active resistance on the part of the client (negative transference, active resistance). Much of the catharsis in such a relationship can be staged. In a co-counselling, democratic set-up, catharsis is more likely to be authentic as transference and resistance are not primary factors in the relationship and the client has no need to 'act in' to a role to either please or anger the therapist. Such a model can readily be transposed to the doctor–patient relationship.

Knowledge of the role of catharsis at both cultural–societal and personal levels is necessary for the practice of cathartic release, management of such release, facilitation of catharsis, and making sense of insights gained during and after catharsis. These are all meta-affect activities, as they encourage both emoting-about-emoting (deep catharsis) and insight gained from catharsis, paralleling a metacognition or thinking-about-thinking. Heron developed courses based around these ideas and practices for general practitioners in the UK and extended these to award-bearing postgraduate programmes. One of us (AB) worked closely with Heron on these developments.

John Heron died in late 2022. In the context of this book, his legacy is central, as reflected on the thread of meta-affect that is woven throughout the coming chapters. Heron's model of meta-affect is grounded in basic human needs: to love and be loved; to understand and be understood; to be at once self-directing and engaged with communal activities. Each of us is innately vulnerable, resourceful, and resilient (our human potential). But human potential cannot be realised without the support of others, and it is best realised through expert technique based on exercising metacognition and meta-affect. Our course of development can be frustrated through illness and emotional distress, and through conflicting values. We can add to the distress of self and others through chronic habits that can be addressed as meta-affective fault-lines remedied through therapies. Patterns of distress are harder to address in chronically defensive societies and sub-cultures (such as medicine) that resist both emotional expression and study of catharsis, but through the meta-affective activities of therapeutic practices, we can learn to gain insight through the discharge of grief, fear, anger, embarrassment, guilt, shame, disgust, boredom, and physical and emotional fatigue. Insight is gained into emotional release therapeutically largely through the balance of attention, where 'free attention' is available for insight and not swamped by catharsis.

Problems with conventional medical education

The issues raised in opening this chapter (what is the 'meta', and specifically, metacognition, meta-affect, and metahumanities) are linked throughout this book to overhauling current practices and philosophies of medical education that can be overly technocratic, dehumanising, and empathy-eroding, introducing artefacts that lead to harm and reproduce inequality and injustice. Use of the arts, humanities, and qualitative social sciences has been pursued as an antidote or balance to these problems (Bleakley 2015, 2023; Bleakley and Neilson 2021). However, such interventions have been used in a largely epidemiological way, with a calculated 'dose' exposure to humanities acting as metaphoric and therapeutic vaccine. Not only has this led to largely unpredictable and mixed outcomes, but such approaches tend to widen the divide between those who enthusiastically embrace its tenets and sceptics who do not (where the latter, in the view of the former, constitute the group that arguably need medical humanities interventions most). Further, while champions of the medical humanities celebrate a 'cure all', they can fail to critically address quality in their interventions where the medical humanities can be applied mechanically, losing their potency. Such medical humanities enthusiasts may also fail to recognise intrinsic qualities in biomedical sciences, such as productive use of metaphor, that provide a readymade resource for medical education. An alternative framing of the issues and opportunities regarding what the medical humanities are and can offer is needed, including a vision of what a 'well-rounded' or 'humanist' physician may look like. But this must be radically adjusted for a posthumanist era concerned about the existential threats and possibilities of climate change, AI, and other developments that could outstrip or diminish humanity. What are the implications of this for medicine and healthcare, and for medical education?

Established humanist frames, regardless of their promise to expand the person, have tended to resort to instrumental techniques, such as information-led, formulaic ways of learning 'communication skills' in undergraduate medical education. Challenging such habitual reduction to the instrumental and mechanical, we develop models of expanding information-led pedagogies to embrace knowledge and meaning as these are augmented by metacognition (thinking about thinking) and associated 'smart' technologies. Here, we consider the importance of satisfying several values perspectives (such as the ethical, aesthetic, political, and transcendental) as these might compose 'metahumanity' beyond the mechanical and instrumental – this, again, in an age of increasingly technologised medicine.

In this Introduction, discussing the etymology of 'meta', we argue that where the meta may reveal the extraordinary: 'It is within the ordinary that meta explodes as the flowering of the extraordinary through deliberate development rather than serendipity'. We don't have to take the lift to the rooftop apartment because the potential for the meta is right here on the ground floor. In other words, we don't have to reach extraordinary heights to reveal the meta, for it may be right under our noses. Our focus in this book is on *how metahumanities can flower in, and through, medical pedagogy*. Our humanities approach is therefore educationally focused and pedagogically rich.

There is an extensive 'critical' medical humanities literature that challenges both extant biomedical and medical education cultures as restrictive (Bleakley 2013, Whitehead and Woods 2016). Where our focus is on medical pedagogy, we follow in the footsteps of recent 'translational' work in medical humanities where biomedical science and the arts can be understood as being in complex, but constructive, conversation with each other rather than in opposition as 'two cultures' (Bleakley 2019, Kristeva et al. 2019, Arnaldi 2022, Bleakley 2023, 2024).

Can we then engage 'warm' humanism and 'cold' technologies to design humane posthumanism futures in medical education and clinical work? There are many differing routes to such metahumanist perspectives, some (but not all) of which we explore in this book. We present these ideas at the verge of simultaneously exciting and terrifying developments in posthumanism and transhumanism. To that end, we have tried to take a bold perspective on these complex topics in outlining a challenging new vision. In the process, we present a critical overhaul of established medical humanities paradigms. We propose a complex 'deep' medical humanities embracing extensions and augmentations of the human that engages values beyond the instrumental. We show how the key to such a transition is the production of embodied metaphor, including the recovery of the intrinsic art and humanity of metaphor-heavy biomedical science, in turn framed by models of dynamic complexity rather than static linearity.

The conservative rhetorician Richard Weavers (1953) introduced the ideas of 'God terms' and 'Devil terms' into everyday speech. They are powerful words or phrases that immediately incite passions. God terms are positive, such as 'freedom', 'self-help', and 'hero'; Devil terms are negative, such as (in an American context) 'communism', 'coward', 'failure', and 'dependent'. We hope that we are not employing our key prefix – 'meta' – as a God term, instead of evidencing through argument that by raising quality, intensity, and value of ordinary states to the extraordinary (cognition to metacognition, affect to meta-affect) we are doing something worthwhile, to be applauded. We do not deny that some of our argument is rhetorical, but we refuse to see 'meta' as a God term, and we reject any idea that 'meta' should be taken as a Devil term!

Overview of chapters

In **Chapter 1**, Alan Bleakley notes current trends in both science and the arts/humanities/qualitative social sciences that propose a 'posthuman' condition in the context of Earth's ecosystems and climate now termed the Anthropocene. Political and ethnic turmoil and climate change have created waves of displacement and migration, and, as science knowledge and practical application in technologies expand exponentially, so the gap between the super-rich and the poor increases. Inequity and inequality are major causes of otherwise avoidable suffering and death. Global political and religious conflicts (implicating nuclear threats), pandemics, and the exponential rise of the use of unregulated AI also pose existential threats. Nevertheless, we remain stubbornly optimistic about the human condition and the use of technology in advancing humanity. For example, globally, around 64% of adults use some form of vision correction (eyeglasses, contact lenses, and/or vision correction surgery), with more than 4 billion wearing corrective glasses. Sixty-six per cent (over 131 million) of all adults in the United States use prescription drugs. More than a million total hip replacements are carried out worldwide in any one year. In everyday life, most of us regularly extend our thinking and problem-solving capacities by using computers. Across the planet, nearly 18% of the population use cars – that adds up to nearly 1.5 billion vehicles radically augmenting our mobility. Where bodies and minds are augmented, our concern is whether this is done humanely, beyond the instrumental and objectifying, to engage moral dilemmas (ethics); beauty, form, and qualities (aesthetics); issues of power (politics); and existential issues and meanings (the transcendental).

The origins of 'metahumanities' are discussed and considered beyond the rather superficial readings that such a perspective critically addresses dualistic thinking, reflecting a move from uniform modernism to deconstructive and reconstructive postmodernisms. Our concern again is not with improvement of the quality of life in general through the humanities (long regarded as an educational seed bed for development of humanity), but with how medical education can specifically benefit from a more holistic understanding of the medical humanities. Can 'deep' medical humanities protect our medical students from the (often-unintended) consequences of a reductive instrumental education? If so, this would embrace a higher and more complex pedagogical experience focused on identity construction through curriculum process rather than production of merely instrumental technicians through an information-led syllabus.

In **Chapter 2**, Alan Bleakley considers multiple issues in medical education and practice, including creativity, complexity, reflective practice, dialectical reasoning, empathy, and capability. Language and metalanguage (the language of language) are central enablers (and potentially also disablers) in all these areas. The many metacognitive aspects of medical education cannot therefore be reduced to linear and predictable statements of fact. The ability to understand and use complex cognitive linguistic constructs – such as metaphor, poetics, and cadence – are central to developing expertise, with reference to issues of guiding values and emergent identities. As such, the medical humanities are also deeply implicated in this work, where '[T]he medical (or health) "humanities" can be read as any intervention that raises the value of biomedical science and clinical and communication skills from the technical-instrumental into other, more complex, registers'. Indeed, a focus on metacognition also shifts the humanities from a matter of instrumental and curative interventions (such as creative writing, art appreciation, and acting) to fundamental issues of mind and thought, and to a reappraisal of identity – what it is to be human and to be an artist, physician, teacher, learner, and patient.

In **Chapter 3**, with illustrative examples in mind, Alan Bleakley considers the role of metacognition in the crucible of the clinical encounter. Attention to subtle details, particularly those associated with non-verbal communication and those afforded by the contexts of such interactions, is central both to learning and to providing meaningful and effective care. Here, '[C]ontext can provide the "meta" in meta-cognition, meta-affect, and meta-sensing, where human activity is shaped by whatever the environment affords in each *umwelt* or ecological niche'. There is a necessary mindfulness in this, an equipoise of mind and action that is attentive, reflective, and interpretive. These come together in critical reflexivity; here, attention is necessarily focused on the patient and the immediate context, but it must also include a metacognitive gaze that attends to emotions as well as to insights gained through both problem-solving and problematising. Again, these capabilities are neither instrumental nor algorithmic; they can only be nurtured and understood using a richer metahumanities frame embracing a wider spectrum of values concerning the nature of humanity.

In **Chapter 4**, and continuing the narrative set up in previous chapters, Alan Bleakley considers the tacit dimension to knowledge of learners and practitioners, noting that a 'cognitive unconscious' is always present, but if it is not acknowledged and examined, it can prove problematic and even dangerous:

> As much as we know more than we can say and we can enjoy the fruits of tacit knowledge, we also know that these fruits are, at the same time, both delicious and poisoned. Tacit knowing is not some mechanical device or instrumental pursuit that we can just turn on and off at will.

Bleakley's argument is predicated on the assumption that we have more knowledge and understanding than our conscious minds entertain. As metacognition, we need to critically and reflexively engage tacit knowledge to understand its value and purposes, for example in processes such as clinical reasoning and the forming of deeper empathy as compathy (see Chapter 12). This engagement includes deliberate mindfulness, emotional engagement, linguistic flexibility, and mobilising intuition, imagination, and differing kinds of creativities (Bleakley 2015, chap. 5). Metahumanities perspectives are needed to both unlock and legitimise such exploration and deliberate practice.

In **Chapter 5**, Quentin Eichbaum explores issues of 'thinking outside the brain' and its implications for metahumanities, particularly in the context of a shared cognition that is a necessary part of teamwork and inter-professional care. In doing so, he discusses how models of shared cognition ultimately led to the concepts of situated, distributed, and embodied cognition (and situativity theory) and how these pertain to the notion of the extended mind. Addressing the evolutionary foundations of both situated and distributed cognition, Eichbaum draws on the work of sociobiologist Edward Wilson and expounds on anthropologist Margaret Wilson's views on embodied cognition. He draws on the ground-breaking work of Andy Clark (2023), who has long argued that cognition is not limited to 'the little grey cells' but can extend to other minds and into our tools and technologies. We can trace this view back to the work of Russian linguist Lev Vygotsky and to socialism which viewed learning not as confined to individual cognition (the dominant model of the individualist, capitalist West) but as extended to the use of artefacts and other persons in collaborative social groups. Clark (ibid.) reappraises these pedagogical models by drawing on contemporary neuroscience and information sciences to demonstrate how thinking, and then learning, is an active *predictive* process grounded in experience. Eichbaum discusses such models of 'active externalism' that take the form of 'dynamic, participatory, self-changing cognition'. He argues that metahumanities afford a necessary integrated knowledge of the extended mind in whatever forms they take and in whatever contexts they are found.

In **Chapter 6**, using a leitmotif of jazz, Rachel Ellaway considers the growing attention to heuristics in professional practice, in particular the heated dispute regarding the appropriateness of heuristic thinking and differing interpretations of expertise. Rather than heuristics being an intrinsic weakness that should be avoided, she outlines the concept of expert heuristics as reflecting a sustained, deliberate, and mindful approach to developing and refining heuristic thinking, including being mindful of its shortcomings that can be considered a form of metaheuristics. From this, she argues that 'metaheuristics can contribute to metahumanities through deliberate engagement in heuristic thinking as an essential part of medical expertise'. From this perspective, heuristics are central to professional development and practice as a way of achieving of metacognitive flow and efficiency from one moment to the next.

In the second section, we focus on new and emerging perspectives afforded by metahumanistic perspectives in pedagogies that could feed contemporary medical education should the latter withdraw from its stubborn reductive, instrumentalist stance.

In **Chapter 7**, Alan Bleakley reprises his arguments from Chapter 3 regarding the centrality of mindful and selective attention. Attention is not simply about what the mind is focused on; it is about a poetic sense of interpretation and possibility that draws together different kinds of knowledge. For instance, attention is the point at which technical biomedical knowledge can be integrated with humanistic understanding of the human condition such as the nature of suffering and the existential challenges of mortality. In following this line of reasoning, Bleakley notes the entangling of burnout and wellness (or the absence thereof) in attending to oneself as the nexus of thought into action. Attention can be lost and compromised and should therefore be strengthened as preparation for the exigencies of practice. This, again, leads us back to metahumanities perspectives on mind and action.

In **Chapter 8**, Quentin Eichbaum explores new perspectives on human perception afforded by metahumanities. Rather than the somewhat reductive and passive theories of perception that inform contemporary practice in medical education, he argues against the notion of an 'immaculate perception' that presents an objective 'veridical' reality. He demonstrates instead how inaccurate, and often flawed and illusory, our perceptions are in helping us navigate the world while subserving evolutionary fitness and our survival. Moreover, rather than perceptions of the outer world impinging on us 'bottom up' towards the brain to be 'objectively' deciphered, perceptions are (drawing again on the work of Andy Clark) seen to be 'predictively' processed (if not intercepted) 'top down' from the brain into the world. Perception is both 'active, participatory, bidirectional, and predictive' and (paradoxically to the naïve – or direct – realist imagination) illusory. Drawing on the work of Anil Seth, Eichbaum explores the implications of an understanding of perception as deeply interpretive (and fundamentally 'illusory'), as well as generative, participatory, and subject to a deconstructive imagination. Indeed, given the close links between perception and consciousness, metahumanistic perspectives are desperately needed to respond to the 'hallucinations' that make up our realities as proponents of representational perception suggest. How then shall we resituate mind, body, and world in configurations that support the values and goals of medical practice? This is particularly pressing where medical practice assumes a naïve realist view of the body, reinforced by medical education's assumptions about reception of ideas in the teaching–learning encounter (what the teacher says or does is what is received by the student).

In **Chapter 9**, Rachel Ellaway considers the thorny topic of 'augmentation' by drawing on Martha Nussbaum's 'human capability approach', which conceptualises capability as a product of the idiosyncratic interaction between an individual's abilities and opportunities. Ellaway expands on this by defining augmentation as changes to human capabilities, and from this 'human augmentation theory' that can be used to explore different ways in which capabilities can change and be changed, and to better understand the entanglements between capability change and metacognition. In doing so, she argues that medical humanities need to be concerned with all aspects of human experience;

experience is inescapably entangled with capability; and we need a more holistic and multidimensional sense of metahumanities grounded in the concept of metacapabilities, the capability to change one's own capabilities and those of others. In doing so, this raises new perspectives on ethics, identity, aesthetics, and politics as related to both medical education and practice.

In **Chapter 10**, Quentin Eichbaum explores several specific principles and strategies for intentionally 'realising' the extended mind that he first discussed in Chapter 5. From these principles, he conceptualises a metacognition of the extended mind. He then discusses implications of the extended mind for medical education, the arts, and metahumanities. Such metahumanities must extend deep roots into the sciences to create more integrated approaches to knowledge and our understanding of the (extended) mind, and to better understand the associations between individual brain-bound cognition and the outer world that is mediated through perception, attention, and ultimately consciousness. Eichbaum merges ideas from the neurosciences with those from the humanities (such as George Lakoff's influential work on metaphor). He also argues that metahumanities need to transcend the orthodox humanities and the sense of isolated individual minds to consider the *distribution* of consciousness, identity, and beauty across and between minds. Again, permeability is key here. The notion of isolated minds itself may be all 'in the mind'!

In **Chapter 11**, Rachel Ellaway builds on her work articulating 'pattern theory' that is based on an understanding of patterns as nexuses of related memories and thoughts in an individual mind that shape how we perceive the world around us. This again reflects issues of metacognition and their entanglements with metahumanities:

> Because we are always seeing the world through patterns the world often seems patterned to us, but what we are really seeing are reflections of our own minds. Indeed, we often struggle to perceive our own pattern thinking, let alone that of others.

Ellaway argues that patterns and pattern thinking are key to learning medicine, and that they play a central role in diagnostics and problem-solving in medical practice. If learners, teachers, and practitioners are not mindful and deliberate in their pattern thinking, then unregarded pattern thinking habits can mislead them and contribute to harm.

In **Chapter 12**, Alan Bleakley explores the little-discussed concept and practice of 'compathy' that he defines as 'empathy that is reflexively and critically examined and interrogated by those who express it'. Widely ignored in the extensive medical education literature on empathy, compathy involves shared feelings rather than a disengaged sense of the other – as a form of situated and extended affect (or meta-affect). Metahumanistic perspectives emphasise the totality of human experience to include shared feelings of a group for its members that again depends on compathy rather than empathy. Bleakley closes by comparing the somewhat superficial, overused, and uncritically received notions of 'empathy' and 'competence' (shaped by a naïve instrumentalism) with the deeper concepts and practices of compathy and capability: 'Just as empathy is superseded by the deeper form of compathy, so competence is superseded by "capability"'.

Our concluding **Chapter 13** offers a manifesto, or position statement, for the entanglements of metacognition, meta-affect, metahumanities, and medical education drawn from the book chapters.

References

Arnaldi, M. 2022. The translational imagination. In: A. Bleakley and S. Neilson, eds. *Poetry in the Clinic: Towards a Lyrical Medicine*. Abingdon: Routledge, pp. 270–2.

Bleakley, A. 1999. From reflective practice to holistic reflexivity. *Studies in Higher Education*, 24, 315–30.

Bleakley, A. 2013. Towards a critical medical humanities. In: V. Bates, A. Bleakley and S. Goodman, eds. *Medicine, Health and the Arts: Approaches to the Medical Humanities*. Abingdon: Routledge.

Bleakley, A. 2015. *Medical Humanities and Medical Education: How the Medical Humanities Can Shape Better Doctors*. Abingdon: Routledge.

Bleakley, A. 2019. The medical humanities: A mixed weather front on a global scale. In: A. Bleakley, ed. *Routledge Handbook of the Medical Humanities*. Abingdon: Routledge.

Bleakley, A. 2023. *Medical Humanities: Ethics, Aesthetics, Politics*. London: Routledge.

Bleakley, A.A. 2024. A Therapeutic intervention for an ailing medical education: The values prism model as proof of concept. *Medical Teacher*, 46, 232–8.

Bleakley, A., Neilson, S., eds. 2021. *Poetry in the Clinic: Towards a Lyrical Medicine*. Abingdon: Routledge.

Brooks, D. 2023. How to stay sane in brutalizing times. *The New York Times International Edition*. Nov 4–5, p. 14, 16.

Clark, A. 1997. *Being There – Putting Brain, Body & World Together Again: Putting Brain, Body and World Together Again*. Cambridge, MA: MIT Press.

Clark, A. 2010. *Supersizing the Mind: Embodiment, Action, and Cognitive Extension*. Oxford: Oxford University Press.

Clark, A. 2016. *Surfing Uncertainty: Prediction, Action, and the Embodied Mind*. Oxford: Oxford University Press.

Clark, A. 2023. *The Experience Machine: How Our Minds Predict and Shape Reality*. London: Allen Lane.

Del Val, J. n.d.-a Metahumanist Manifesto: its genealogy, evolution and relevance 10 years after. Author's website: https://metabody.eu/metahumanist-manifesto-10-years-after/ Last accessed: 5th Feb 2024.

Del Val, J. n.d.-b Metahumanism. Author's website: https://metabody.eu/metahumanism/ Last accessed: 5th Feb 2024.

Engeström, Y. 2008. *From Teams to Knots: Activity-Theoretical Studies of Collaboration and Learning at Work*. Cambridge: Cambridge University Press.

Engeström, Y. 2016. *Studies in Expansive Learning: Learning What is Not Yet There*. Cambridge: Cambridge University Press.

Engeström, Y. 2018. *Expertise in Transition: Expansive Learning in Medical Work*. Cambridge: Cambridge University Press.

Heron, J. 1977. *Six Category Intervention Analysis*. Guilford: University of Surrey.

Heron, J. 1989. *Catharsis in Human Development*. Guilford: University of Surrey. Available at: https://co-counselling.info/en/ref/catharsis-human-development. Last accessed: 25/03/2023

Heron, J. 1992. *Feeling and Personhood: Psychology in Another Key*. London: Sage.
Heron, J. 1998, *Sacred Science: Person-Centred Inquiry into the Spiritual and the Subtle*. Monmouth: PCCS Books.
Heron, J. 1999. *The Complete Facilitator's Handbook*. London: Kogan Page.
Heron, J. 2001. *Helping the Client: A Creative Practical Guide*. 5th ed. London: Sage
Kneebone, R. 2020. *Expert: Understanding the Path to Mastery*. London: Penguin.
Kristeva, J., Moro, M.-R., Ødemark, J., Engebretsen, E. 2019. The cultural crossings of care: A call for translational medical humanities. In: A. Bleakley, ed. *The Routledge Handbook of the Medical Humanities*. Abingdon: Routledge, pp. 34–40.
Polanyi, M. 1966. *The Tacit Dimension*. Chicago, IL: University of Chicago Press.
Reber, A.S., Allen, R., eds. 2022. *The Cognitive Unconscious: The First Half Century*. Oxford: Oxford University Press.
Sand, M. 2013. *Transhumanism: at the Rim of Science*. Report from the Conference "The Posthuman: Differences, Embodiments, Performativity", *the 5th Beyond Humanism Conference*, Rome, Italy, September 11–14. Available at: https://www.google.com/url?sa=t&rct=j&q=&esrc=s&source=web&cd=&ved=2ahUKEwiQ_-2ryp6EAxVpW0EAHbhrDeQQFnoECCkQAQ&url=https%3A%2F%2Fwww.tatup.de%2Findex.php%2Ftatup%2Farticle%2Fdownload%2F581%2F1028%2F1354&usg=AOvVaw0Vfy50b9U0S_rPo-vJu_3s&opi=89978449 Last accessed: 13 Feb 2024.
Schön, D. 1983. *The Reflective Practitioner: How Professionals Think in Action*. New York, NY: Basic Books.
Schön, D.A. 1990. *Educating the Reflective Practitioner: Toward a New Design for Teaching and Learning in the Professions*. San Francisco, CA: Jossey-Bass.
Splete, H. 2023. Double lung transplant uses double D breast implants. *Medscape Psychiatry*. Available at: https://www.medscape.com/viewarticle/998277?ecd=wnl_tp10_daily_231109_MSCPEDIT_etid6042465&uac=281358AK&impID=6042465#vp_2. Last accessed: 21/03/2024
Taleb, N. 2012. *Antifragile: Things That Gain from Disorder*. New York, NY: Random House.
Tarricone, P. 2011. *The Taxonomy of Metacognition*. London: Psychology Press.
Tuncel, Y. 2023. Reflections on Trash-humanism as Performed by Jaime del Val. *Dossier: Metahuman Futures*, 3 (2). Available at: https://journals.tplondon.com/jp/article/view/2968 Last accessed: 12 Feb. 2024.
Weavers, R.M. 1953. *The Ethics of Rhetoric*. Chicago. Ill: Henry Regnery Co.
Whitehead, A., Woods, A. eds. 2016. *The Edinburgh Companion to the Critical Medical Humanities*. Edinburgh: Edinburgh University Press.

Part I

1 Forms of metahumanism

Alan Bleakley

Warm carbon hearts meet cold silicon technologies

An emergent movement of 'morbid environmentalism' and 'Anthropocene antihumanists' suggests that humanity is a parasitic force that has been disastrous for planet Earth (Benatar 2006, MacCormack 2020, Kirsch 2023). As humanity continues to pursue its destructive path towards final annihilation, taking other species with it, would it not be better in a moral–ecological sense to stop having children, thus turning off the taps of human ambition and greed that have provided such poisonous waters for life on Earth?

Such morbid environmentalism is echoed somewhat in existential concerns over artificial intelligence (AI) turning rogue, as we touched on in the previous chapter. But AI enthusiasts are more likely to follow a 'transhumanist' view, where human qualities are radically extended and deepened by artefacts. In medicine, there is abundant optimism along these lines (van der Niet and Bleakley 2021, Kolata 2023, Lee et al. 2023). Peter Lee and colleagues (2023), in their recent *The AI Revolution in Medicine: GPT-4 and Beyond*, paint an optimistic picture of the 'momentous potential' for GPT-4 (Generative Pre-trained Transformer-4) in medical areas such as consulting, diagnostics, and recording information.

Such optimism is founded on the notion that GPT-4 demonstrates genuine empathy and concern and that this could become reflexive. Here, the AI technology not only thinks about what it does (reflection), but also changes its values for the better, through such reflection (reflexivity) – in other words, a meta-AI. This implies a machine with affect, even intuitive qualities. Given the alarming condition even today that flesh-and-blood medical students characteristically lose empathy and gain cynicism by year 4 of their undergraduate careers, that AI may be more effective in these areas of so-called soft skills in medicine is quite alarming. However, we should not get carried away with the rather simplistic notions concerning connections between so-called 'empathy' and patient consultations in the picture painted by Lee and colleagues in discussing developments of GPT-4. This is because flesh-and-blood humans themselves are still thrashing out quite what they mean by 'empathy' and 'emotional labour' in the context of healthcare (Eichbaum et al. 2022, this volume Chapter 12).

DOI: 10.4324/9781032687339-3

As we fantasise about fleshly and sensual aspects of the AI and robotics revolutions, at the outer limits of AI thinking, Robin Mackenzie (2020) considers the ethical conundrums raised by having sex with 'sentient, self-aware sex robots' (sexbots). Designed as intimacy partners, what ethical implications will be raised by sentient AI in spheres such as sexual health (of sexbots, not just of their human partners)? Will we need hybrid relationship/sexuality counsellors? Does robot gender matter in an age of gender fluidity and transgender expression? What might a robotic sexually transmitted disease look like and how will a medicine of the future wrestle with this? Antihumanist pessimism could quickly gain a foothold here!

From a humanist perspective of course, morbid environmentalism and antihumanist pessimism appear deeply callous, a form of scaremongering. By the same token, cognisance of the dangers of AI autonomy is already leading to co-ordinated prophylaxis. In the *Guardian*, Geneva Abdul (2023) reports that 'Experts join forces to warn over AI's threat to humanity'. The existential threat created by what is perceived as poor or piecemeal regulation of AI has led to the formation of a global expert group concerned with the need for close monitoring and regulation. AI is then bracketed with pandemics and nuclear wars as primary existential threats. Stripped of moral reasoning and emotional sensitivity, a collective, superior cold intelligence working at extraordinary power that can be exponentially enlarged can outstrip the limits of human reasoning. Non-regulation may lead to a future scenario differing little from the dystopia shared by the antihumanists and morbid environmentalists, where humanity is redundant, doomed. Such 'extended human' entanglements warrant close, critical inspection, and we suggest that this is best done from the perspective of metacognition – thinking-about-thinking – as a species of medical humanities, thus guaranteeing that extended cognition is interlaced with extended affect and sensibility or aesthetic concerns. This adds up to a complex and multifaceted 'metahumanities', where disciplinary concerns (history, art, design, literature, etc.) are displaced for values concerns: aesthetics, ethics, politics, and the transcendental.

Natasha Brie Beranek (2021) synthesises recent thinking about metahumanities. She notes that the term was coined by Stefan Lorenz Sorgner in the context of the development of the transhumanist movement, discussed above specifically in relation to AI. Beranek continues: 'Sorgner defines the metahumanities as a further development of the traditional humanities through the inclusion of non-dualistic insights'. This doesn't get us very far, as such a definition could well describe the shift from structuralism – based on dualities or oppositionalist thinking – to post-structuralism, where thinking in dualities is *sous rature* or 'under erasure' as Martin Heidegger and then Jacques Derrida put it (~~thinking in dualities~~). This 'strikethrough' means that dualism is 'suspended', or its presence is inadequate yet necessary. It is impossible to exclude it from language and thought, and new forms of thought replace it such as tolerance of ambiguity. Dualism is the modernist way of resolving ambiguity ('you're either with us or against us') recapitulated by authoritarian regimes and their leaders in contemporary times – all unreconstructed modernists.

This is also the logic of neoliberal capitalism. The snowclone 'it's the economy, stupid', while originating with one of Bill Clinton's advisors, James Carville, in 1992, readily feeds into right wing sentiment. Economic and instrumental values define the political and overshadow aesthetic, ethical, and transcendental values. The humanities in universities have suffered in this political climate that favours functional science and technology over the arts and humanities, the latter seen as having little economic knock-on (despite the arts and entertainment cultures being a major contributor to economies). The guiding value behind such polarisation is what William James called 'tough-mindedness' as opposed to 'tender-mindedness' (the former being the domain of conservative politics, the latter of liberal politics). A knock-on effect of this is that managerial functions in universities are privileged over academic studies. This is echoed in medicine, where managerialism prevails on the basis that the economy of a health system (its resource allocation) is more important than its healthcare functions. Finally, 'cognitive capitalism' prevails, where cognition is treated as private property and collaborative cognition is discouraged.

Beranek (2021) suggests that where metahumanities amplify humanity positively, this is achieved not by introducing transgressive values, but 'Overall, the metahumanities will be hastened by shifts in mainstream perceptions about how biotechnologies and posthumanist theories often amplify rather than contravene common ideals and values'. While posthumanism and transhumanism appear to create territory for intellectuals, they describe everyday increases in quality of life through supplements such as smart technologies (personalised education, safer driving, better healthcare, and cleaner transport), although the horizon for such enhancements includes controversial technologies such as gene enhancement.

Where science and technology are perceived as more important to culture than the arts and humanities, they attract greater funding for research and development, as funding for the humanities is (dis)proportionately cut. But it is the arts and humanities that provide a critical eye to shape the direction of science. We might see the arts and humanities not primarily as decorative or providing entertainment, but as the 'values carriers' for ethics, aesthetics, politics, and the transcendental beyond the instrumental or functional. These value perspectives embody critique.

Metacognition embraces such values perspectives beyond the instrumental such that reduction of life purely to information is stemmed, where meaning is sought. However, we are cautious here to not demote 'information' to mere instrumental status where information is not meaningless – for example information can form patterns that are highly meaningful (see Chapter 11). Metapatterns include fractals – repeated patterns at differing levels of magnification that show complexity operating at differing levels of expression in matter. Or the parts repeat the whole. Information, such as DNA, is patterned.

Medicine is at the forefront of technological innovation, already drawing heavily on AI. At the other end of the scale to cold technologies, a warm humanist movement within medicine – imported from Carl Rogers' (1951) 'client-centred' and 'person-centred' counselling and psychotherapy model – has long promoted an embracing 'patient-centred' practice. Here, empathy (itself a complex notion open to critique) is at the core of practice (see Chapter 12). This has been the anchor and touchstone for conventional medical humanities in medical education since the first forays into art therapy in the UK by Adrian Hill in 1945. But it is an anchor that now drags.

'Person-centredness' in Rogers' model is a regression to Renaissance humanism and essentialism of the 'I', rather than a forward-looking account of persons as contextualised in culture and history and extended by technologies – from reading glasses to advanced computers, prescription drugs, gene splicing, and embedded microchips. 'Patient-centredness' still has currency, with its central pillars of empathy and *parrhesia* or truth-telling, but again we can no longer look back to Renaissance humanism to make sense of an emergent humanity yoked to, and extended by, rapidly advancing digital technologies. We now live in a posthumanist age (Nichols 1988, Haraway 1991, Lorimer 2009), where humanity is part of a symbiotic democracy of both carbon- and silicon-based life forms. The graphic artist Mathieu Bablet (2021) riffs on this theme in his *Carbon and Silicon*, where 'two androids crisscross the planet for centuries in search of themselves and each other while civilization crumbles around them'.

The most radical perspective of posthumanism is perhaps Object-Oriented Ontology (OOO) (Harman 2018) in which artefacts are afforded the same ontological status as humans. The patient undergoing surgery, the surgeon, the scalpel she uses to open the patient's flesh, the monitoring machines used by the anaesthetist, the bed that the patient lies on, and even overhead lights and the floor that everybody treads are democratic participants in a circle of Being. This is true Theatre.

Where the medical humanities in medical education have looked backwards to classical humanism and promoted patient-centredness and empathy as the primary products of their influences, medical humanities must surely be dragged into the near future to converse with developments such as AI and OOO. Here, however, is a potential trap. The 'transhumanist' movement emanating from Silicon Valley, California – in contrast to the antihumanists above – is naively optimistic about a cyborg future, where humans are happily augmented by AI, or vice versa, with extravagant aims such as eliminating disease and suspending death (More and Vita-More 2013, Sorgner 2022). Transhumanists tend to think, or imagine, materially, so that the future of mental illness and neurodiversity, for example, are left to speculations of science fiction writers. Transhumanist materialism fails to grasp contextual factors in emotional life (such as the power of embodied metaphor) that are irreducible to brain process, where they claim material substrates for all conditions.

We wish to remain critically responsive to developments of the augmented doctor and the augmented medical educator. We are at once fascinated and repelled by conundrums such as the similarity between medicine's commitment to maintaining life, practically at all costs, and the transhumanist Peter Thiel's comment that a future technologically sophisticated medicine will 'reverse all human ailments … where Death will eventually be reduced from a mystery to a solvable problem' (in Sample 2022). This is the ultimate expression of medicine as technological fix, grounded entirely in instrumental values, ignoring the ethical, aesthetic, political, and transcendental values that make medicine and medical education so complex, rich, and worthy. Thiel was the founder of PayPal, a supporter of Donald Trump, and has invested heavily in cryogenics; so what kind of future does he imagine for the 'never dying'?

In this book, we resist the lure of such utopian, near-future science fictions for what we see as emerging metahumanity trends nevertheless grounded in longstanding traditions of clinical practice such as concern and care for patients and colleagues. We see this future-facing but sensitive transition of the medical humanities, a shift into 'meta' thinking, as reconfiguring what we mean by 'learning' within medical education and 'application' within clinical practice. Where 'meta' literally means 'beyond' or 'greater', it is then expansive and potentially boundary breaking. These are useful metaphors. A better metaphor may be 'deepening' of the current state of thinking and practice in the medical humanities in medical education. We thus coin the term 'deep medical humanities' to refer to this innovation, moving beyond, but incorporating, current terms such as 'critical' medical humanities and 'translational' medical humanities. Here, we are reminded by Laurence Kirmayer (2024) that '4E cognitive sciences have revealed some of the secrets of how metaphor mediates the immediate by focusing on processes of embodiment, embedding, enactment and extension'. For us, the near future, as neither morbid antihumanism nor ethically unsound transhumanism, is one of creative multiplication of embodied metaphors. Is this not a poetics, or an improvisatory jazz, of medicine?

What's in a name?

The term 'medical humanities' is, unfortunately, as clear as mud. As keen participants in, and acute observers of, trends in medical humanities cultures, we are bothered by the continuing loose, uncritical use of this collective term (sometimes used in the singular and sometimes in the plural). We do not crave a definitive definition (there is none), but rather a better scoping of the territory that resists listings or typologies for a fluid 'territorializing' or 'nomadism' (Deleuze and Guattari 1972).

Currently, the field of medical humanities suffers from oppositional categories, with two fundamentally different readings across two cultures. First, 'medical humanities' are read as the academic study of medical culture through the arts and humanities, such as the history of medicine and medical bioethics. Here, disciplines such as history, moral philosophy, and literature turn their critical gazes upon medical culture and medical identities. And here, the humanities act not to shape 'humaneness', but as critical lenses. Sometimes, this culture refers to itself as 'applied medical humanities', as the academic study of clinical practices (rather than the overarching culture of medicine), often drawing on medical memoirs or autoethnographies as primary source material. Second, 'medical humanities' are read as the application of arts, humanities, and qualitative social sciences to medical education, or the shaping of medical pedagogies. This includes curriculum design and ways of teaching and learning. Here, the humanities act to shape 'humaneness' and 'professionalism' that Maureen Dowd (2023) refers to as '(H)igher principles – dignity, civility, patience, respect, tolerance, goodness, sympathy and empathy'.

Medical humanities in medical education generally read 'humanities' as 'humanising', or countering the tendency for empathy decline, emotional insulation, and cynicism that tend to set in towards the end of a medicine undergraduate degree. This can be seen as a regression to the person-centred models referred to earlier, now challenged by the extended and augmented person. Or humanising is an essential process but is complicated by embedding in technologies that extend humanity. For example, a new definition of empathy emerges from OOO as respect for the identities and qualities of all objects seen from within their own worlds (is this not what empathy promises – standing not just in the shoes of your patient, but also in the mechanical work of that patient's newly placed stents?) The most popular version of traditional humanising medical humanities is narrative medicine – again a complex of approaches that focuses upon 'honouring the stories of illness', to borrow Rita Charon's (2006) descriptor. But we must also attend to the life and function of the story itself, its structures, and possibilities (which of course literary techniques such as close reading demand). Conventional narrative medicine has failed to engage the metacognitive as we understood it, where the descriptor 'machines' is used in the sense that Deleuze and Guattari (1972) describe humans – as 'desiring machines' – open complex, adaptive, dynamic systems that form 'assemblages' with other 'machines' in a series of 'flows'. To apprehend the individual and social body as flow rather than static entity is to treat such bodies as embodied metaphors, or bodies-beyond-bodies (metahumanity as process). Traditional narrative medicine is too focused on person as text to pay close attention to matters of subtext, context, and para-text (storying is disembodied and then reconstituted by giving equal ontological status to the person – characters – and the word processing software and associated hardware that creates the artefact, for example, where designers strive to recreate the 'feel' of pen on screen as imitating writing on paper).

A 'medical humanities' of the future may strive for this same simulated effect – to bring skin and machine, cognition, and information, affect and AI-engineered empathy, into productive conversation. And there is a set of topics and ground-rules here that can provide a frame for such a discussion: the tacit dimension, forms of attention, kinds of complexity, collective sense-making, catharsis that leads to insight, capabilities, augmentation, meta-heuristics, pattern thinking, and so forth. Such topics make up the chapters of this book.

Thinking with immense particulars

The use of the arts and humanities (as 'medical humanities') in medical education has been justified as compensation for a dehumanising biomedicine, while educating for tolerance of ambiguity. Throughout their undergraduate careers, medical students are characteristically socialised into objectification of patients or show a decline in empathy (Howick et al. 2023). We should, however, expect incremental increases in empathy where medical education is effective. Such objectification is advertised by patients being reduced to their symptoms, rather than appreciated in a holistic way. Further, and paradoxically, decline in sensitivity is shown towards the biomedical sciences themselves, treated as instrumental, functional, and information driven, mirroring the way that such science is typically taught. This, rather than developing an appreciation for bioscience as imaginative, aesthetic, and full of wonder.

Medical students worldwide are still dutifully sitting formal examinations based on regurgitation of memorised information, rather than engaging with scaffolded learning of advanced thinking strategies grounded in work-based experiences. Such dulling functionalism also readily bleeds out into learning clinical and communication skills, so that the very heart of the clinical encounter is often (mis)learned in formulaic ways. Finally, early decline in empathy often develops into cynicism, a major factor in physician burnout (Bleakley 2020).

Again, the medical humanities have often been advertised as a cure for such a range of ailments in medical education (Bleakley 2015). But medical schools, underfunded and with over-stretched curricula and faculty, generally pay the medical humanities lip service, as surplus to core requirements. While many medical schools claim to have developed medical humanities programmes, these are often electives taken by relatively few students (rather than core and compulsory curriculum elements) that are not formally assessed. Further, medical humanities themselves can be reductive and instrumental, framed as functional 'fixes' for an impoverished biomedicine while, ironically, remaining functional themselves.

While some arts- and humanities-based innovations have been successful, even remarkable, the focus on the medical humanities as compensation for reductive biomedical and clinical sciences fails to attend to the root issue: how can the extraordinary intrinsic qualities of biomedical science and clinical and communication skills flourish within an ordinary medicine and surgery undergraduate curriculum? This presents a dual challenge: first, realising that biosciences and clinical and communication skills are not restricted to instrumental values (as pure information), but as already noted can embrace ethical, aesthetic, political, and transcendental values (as meaning); and second, that this shift in values, qualities, intensities, and complexity offers a pedagogical challenge – first, of curriculum planning; and second, of methods of teaching and learning.

Recent advances in thinking about the medical humanities as translational media discuss how the biosciences (and information sciences) can engage the arts, humanities, and qualitative social sciences in productive conversation

(Kristeva et al. 2019, Arnaldi et al. 2022, Bleakley 2023). Such advances challenge the (tired) 'two cultures' debate advertising an oppositional model where arts and sciences are seen as having fundamentally different epistemologies. The translational process raises the quality, intensity, and complexity of all disciplines through appropriate pedagogies. The key translational media are linguistic tropes, particularly metaphors, but also embodied semiotics. A key claim of the medical humanities – leading to the development of narrative medicine – is that clinical biomedicine reduces patients to facts usually notated numerically (charts, test results), so that patients' 'stories' must be retrieved for them to be considered holistically. But this ignores the fact that bioscience can be as metaphorically rich and imaginative as narrative (e.g., Ramon y Cajal first calling synapses 'protoplasmic kisses'), despite its modern tendency to reduce language to functional terms, overriding the poetic (Bleakley and Neilson 2022).

The overall translational project sets out to transcend purely informational cultures of medicine and medical pedagogy to embrace 'meaning'. This process, in turn, embraces metacognition (thinking about thinking, or reflexivity) (Quirk 2006), meta-affect (gaining insight into catharsis, rather than being swamped by emotion, through cultivating 'free attention') (Heron 1977), meta-sensing (shaping acute sensibilities) (Bleakley 2020), and clinical metaphysics (thinking philosophically about the meaning of medical practice) (Braude 2012).

In this book on use of the 'meta' in medical pedagogy, we ask not how core science is *used* in medical education, but how it is *produced* or shaped by its informing values. In a meta-turn, we also ask how instrumental curriculum thinking and related emergent practices can be elevated to greater finesse (complexity, quality, and intensity). These transitions and translations can also be thought of as values-led initiatives that transform information into meaning (Tomlinson 2023). A more complex and aesthetically interesting science can be excavated from years of over-layering with functional forms where science is reduced to mere information. Further, a pedagogical layer can be excavated from the ruins of years of instrumental medical education.

It is perhaps how medicine is learned, and not medicine itself, that leads to a culture of reductive, instrumental biomedical science; and to a scientising of clinical and communication skills that calcifies the latter two areas of study grounding them in quantities rather than qualities. With these observations in mind, we suggest that a fruitful way to frame the medical humanities is to (i) place greater emphasis upon the value of qualitative social sciences in medical education (this includes embracing population and global health issues such as health inequalities and the impact of climate change and mass migrations) and (ii) to inquire more deeply into the ways that learning agility – such as 'learning-to-learn' – can be intensified in medicine and surgery curricula. We see this, in short, as the deepening of understanding of metacognition and meta-affect. To flesh out this argument, we offer two illustrative case studies: early 2000s' pedagogical innovations at two medical schools.

Vanderbilt and Peninsula: pioneers in using strategies of 'learning-to-learn'

How can the 'medical humanities' (a sprawling and ungainly territory) best be introduced pedagogically into a medicine and surgery undergraduate curriculum (perhaps as a meta-pedagogy, facilitating reflexivity and critical inquiry amongst medical students as they face a possible tsunami of rote learning)? As far as we know, in the early 2000s, Vanderbilt University School of Medicine, Nashville, USA (Eichbaum 2014), and Peninsula Medical School (Universities of Exeter and Plymouth), UK (Bleakley 2020, 2023), were among the first medical schools globally to embrace the idea that the medical humanities were best not introduced as compensation to an instrumental biomedical science but as a filter, lens, or prism through which a standard scientific medical education (embracing anatomy, basic biomedical science, applied clinical and information science, and applied clinical and communication skills) could be radically improved in quality, intensity, and scope. The two innovations shared the fundamental idea that learning tolerance of ambiguity is essential to a medical education.

At Vanderbilt, using pedagogies of intensive small group learning, the model developed to achieve this end was translational, as

> an approach that integrates the humanities with the basic and clinical sciences, based on metacognition. This metacognitive approach to the humanities … has three goals: 1) to develop students as flexible thinkers and agile learners and to provide them with essential cognitive and emotional skills for navigating medical complexity and uncertainty; 2) to elicit in students empathy and tolerance by making them aware of the immense diversity in human cognition (and emotion); and 3) to integrate the humanities with the basic and clinical sciences.
>
> (Eichbaum 2014)

Importantly, metacognitive abilities were seen as necessarily intertwined with 'emotional monitoring and regulation', where '[T]hinking and learning in the group setting of the colloquium ultimately also fosters the student's professional identity'. Students would become 'flexible thinkers and agile learners' through 'perspective taking' (Eichbaum 2014). What is important here are the metaphors describing these pedagogical aims, such as 'flexible' and 'agile'. This shifts pedagogic outcomes from instrumental objectives centred on memorising information to qualities of being centred on meaning, with metaphor as the productive translational device. The Vanderbilt approach encourages students to develop a deeply nuanced knowledge of how the mind works – not just to imbibe information, but to afford meaning for that information. This is the heart of 'meta' – not *what* we know, but *how* and *why* we know.

At Peninsula, there was the luxury of designing a curriculum from scratch. Three key issues were identified. First, medical students must learn to tolerate ambiguity and uncertainty; second, they should not suffer from characteristic empathy decline and increasing cynicism; and third, they should learn anatomy, biomedical science, and clinical and communication capabilities as approaches not restricted to the instrumental and functional but embracing a range of values (Bleakley 2023). This approach again shifts medicine from a study of information to one of meaning, focusing on the needs of patients in the context of wider cultural issues such as deprivation, inequity and inequality, the climate crisis, and mass migrations. In turn, this would cultivate an identity formation replacing older initiation-led traditions such as the rituals of cadaver dissection, humiliation at the hands of seniors in bedside teaching, and white coat ceremonies.

Central to such an approach was educating core science and social science faculty to frame learning beyond instrumental concerns to embrace other values. This required imaginative use of metaphor, mobilisation of complexity theory, and sophisticated pedagogical strategies of learning-to-learn. The approach was at once metacognitive, meta-affective, meta-sensory, and meta-pedagogical. This drew heavily on the ideas and practices of the Curriculum Reconceptualisation movement (Doll 1993, Pinar 2019) to shape a staff development programme. The key principles of this movement are that education is a form of character building or identity construction and that curriculum is not restricted to *content* (syllabus) but refers to a *process* of learning. Thus, curriculum is read as a verb (*currere*) meaning, literally, ‘to run the course’. How the course is negotiated (with the help of tutors through ‘scaffolding’ learning) shapes character.

Key to the approaches adopted at Vanderbilt and Peninsula were, again, that sciences and humanities do not constitute ‘two cultures’ at war. Rather, science at root can be both humane and artistic or imaginative, while humanities can readily be pedestrian and instrumental, although it is often peddled as the best way to educate for tolerance of ambiguity. Indeed, one of the great qualities of both good, inventive science and arts/humanities is to be disruptive, upsetting norms and established habits. The metacognitive, meta-affective, meta-sensory approach provides the conditions for thinking ‘slant’ (or ‘slantwise’) about medicine.

Given this background, the three authors of this book suggest that we might look at medical humanities traditions from the angle not of how we might rescue biomedicine from its tendency to resort to instrumental values (through literal scientific descriptors), but how we might raise the value of *both* biomedical sciences and arts/humanities approaches (through metaphor and complexity, or as quality, intensity, and depth). Again, we do this by invoking the ‘meta’ (the greater than) of both cognition and affect/sense. This leads us into the territory of cognitive science, where meanings of metacognition and meta-affect have been hot topics of discussion and experimentation for many years, as cognition-in-the-head is extended, embodied, enacted, and embedded (the ‘4 Es’). To this, we might add ‘entangled’ as a fifth E. Readers will gain a new understanding of possible futures of the medical humanities as we ‘think with immense particulars’ – moving from neuroscience’s specificities to the philosophy of Externalism's reach to consider medical work as metacognition and meta-affect grounded in both brains and expansive environmental contexts. Our thesis is that symptoms have – simultaneously – both no boundaries and the tightest of personal boundaries. It is managing this paradox that makes medical work complex.

In the concluding chapter, we set out a manifesto for metahumanities in medical education based on increasing the quality, intensity, and reach of the biomedical sciences, or the field of 'meta'. We note that metacognition has a troubled existence in the cognitive psychology space because it is not something 'other' in the mind, but is a result of layered, patterned, and disciplined minds that are also strange to themselves (see Chapter 11). This is something AI research is starting to demonstrate – you cannot design minds, but you can design substrates that can develop idiosyncratic mind-like behaviours that the designers do not fully understand. So, we ask: is there a more holistic term than 'metacognition' or is this a matter of liberating the term or 'making it strange'? Theory of mind and research into the nature of consciousness are both important here. Subsequent chapters will interrogate these issues.

References

Abdul, G. 2023. AI experts warn of its threat to humanity. *The Guardian*. 31 May 2023. Available at: https://www.pressreader.com/uk/the-guardian/20230531/281500755632106. Last accessed: 28 June 2023.

Arnaldi, M., Engebretsen, E., Forsdick, C. 2022. Translating COVID-19: From contagion to containment. *Journal of Medical Humanities*, 43, 387–404.

Bablet, M. 2021. *Carbon and Silicon*. London: Magnetic Press.

Benatar, D. 2006. *Better Never to Have Been*. Oxford: OUP.

Bleakley A. 2015. *Medical Humanities and Medical Education*. Abingdon: Routledge.

Bleakley A. 2020. *Educating Doctors' Senses Through the Medical Humanities: "How Do I Look?"* Abingdon: Routledge.

Bleakley, A. 2023. *Medical Humanities: Ethics, Aesthetics, Politics*. London: Routledge.

Bleakley, A., Neilson, S. 2022. *Poetry in the Clinic: Towards a Lyrical Medicine*. Abingdon: Routledge.

Braude, H. 2012. *Intuition in Medicine: A Philosophical Defence of Clinical Reasoning*. Chicago, IL: University of Chicago Press.

Beranek, N.B. 2021. The Metahumanities. *Deliberatio*, 1, 97–108.

Charon, R. 2006. *Narrative Medicine: Honoring the Stories of Illness*. Oxford: OUP.

Deleuze, G., Guattari, F. 1972. *Anti-Oedipus: Capitalism and Schizophrenia*. Ann Arbor, MI: University of Minnesota Press.

Doll, W. 1993. *A Post-Modern Perspective on Curriculum*. Columbia University, NY: Teachers College Press.

Dowd, M. 2023. Don't kill 'Frankenstein' with real Frankensteins at large. *The New York Times*. May 27 2023. Available at: https://www.nytimes.com/2023/05/27/opinion/english-humanities-ai.html. Last accessed: 28 Jun 2023

Eichbaum, Q.G. 2014. Thinking about thinking and emotion: The metacognitive approach to the medical humanities that integrates the humanities with the basic and clinical sciences. *Permanente Journal*, 18, 64–75.

Eichbaum, Q., Barbeau-Meunier, C.-A., White, M., et al. 2022. Empathy across cultures – one size does not fit all: from the ego-logical to the eco-logical of relational empathy. *Advances in Health Sciences Education*, 28, 643–57.

Haraway, D. 1991. *Simians, Cyborgs and Women: The Reinvention of Nature*. New York, NY: Routledge.
Harman G. 2018. *Object-Oriented Ontology*. London: Pelican.
Heron J. 1977. *Six Category Intervention Analysis*. Guilford: University of Surrey.
Howick, J., Dudko, M., Feng, S.N., et al. 2023. Why might medical student empathy change throughout medical school? a systematic review and thematic synthesis of qualitative studies. *BMC Medical Education*, 23, 270.
Kirmayer, L. 2024. Metaphor and the poetics of illness and healing. In: A. Bleakley and S. Neilson, eds. *Handbook of Medicine and Poetry*. Abingdon: Routledge.
Kirsch, A. 2023. *The Revolt Against Humanity: Imagining a Future Without Us*. New York, NY: Columbia Global Reports.
Kolata, G. 2023. For bedside warmth, consult the program. *The New York Times International Edition*. June 15, 7
Kristeva, J., et al. 2019 The cultural crossings of care: A call for translational medical humanities. In: A. Bleakley, ed. *Routledge Handbook of Medical Humanities*. Abingdon: Routledge, p. 34.
Lee, P., Goldberg, C., Kohane, I. 2023. *The AI Revolution in Medicine: GPT-4 and Beyond*. London: Pearson.
Lorimer J. 2009. Posthumanism/Posthumanistic geographies. In: R. Kitchin, N. Thrift (eds.) *International Encyclopedia of Human Geography*, Volume 8. Oxford: Elsevier, 344–54.
MacCormack, P. 2020. *The Ahuman Manifesto*. London: Bloomsbury Academic.
Mackenzie, R. 2020. Sexbots: Drawing on Tibetan Buddhism and the Tantric tradition. *Journal of Future Robot Life*, 1, 65–89. Available at: https://content.iospress.com/download/journal-of-future-robot-life/frl200003?id=journal-of-future-robot-life%2Ffrl200003. Last accessed: 28 June 2023.
More, M., Vita-More, N. eds. 2013. *The Transhumanist Reader*. Chichester: Wiley-Blackwell.
Nichols, S. 1988. *The Post-Human Movement Manifesto*. Available at: http://dpya.org/en/index.php/1988_-_The_Post-Human_Movement_Manifesto_-_Steve_Nichols. Last accessed: 28 Jun 2023
Pinar, W. 2019. *What is Curriculum Theory?* 3rd ed. Abingdon: Routledge.
Quirk, M. 2006. *Intuition and Metacognition in Medical Education*. Dordrecht: Springer.
Rogers, C.R. 1951. *Client-Centered Therapy*. New York, NY: Houghton-Mifflin.
Sample, I. 2022. If they could turn back time: how tech billionaires are trying to reverse the ageing process. *The Guardian*. 17 Feb 2022. Available at: https://www.theguardian.com/science/2022/feb/17/if-they-could-turn-back-time-how-tech-billionaires-are-trying-to-reverse-the-ageing-process#:~:text=As%20powerful%20computation%20is%20brought,than%20old%20age%2C%20of%20course. Last accessed: 13/03/2024.
Sorgner, S. 2022. *On Transhumanism*. University Park, PA: Penn State University Press.
Tomlinson, G. 2023. *The Machines of Evolution and the Scope of Meaning*. Princeton, NJ: Princeton University Press.
Van der Niet, A., Bleakley, A. 2021. Where medical education meets artificial intelligence: 'Does technology care?' *Medical Education*, 55, 30–36.

2 Metacognition and the making of meaning

Alan Bleakley

Where life gets meta

'Your love keeps lifting me higher/Than I've ever been lifted before' sings Jackie Wilson in the 1967 soul classic 'Higher and Higher'. 'Let's Get Higher' sing Arling and Cameron in 2000, a floor-filler from the rave era. The former refers to the elation of first love, the latter to the effects of the drug Ecstasy. Both reflect the search for 'meta' albeit by very different routes. As an adjective, 'meta' has entered slang vocabulary to refer to someone being 'extremely self-aware or self-reflective' or 'self-referential'. Indeed, the criticism that 'that's so meta' more often refers cynically to extreme self-reference than to savvy knowing or insight beyond the norm. Of course, Meta (referring to the 'metaverse') is the rebranded name of Facebook, perhaps the most widely used social media platform. Through using Meta, Mark Zuckerberg wanted to take us higher in yet another sense. However, in Hebrew, 'meta' means 'dead' (referring to the 'beyond'), perhaps ironically presaging Meta's plummeting share prices following the name switch from Facebook. Clearly, Meta is not necessarily better in the world of business. But in philosophy and pedagogy, meta is at the very heart of thinking at higher levels.

Metacognition – thinking-about-thinking – covers a wide conceptual territory and embraces a huge literature, albeit one dominated by literature on how children learn in schools and by various 'pop' psychologies (Metcalfe and Shimamura 1996, Dunlosky and Metcalfe 2008, Fleming and Frith 2014, van Velzen 2016, Webb 2021). As we saw in the previous chapter, Pina Tarricone (2011) provides a comprehensive overview of kinds of metacognition within a psychological framework. The simplest level of metacognition, or 'cognitive reflection' (Shtulman and Young 2023), is advertised by children learning to reflect on how they make counterintuitive decisions:

> What do cows drink? The correct answer is water, but many are tempted to say milk. The disposition to override an intuitive response (milk) with a more analytic response (water) is known as *cognitive reflection*. Tests of cognitive reflection predict a wide range of skills and abilities in adults. … cognitive reflection may be a prerequisite for developing, and improving, analytic thought, thus highlighting the value of studying cognitive reflection from a developmental perspective.

DOI: 10.4324/9781032687339-4

In medical education, where – as we shall see – metacognition and meta-affect are of central concern, there is sparse literature. One title on intuition and metacognition stands out in medical education (Quirk 2006) and one in surgical education (Schiralkar 2023). As noted in the previous chapters, there is an exponential development in the field of artificial intelligence (AI), reflected in both popular and specialist journalism, where articles on the proliferation of AI were once celebratory but now add to a posthumanist 'doom' literature. This teams up with (appropriately) pessimistic accounts of the trajectory of global warming and the climate disaster. AI in general is in danger of becoming a rogue or runaway member of the 'meta' family, but, as already noted, is a stable addition in both medical education (largely in the realm of learning clinical skills through simulation) and medical practice (largely in diagnostic imaging).

Our focus in this book is medical pedagogy. Some of the metacognitive topics highlighted by medical education scholars include the following:

- *Creativity*. An overused and undervalued term, 'creativity' can cover a wide range of activities from moderately unusual or novel configurations of existing things to mind-blowing innovation as invention of new concepts, activities, or products (Bleakley 2015). We should then talk of multiple 'creativities'. These are impossible without metacognition; not only do creativities, of necessity, raise ordinary thinking to extraordinary levels, they also require a degree of reflection and mental poise that is inescapably metacognitive.
- *Complexity* in its nonlinear and emergent sense. There can be no creativity in linear processes, however complicated, other than by diverging or departing from them. As an illustration of this, the criticism of 'it's not rocket science', implying that something is readily achievable or understandable, is an oxymoron (Regehr 2010). Rocket science is highly complicated but not complex. If it were, then there would be too many intangibles to send anyone or anything into space. Rocket science works as a closed system with known parameters. By comparison, an open, dynamic, and complex system is subject to a host of unpredictable factors due to its fluidity. This is not to say that metacognition does not apply to complicated linear thinking. Thinking about decisions and reflecting upon their consequences is vital to such activity. But the value of metacognition is more fully realised when working with complex systems, and indeed metacognition at its best – where it embraces intuition – can be considered as a dynamic, open, complex, adaptive system close to chaos and capable of reordering spontaneously at higher levels of complexity.
- *Reflective practice* includes reflecting *on* practice after the event, reflecting *in* practice during the event, and reflecting *with* practice where practice itself is an act of reflection (Schön 1990). Reflecting on reflection constitutes 'critical reflexivity' (Bleakley 1999), where reflecting collectively (as in a team debrief) constitutes 'refractive practice' as personal opinions and habits are refracted through the collective's norms thereby affording new and

unexpected perspectives. Critical reflexivity can also be considered as an in-the-moment consideration of the quality and implications of practice common during expert practice (Kneebone 2016, 2020). Such reflexivity involves tacit knowledge (Polanyi 2009) or a cognitive unconscious (Reber and Allen 2022) discussed in Chapter 4. Reflective practice is also discussed in our Preface.

- *Dialectics* is the conscious and deliberative method of putting forward a thesis, offering an antithesis in response, and then, in addressing the paradoxes and contradictions the two positions create, reaching a higher-order synthesis that in turn becomes a new thesis, where the cycle can be repeated. For Hegel, dialectic describes a philosophical movement that in principle has an end point, typically a single, shared humanitarian idea or ideal, that Hegel called 'identification with Spirit'. Marx took Hegel's dialectical idealism and stood it on its head to propose a dialectical materialism based on the struggle between labour and capital from which workers would end up owning the means of production of capital and sharing profit equitably. In postmodern thinking (that transcends thinking in opposites), contradictions emerging from the meeting of theses and antitheses need not be 'resolved' but can be tolerated and may provide a source of innovation.
- *Empathy* is perhaps the most common form of metacognition (or meta-affect) and it is the closest we may come psychologically to Hegel's ideal of Spirit. Empathy moves beyond simple recognition of another's values, opinions, feelings, thought, and behaviours to identification with these states. This is what Marx referred to as shared emotional capital. Sympathy is not the same as empathy, whose highest state is compathy or ideal identification, discussed at length in Chapter 12.
- *Ambient free attention* is perhaps the most undervalued aspect of metacognition, where free-floating attention can be distinguished from consciously directed attention. The latter affords a frame of reference and, in Gestalt psychology, is the figure (foregrounded) as opposed to the ground (backgrounded). As one concentrates on a situation through focused or directed attention, in parallel an ambient or free-floating attention operates that is open to conscious recognition. This is a 'twilight' attention, or suspended state, lingering between consciousness and unconsciousness, working at a less concentrated and more diffuse level than focused attention. Ambient free-floating attention lives in an ecological space of *umwelt* or immediate surroundings, or indeed *is* that space. Such attention is ecological rather than ego-logical (Bleakley and Neilson 2021). By ecological, I mean an attention of affordance, one generated by the environment or immediate context and not directed outwards from person to environment; by ego-logical, I mean an attention generated by the person and directed out to the environment. Forms of attention are discussed at length in Chapter 7.
- *Predictive processing*. Consciousness involves a loop between forward thinking or prediction and memory as experience of the past (Clark 2016). Experience clearly shapes activity through memory, but also prepares one

for future activity by projecting possible near futures. Every action then can be understood as being based on a split-second future-facing prediction of the outcomes of chosen actions. Expertise, for example in elite sports or medicine, demands that we can approximate what might happen next and improvise accordingly. This describes a kind of intuition, but one that is not mysterious. Prediction is every day. Andy Clark's work is referred to throughout this book.

- *Abduction*. Charles Sanders Peirce (1839–1914) is known as the 'father of pragmatism', a philosophy that resists abstraction for concrete action or practical application. Peirce was the originator of the pragmatic research approach of 'abduction'. Where induction draws general conclusions from variable data, deduction posits a hypothesis and collects data to test it. Abduction proceeds by way of iteratively developing 'best fit' ways of making sense of our experiences that can include inspired insight and intuitive grasp. As Perez (2020) suggests, 'Abduction comes from imagination. But imagination cannot happen without the vocabulary to imagine'. This vocabulary is metacognition. I would suggest that the 'vocabulary to imagine' is or can be, in great part, poetic or based on inventive metaphor. Perez thus describes abduction as 'inductive thinking but at the meta level'. Now I have invoked creativity, intuition, and imagination. These are the most unstable but powerful aspects of a metacognition and meta-affect working in unison as a 'bodymind' and speaking in embodied metaphors, or poetically.

Here, I concentrate on metacognition in the sphere of medical education. Medical education remains fascinated with the mundane where it values information over knowledge, competence over capability, and training over education. These positions reflect reductive instrumental values. 'Competence' means 'good enough', and 'training' (from the Latin *trahere*) to 'drag behind', as in the 'train' or 'trail' of a dress, or a set of train carriages. This has a sense of dragging students into medicine rather the more noble aspirations implied by vocation (a calling). Is this really what we want a medical education to do, to drag our students behind us, and in doing so to make them (or help them to be) no more than 'good enough'? Education (from the Latin *educare*) means to 'draw out' or 'lead out', where education is a drawing out of capability. 'Capability' is more complex than 'competence' because it embraces not just what can be demonstrated at a certain point in time, but what potential is also latent in the learner that could be drawn out through sensitive and appropriate facilitation (Neve and Hanks 2016). Proponents of capability point to the short-termism of 'competence' as a here-and-now content demonstration, where capability embraces process focused on indicators of development and potential (Fraser and Greenhalgh 2001, Quirk 2006).

'Capability' has become a key concept in social justice debate. Following Amartya Sen's pioneering work, Martha Nussbaum (2013) argues that human welfare should be judged not on normative standards (e.g., Western ideas of equality as distribution of wealth) but on local needs (what it takes for this person in this context to lead a 'good life'). Such capability embraces the rights and freedoms to make choices as well as what is needed in the way of material resources to lead a fulfilling life. 'Poverty' is then understood as relative to capability deprivation (Vollmann 2008). Importantly, capability deprivation involves false consciousness, or the following of a dogma that impoverishes rather than empowers – see Chapter 9 for fuller exposition of capability.

Inhibiting metacognition through defaulting to a mundane instrumentalism (competence and training mentality) can be seen as producing a kind of poverty. Paradoxically therefore, we might see the current hegemony of competence approaches in medical education as depriving students of capability opportunities. Myopic focus on current outcomes or objectives fails to recognise the larger, more fluid, picture of potential. In this reductive approach, competence erodes capability – providing a longer-term peril for medical education. Blocking metacognition in medical education is a primary side-effect of short-term training approaches, as opposed to longer-term education, where information is promoted over meaning and instrumentalism is the dominant value approach. How did medical education get into this mess of adopting reductive instrumentalism as its key framework?

Language and metaphor matter, as we shall see, in shaping practices and activities. If we privilege instrumentalism, we will never embrace 'meta', for we can never get beyond the reductive baseline of the functional (if it 'works', why try to sophisticate it?). The imperialism of the instrumental is like driving with one foot hard on the accelerator and the other pressing just as hard on the brake. It is like a ship trying to leave port without raising the anchor. Part of the reason for this would seem to be risk-reduction, in particular a systemic avoidance of ambiguity and uncertainty (despite this being everyday terrain for clinical practice). As a result, we by-pass the more complex and enriching values of the ethical, aesthetic, political, and transcendental, so necessary for intensity and depth of learning.

The 'transcendental' – the realm of 'meaning' – here refers to values beyond the mundane, but particularly metacognition and intuition, as well as aspects of spirituality and wider senses of meaning. 'Meta' is not just 'higher', but deeper and wider. It embraces what Yrjö Engeström (2018) refers to as 'expansive learning' that crosses barriers, opens the imagination, and provides fertile ground for speculation. Without 'meta', there is no creativity – or what Engeström (Engeström 2018) calls 'spearheads of innovation' that demand risk – but rather a constant recursion to the safe ground of the known and habitual or a 'will-to-stability' (Engeström 2018). Paradoxically, it would seem, such metacognition is mundane – as the exercise of the mother tongue, vernacular, or ordinary speech. This is because such speech is inordinately inventive (especially through local idioms) and the vehicle for such invention is metaphor. As previously noted, for the ancient Greeks, 'meta' meant any place but the here-and-now mundane, whether it be 'beyond', 'behind', or 'after'. Metaphor is a figure of speech (or trope) that expands (Greek *pherein* – 'to carry') beyond the bearer to indicate something more extensive or imaginative

(Greek *meta*), such as 'drowning in work'. Work does not literally drown you but does so figuratively. The meta in speech is refused where language becomes technical or literal. For example, in medicine, the reductive technical terms 'tachypnoea' and 'haematemesis' refer to, respectively, 'panting for breath' and 'vomiting blood'. The vernacular is embodied and poetic, where the technical terms are dry and functional. I expand this point later in the chapter.

To return to the general use of 'meta', the meta in metacognition means that the cognitive gaze is both deepened and widened: turned in on itself (planning, monitoring, and evaluating one's ongoing activities) and expanded to embrace others (social learning) and artefacts key to learning (such as computers). Thus, metacognition is a higher form of cognition, a step up for a more encompassing and critically aware purview. The spatial metaphors are misleading, because the more complex purview may be from below – for example in a psychoanalytic gaze that grasps a particular function of once unconscious, repressed material now emergent or made plain. To that end, metacognition can be defined as any process of thinking, feeling, intuiting, and/or sensing that raises value of experience from the mundane level of 'information' to the transcendental level of 'meaning'. However, some caution is also required. Almost all my references to 'meta' up to this point have been positive – meta as bigger, better, deeper, and wider. But meta can be applied as a descriptor of pathology. Metastatic tumours grow and cancers spread, as do viruses, both in vitro and in silico. Egos inflate and some people expand by controlling and bullying, or terrorising and conquering, dominating space and speech. Imperialism, colonialism, authoritarianism, and totalitarianism are all meta forms of politics, as oppressive inflations of power.

Kant's ethical imperative

Metacognition is grounded, in part, in the liberty to be able to think for yourself with others in mind. We might just take this for granted, as a natural process of thinking. But metacognition is not 'natural' at all, particularly where it is culturally and historically shaped or determined. For example, enslaved persons, members of cults, or the citizens of totalitarian states are not free to think for themselves. They must subsume their thought to dogma and creed. Indeed, much current populist politics is also driven by dogma, conspiracy theories, and 'alternative facts', while thinking for yourself is deprecated or even punished.

The modern Western notion of metacognition is grounded in Immanuel Kant's rebuttal of why the populace is not allowed to think for itself, particularly where it is driven by class and religious orthodoxies. Kant's 1784 groundbreaking essay, 'An Answer to the Question: What Is Enlightenment?', that promoted metacognition as thinking for yourself in ways that transcend ideology, was predated by a 1783 lecture given in Berlin by the personal physician of Fredrick the Great, Johann Karl Wilhelm Möhsen, entitled 'What Is to Be Done toward the Enlightenment of the Citizenry?'

Möhsen was a member of a secret society that discussed libertarian ideas – such as freedom of the press – of the sort that Kant was to publicly advertise. In 1784, Kant wrote that '*Enlightenment is mankind's exit from its self-incurred immaturity. Immaturity* is the inability to make use of one's own understanding without the guidance of another. … Have the courage to use your *own* understanding! is thus the motto of enlightenment' (ibid., italics in original). Kant was thinking of both Church and State as authorities shaping the thoughts and values of citizens, cast in a rigid class system so that meta-thinking was denied to individuals. The 'tedious business' of thinking, said Kant, is readily taken over by another: the pastor provides conscience through scripture, the doctor prescribes diet, and so forth. 'Immaturity' becomes the by-word for lack of courage to innovate. In other words, what prevails is Engeström's 'will-to-stability', referred to earlier, embedded in a dominant discourse of reductive instrumentalism.

Why is metacognition of importance to medicine and medical education? Primarily because, again, it is the step away from instrumental activity that creates meaning. Without metacognition, there would be no innovation or progress, no blue-sky thinking. But metacognition is not on tap. The shift from ordinary cognition to metacognition requires sustained application. The work is primarily to release the anchor of the instrumental in order that the ship can leave port and sail. In fact, two main anchors need to be hauled in: first, thinking in linear rather than complex ways, and second, thinking through language that is denotative and indicative, rather than connotative and subjunctive. To denote is to point directly to something ('homework' is what you do out of school hours) whereas to connote is to imply a range of meanings ('if you want to get up to speed, you'd better do your homework'). The indicative mood is to talk about facts or information (e.g., referring to surgical instruments, 'it looks like a retractor') and is often linked with the imperative mood ('pass me the retractor'), where the subjunctive is to talk in terms of possibilities and moods ('I feel uncomfortable about using a retractor, what do you think?').

Complexity

Refusal of complexity for linearity

In an instrumental climate where linearity is privileged over complexity, medicine and medical education are configured as a jigsaw, or a clockwork mechanism. Once all the parts are in place, then we (presumably) have a closed, functioning system that can be readily maintained. For example, linearity works most of the time for an interventionist cardiologist fitting a stent, but not for a psychiatrist deciding whether to prescribe anti-psychotic drugs or a course of talking therapy, where complexity reigns. You can point out the virtues of democratic habits to an authoritarian, but this will not necessarily persuade them to abandon allegiance to hierarchical structures.

Medicine and medical education are not static and closed; they are dynamic, open, complex systems working at the edge of chaos and capable of reformulating at higher orders of complexity rather than falling into chaos (Bleakley 2023: chapter 6). The main dilemma facing medicine is that the work is full of ambiguity, yet elimination of uncertainty is necessary for accurate diagnoses and related treatments, while fear of failure is a dominant trait. A reductive, mechanistic point of view is therefore at odds with the reality of clinical medicine. Thus, there is an ever-present dilemma in undergraduate medical education: how to prepare students for the realities of practice who crave certainty and are generally intolerant of ambiguity. Faced with the need to come up with a definitive diagnosis, medical students feel that uncertainty and doubt are professional failures. Yet, as Voltaire said, 'Doubt is not a pleasant state of mind, but certainty is absurd'.

While embracing complexity theory is demanding, resorting to bottom-line, reductive approaches such as framing processes as training or goals in terms of competences is, frankly, lazy. Where complexity and chaos theories have long enjoyed a high profile in biological and biomedical sciences (Capra and Luisi 2014), you might expect that complexity thinking would be at the forefront of medical education theory, practice, and research. However, Christancho et al. (2018) synthesised the medical education and health sciences literature on the 'use of complexity science in medical education' from 2000 to 2017 and found only 46 papers. Further, 'complexity' is not well articulated or understood as either concept or activity and takes on differing meanings in different disciplines such as the biological sciences, physical sciences, information sciences, mathematics, social sciences, arts, and the humanities.

When Christancho and colleagues asked: 'Do medical education scholars understand that there are multiple legitimate orientations to complexity science, deriving from distinct disciplinary origins, drawing on different metaphors and serving distinct purposes?' They found that not only is there a paucity of literature drawing on complexity as a research paradigm in medical education, but also there is paucity in scholarship embracing innovation. 'Complexity', like 'creativity', tends to be used as a catch-all where differing kinds of complexities and creativities can be mapped both phenomenologically and in the abstract. It seems that complexity thinking is still fringe to medical education and is poorly conceptualised, even as we explicitly acknowledge that both medicine and medical education are complex, adaptive systems. It is as if medical educators and education scholars desperately want to reduce complexity science to linear concepts, a fruitless exercise. One characteristic way in which this manifests itself is in mistaking a syllabus (what is to be taught) for a curriculum (the system of processes and complex encounters through which the syllabus is brought to life), a common symptom of mundane cognition rather than the more complex metacognition.

Curriculum is derived from the Latin *currere* – 'to run a course', referring originally to Roman chariot races and then to a course of study – this, as a *process* of learning, experiencing, and becoming (as identity construction).

Content within a curriculum is a 'syllabus'. A collection of syllabi forms a closed system and not an open, complex system. William Pinar (2019), a major voice in the field of Curriculum Reconceptualisation, insists that curriculum is process, complex, and inscriptive (not just of personal identity, but of wider collective identity as democracy). As noted previously, this work is sadly neglected in the mainstream medical education literature (Bleakley 2020). Thus, in medical pedagogies, we can think of syllabus (content) interests as mundane in comparison with the more complex 'meta' issue of curriculum (process) interests.

Production of metaphors

Metacognition is grounded in metalanguage. Again, to think metacognitively is to think with something beyond the baseline, mundane and literal. As noted, such reductive language is denotative; it points to something concrete with no added implication (e.g., 'sulphur' as a chemical substance or a symbol [S] in the Periodic Table pointing to that substance). Where language draws on tropes or figures of speech (primarily metaphors), the register shifts from denotation to connotation. To connote, again, is to imply a range of meanings. After killing Desdemona and realising his tragic mistake, Othello says 'roast me in sulphur/ Wash me down in steep-gulfs of liquid fire', giving himself up in contrition to terrible torture. 'Sulphur' here has multiple connotations – not just intense flame and heat, but also stink. Something spewed from the guts of the earth as simultaneous cleanser and pollutant.

In medicine and medical education, positivism tends to reduce everything to a literal or technical expression, and in doing so acts as a cultural mechanism for socialisation, an 'insider's' vocabulary. As noted earlier, this shows in medicine's cultural preference for reductive, technical words rather than the vernacular used by patients. An example given earlier is that 'tachypnoea' and 'haematemesis' refer to, respectively, 'panting for breath' and 'vomiting blood'. The latter, vernacular, phrases are embodied metaphors – just soundlessly voicing them imitates symptoms (try it), while the former are literal technical terms. Another example is 'synapse' (from the Greek *sunapsis* as 'point of contact'), originally named 'protoplasmic kisses' by its founder Santiago Ramon y Cajal.

Cajal was a dedicated scientist – in 1906, he won the Nobel Prize in physiology for his work on the structures of the nervous system – yet he was also a Romantic who wrote down his dreams to create an atmosphere of metaphor upon which he fed. He despised and ridiculed Freud's work at the same time as he saw symbolic meaning in dreams, surely metaphors for his own work. For example, he dreams of humiliating circumstances, where he attends a diplomatic event, and as he turns to leave, his pants drop. Thieves enter his house and threaten him with a gun, but when he pleads with them not to kill him, the gun turns out to be a harmless toy (Wilkinson 2023). Do such metaphorical contexts not raise the value of instrumental science to that of an art – full of uncertainty and ambiguity, pun, surprise, and even humiliation?

While biomedicine is awash with metaphors, these are often displaced by literal terms. Michael Dustin (2003), noting similarities between viral spread and synapse functions, celebrates the use of metaphor ('Cajal described the neural synapse as a "protoplasmic kiss," and this metaphor applies equally well to the immunological synapse'), but appears to be anchored by a mechanical imagination where 'Viruses are masters at co-opting the machinery of the immune response'. Is the body really a 'machine', as Vesalius described it? Only if your guiding perspective is instrumentalism. Dustin too is caught with his pants down.

As Robert Taylor (2017) shows, medical language operates in two valences simultaneously: for medical audiences and for public consumption (patients). Technical terms, usually derived from the Greek or Latin, are employed in medical contexts for clarity and precision, and as socialisation devices, where the vernacular is used with patients. Again, the latter can be metaphor-rich where the former are instrumental or technical, their metaphorical potential bled out. For example, doctors use 'ichthyosis' where patients understand 'scaly skin', the latter doubly resonant as its alliterative. The metaphoric route, that I celebrate here, embraces aesthetics. This includes 'echoic words' (technically, 'onomatopoeia') where the sound of utterance simulates the description, such as 'cough', 'hiccup', 'murmur', and 'sneeze', or resonant phrases such as 'thunderclap headache'.

Sometimes, these metaphors are right under our noses, but we do not register them as we approach through the lens of literalism. For example, the physician Joseph Wassersug (1987), in an article deriding the medical humanities, said: 'real medical progress has not been made by humanitarians but by doctors equipped with microscopes, scalpels, dyes, catheters, rays, test tubes, and culture plates'. Wassersug seemingly fails to see that everyday medical equipment affords a poetics, a feast of forceful metaphor, alliteration, and consonance: for example, the common surgical equipment 'grasping forceps', 'skin hook', 'locking forceps', and 'rake retractor'. Here, the metaphors are in plain sight, but the value complex of instrumentalism unsights us, overriding other values such as the aesthetic. If you think literally and functionally, then looking at the image of the rake retractor will probably not stimulate an aesthetic response. However, these surgical instruments are elegant, minimalist objects of beauty.

The Values Prism

I have indicated how an instrumental discourse refuses the meta. How we might address this is a complex task, but it has a unifying procedural solution: in each case that instrumentalism shows – such as resorting to functional pedagogies, purely technical biomedical science, and formulaic approaches to clinical and communication skills – we can raise the value of the phenomenon by introducing aesthetic, ethical, political, and/or transcendental (meaning) approaches, *as embracing metacognition.* I have already described such a shift but let me now explore its anatomy. This shift in meanings (through values orientations rather than bounded disciplines) can be described as a 'translational' approach (Bleakley 2023). Such translations can be achieved through the media that make up the medical humanities – the disciplines and inter-disciplines of the arts, humanities, and qualitative social sciences – but it is no secret that the medical humanities can also be employed in the service of reductive instrumentalism. Indeed, the normative use of the medical humanities as a compensation for a reductive biomedicine can itself constitute a resort to functionality or the instrumental. Here, the medical humanities act as both tool and dose to fix an ailing biomedicine, but paradoxically add to the instrumental burden.

In the model presented here, the medical (or health) 'humanities' can be read as any intervention that raises the value of biomedical science and clinical and communication skills from the technical-instrumental into other, more complex, registers. This increases intensities and expands qualities, as illustrated in Figure 2.1, the 'Values Prism' (Bleakley 2023, 2024). This avoids framing the medical humanities as 'saviour' (or regulated dose) for conventional biomedicine as noted. Expressive biomedicine, mindful of the intrinsic humanity and artistry of both laboratory science and clinical practice, is already a member of the medical humanities stable.

Key to this translational model is the strategy of increasing the productive metaphor count, thus enriching language, semiotics, and semantics, and providing greater depth of meaning. Some established metaphors are not productive, but tired and overused – such as martial metaphors (medicine as war or combat) or engineering metaphors (the body as machine), although Anita Wohlmann (2022) puts forward a persuasive argument that such metaphors can be 're-cycled' and then still have purpose. As we saw earlier, technical language in medicine (such as 'tachypnoea') can quash the metaphor available in the vernacular ('panting for breath') that raises the value of the language from

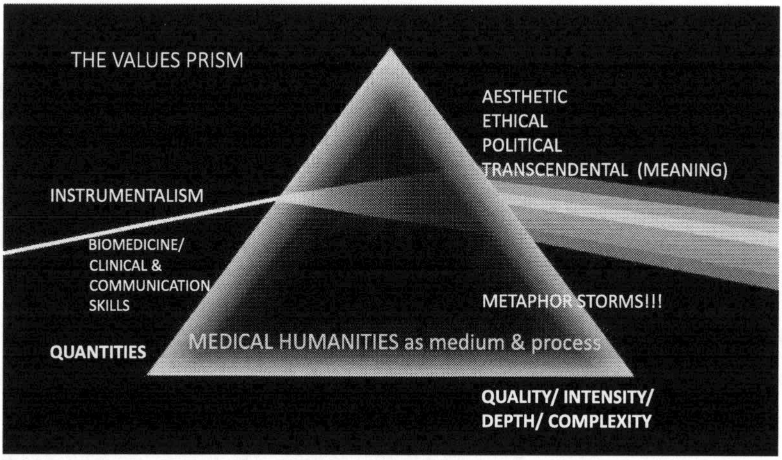

Figure 2.1 The medical humanities Values Prism.

technical-instrumental to aesthetic. A technical descriptor, such as 'rake retractor', is taken literally and heard functionally where in fact it is alliterative and poetic. This is a beautiful example because its functional value in surgery (acting as rake and retractor in pulling back skin, tendons, or soft tissue) is already poetically enhanced through intonation imitating that function. The aesthetic is already apparent in the function.

The Values Prism (Figure 2.1) configures the purely instrumental (and generally quantitative) as a white light that is scattered into colours as qualities, possibilities, and intensities (the spectrum of values) as it is mediated by appropriate and carefully constructed 'medical humanities' opportunities or interventions. (My colleague Rachel Ellaway points out that there is another way of looking at the work of the prism in refracting white light into component colours, where the prism 'deconstructs the wild chaos of white light' [personal communication]. Rachel is technically right about white light, but this is not how we *experience* it.) Again, the primary intervention is to raise biomedical science pedagogy from information-based, instrumental framing and teaching to meaning-based approaches engaging other values. This, again, moves focus from quantities to qualities. The next level of intervention is to raise clinical and communication skills teaching to higher levels of value. A third level is to introduce high-quality arts, humanities, and social sciences interventions to raise intensities (such as seeding democratic habits). These processes are, again, facilitated by production of innovative metaphors.

Tracey Moniz et al. (2021) developed a 'Prism Model' of medical humanities interventions in medical education. (This is quite different from the Values Prism model that I propose here, first developed at Peninsula Medical School UK in the early 2000s.) From a systematic literature review, Moniz and colleagues articulate three discursive positions for the medical humanities: 'art as intrinsic to, additive to or curative for medicine'. Intrinsic means a natural, essential part of medicine; additive means a complement to medicine; and curative means 'a remedy that can address shortcomings of medicine and medical education'. These positions are echoed in the purposes of the Values Prism model articulated here. Biomedicine is intrinsically artistic, artful, and humane as it embraces value positions beyond the instrumental. While art and the humanities can add value to instrumental biomedicine, so a fulsome biomedicine can cure an ailing art or humanities. But can we say the same for medical education? Can we look forward to the day when medical pedagogies are truly cultured, as meta-pedagogies fed by both metahumanities and metascience? (A metascience being a science that reflexively investigates its own values and practices moulded by such values, for example the extent to which 'facts' claimed by science are social constructs).

Values positions

So, the leap from cognition to metacognition (embracing valuing, thinking, feeling, sensing, and intuition/ imagination) is posited as passing the instrumental (that is closely aligned with economic values) through the prism of the 'medical humanities' perspective and process so that a range of other values positions emerges, constituting the 'meta'. It is worth repeating that, while the instrumental usually aligns with biomedical sciences and technical approaches to clinical and communication skills in medicine under the dominant discourse of competence and training regimes, this is not always the case. First, the biomedical sciences may be taught and learned embracing a wider range of values beyond the instrumental (anatomy learned through life drawing, the body viewed as a complex system, pharmaceuticals treated as living devices, and so forth). And second, the medical humanities themselves can be conceived and applied instrumentally, as noted above.

The ethical

Ethics is already metacognitive because we are thinking-about-thinking (or acting) in terms of the moral consequences of our actions. Conversely, ethics informs us about lack of metacognition – not thinking about consequences, or acting in haste, or under the influence of passions, exhaustion, mind-altering substances, or interpellation into a dogma (a position of faith for example). Nietzsche famously points to the need for metacognition in 'the transvaluation of all values', a position of deep perspective. He did not say that such a position is only obtained by stripping away all held values positions – an ontological impossibility. Rather, his point is about axiology or values in relation to one another. We can hold a values position such as democracy that judges autocracies, for example, to be misguided and repressive, while still understanding the conditions under which an autocracy may exist. The most obvious example here is that we know from research evidence (and intuitively) that collaborative, democratic inter-professional teamwork leads to improved patient safety and work satisfaction, yet we understand why hierarchies linger in healthcare, due to historical legacies. These privilege a 'masculinised' heroic individualism (Bleakley 2020). This is a comfortable fit for more autocratic medical students who are less tolerant of ambiguity (and male), but uncomfortable for more collectively oriented students more tolerant of ambiguity and supportive of democratic teamwork (usually women).

Within healthcare ethics, metacognition can inform a shift from less to more powerful moralities as we note historical factors that privilege certain models. Thus, the Principles approach developed by Beauchamp and Childress (1979) has been the dominant discourse in medical ethics for many years. This approach posits four universal values that must be considered in any ethical judgement: autonomy (to respect individual choice), non-maleficence (to do no harm), beneficence (to act with the best interests of the other in mind), and justice (fairness and equality). This model was extended to a 'principles plus attention to scope model' by Gillon (1994) (who first introduced the North American-derived Principles approach to a UK audience), where the limits to principlism are noted, such as one moral principle conflicting with another (the classic case is autonomy clashing with medical beneficence – for example an individual's religious beliefs [such as a Jehovah's Witness] leading to refusal of blood transfusions). Informed by nursing practices as well as medicine, the four principles have been extended to seven: accountability, justice, non-maleficence, autonomy, beneficence, fidelity, and veracity (Faubion 2023); and then nine, to include privacy and confidentiality (Byrd and Winkelstein 2014).

Universal principles, by definition, suffer from issues of application to unique individuals and idiosyncratic circumstances (Macklin 2003), but also lack of attention to cross-cultural differences (e.g., impacting ethnicity and gender) and shifting historical conditions. How do you apply the principle of autonomy to a culture that only recognises collectivism? For such reasons, context-sensitive approaches to individual cases are posited as a more appropriate ethical approach. This is pluralism that comes in many guises. Principlism is confounded where ethics meets politics for example. The repeal of *Roe v. Wade* in the 'abortion wars' in North America is a recent example. Whose justice and autonomy are we talking about when women who require abortions (e.g., in conditions of pregnancy through rape) and principled doctors prepared to offer abortions are restricted in choice by ideological politics? Casuistry (individual or case-based ethics) works in the opposite direction to principlism, where an individual case is considered in context for its unique presentation.

The aesthetic

'Aesthetic' at root means 'sense impression' and is strictly a study of how the senses form us as individuals and as cultures. Unfortunately, aesthetics has become associated with 'taste', as in 'high art' rather than popular culture. In medicine and medical education, aesthetic values can be recovered through reference to how well the senses (to embrace sensibility or physical qualities, and sensitivity or emotional qualities) can be educated for general medicine but especially for specialties (Bleakley 2021). This tuning of the senses in relation to embodied knowledge and affect embraces metacognition as meta-sensing and meta-affect. Both are marks of the 'expert' (Kneebone 2020).

A systematic (mis)education into insensibility

Medical education should educate for sensibility – tuning students' awareness through the senses so that they become acutely aware of cues and clues given off by patients as they engage in diagnostic clinical reasoning and expert communication. However, despite this promise, medical education can be seen to offer a systematic miseducation into insensibility, a dulling of sensibility and sensitivity, or body and affect (Bleakley 2020). Instrumentalism, literalism, and linearity serve to frustrate sophisticated education of the senses as they an-aesthetise (again, 'aesthetic' means 'sense-based').

Emotional insulation

In the face of meeting trauma, suffering, and death, medical students undergo a progressive de-sensitising and dampening of affect, as 'emotional insulation'. This serves as a protective mechanism against emotional overload. But emotional insulation is overdetermined in initial medical education (as compared with the fine-tuning of affect sought in education for counsellors, psychotherapists, and clinical psychologists). Here, the ego defence of emotional insulation becomes more a clinical armour as it hardens into empathy decline and increasing cynicism. In contrast, psychotherapists know about maintaining a balance of attention, where empathy does not tip into over-identification. This is couched in the language of countertransference. Medical students could engage with the basics of such psychotherapeutic acumen early in their careers as a form of metacognitive learning, embracing the knowing of affect and its flux. The latter is a quality that John Heron (2001) refers to as the 'balance of attention' – or learning to maintain 'free attention' where affect may overwhelm embodied knowing so that affect is essentially 'managed' through metacognition as 'thinking about feeling'.

Learning anatomy through cadaver dissection

While a longstanding convention, cadaver dissection is increasingly seen as an initiation rite rather than the best way to learn anatomy (McMenamin et al. 2018). Preserved corpses afford another way to dull the senses in medical education (Bleakley 2021). Cadavers used for anatomy teaching are also becoming scarce, and unless students want to be surgeons, pathologists, or radiologists, anatomy is best learned by how you will meet it in practice – as surface anatomy in living and moving bodies (McLachlan and Patten 2006).

This can involve, for example, peer-to-peer examination amongst medical students where ethical and political considerations, such as gender, are paramount (Singh et al. 2020); life drawing (where students are exposed to the arts); use of live 'medical models' paid to coach serial intimate examinations (Kulze 2015); the longstanding tradition of using actor patients; sophisticated virtual anatomy teaching systems (Zhang et al. 2019); drawing on readymade educational opportunities such as plastination exhibits; and attending autopsies. Each of these activities can raise value from the purely instrumental level of passing information to the more complex gaining of meaning – this, through for example the ethics of body donations in plastinated specimens, or of peer-to-peer examinations; the aesthetics of virtual anatomy; the gender politics of intimate examination; and the transcendental issues of attending an autopsy.

Use of simulation

Where cadaver dissection is the oldest rite of passage in medicine, the most recent involves the rituals of the simulation laboratory. Clinical and communication skills are largely initially learned through simulation, but this – as noted earlier – has drawbacks based in problems of transferability. Many clinical skills of course cannot be learned *in vivo* and must be practised *in vitro* using both lo- and hi-tech models. Clinical skills simulation is often approached and taught from a reductive instrumentalist perspective so that ethical, aesthetic, political, and transcendental issues are by-passed (except, for example, in a debrief on a 'failed' resuscitation attempt that may discuss death). Sometimes, this is a glaring howler, such as the longstanding tradition of hi-tech manikins being male and having pink skin; and never mind the dulling of the senses where touch and smell are entirely compromised – or, aesthetic, ethical, and political issues are suspended or by-passed.

Is there anything that can be done about stripping back experiences in simulation, even when, paradoxically, using a hi-tech, bells-and-whistles manikin? Roger Kneebone's (2016, 2020) ground-breaking work shows that much *in vitro* learning for clinical skills is poorly thought out where fidelity is low, and context is ignored. Working with technicians who make realistic models for television medical soap operas (such as flesh wounds), while setting learning experiences in contexts approximating *in vivo* environments, introduces values beyond the instrumental. Scenarios such as wound debriding and dressing can be simulated with a high level of fidelity, introducing aesthetic and ethical values to an otherwise de-sensitising instrumental scenario. For example, an entire operating theatre context can be simulated using props. Better, an operating theatre can be set up as a learning environment using simulation, so that fidelity is maintained, for both technical procedures and non-technical team communication (Robertson et al. 2017). Further, as Kneebone's work amply illustrates, simulation scenarios can engage the public for educational purposes, thus raising value from the instrumental to engage the ethical and political (by addressing power issues). For example, Kneebone has devised a 'blow up' portable 'theatre' space that can be erected anywhere readily, to carry out simulation scenarios in which the public can be directly involved. For example, television medical soap opera make-up personnel provide virtual flesh wounds or open abdomens, so that procedures such as stitching and retracting of organs can be tried out by members of the public. This is meta-simulation at its best, primarily embracing aesthetic values. Kneebone also shows that while hi-fidelity reproduction is necessary for immediate contexts in simulation (such as an operating theatre team around a table), aspects of the theatre room that are not part of immediate focus (such as anaesthetic equipment) can be lo-fidelity.

The political

Failure to educate for democratic habits

Another historically conditioned failing of medical education is that it has been so tightly focused on masculinist, heroic individualism at the expense of contributing to the collective good. Here, medical pedagogy has been tainted by traditions of medical culture. An unintended consequence of Abraham Flexner's 1910 Carnegie Foundation report was that underperforming or under-resourced medical schools were closed while these were the very schools serving women and minorities. Medicine too was embedded in, and shaped by, the bigger cultural influence of the North American fetishising of heroic individualism. This embraces a 'frontiersman' mentality of autonomy, grounded in Protestant–Capitalist values of self-help. All of this frustrates collectivism or authentic democracy, historically badged as a socialist aberration in North America.

This resistance to the collective good matters because healthcare is practised in inter-professional teamwork settings. Where poor teamwork makes a major contribution to medical error (Herzberg et al. 2019), authentic democratic habits must be established. One such habit is peer assessment (formalised as judgement against agreed criteria), glaringly absent as a key aspect of assessment in medical education yet key to establishing democratic habits (Heron 2001). Also, is medical education moving quickly enough to facilitate transitions to authentic democracy in an era of rising health inequality, particularly as these relate to health issues brought on by a global refugee crisis and the climate emergency (Bleakley 2020)?

The transcendental

Metacognition itself is a transcendental value, aiming for Nietzsche's transvaluation of all values that promises meaning free from dogma. The transcendental is usually read as spiritual, particularly important in end-of-life care. But this can also embrace the humanistic at the highest level of empathy famously described by Carl Rogers as 'unconditional positive regard' – perhaps a value too far, a condition of angels rather than mortals.

Summary

I have suggested a revisioning of metacognition, conventionally thought of as 'thinking-about-thinking', to place emphasis upon values. In particular, the meta is read as the shift from mundane, reductive instrumentalism to embrace a range of other values: the ethical, aesthetic, political, and transcendental. In the context of medicine and medical education, the mundane is functional biomedicine and clinical and communication skills at the level of information rather than meaning. This is embodied in reductive pedagogical approaches that value competence and training over capability and education. The translation of the instrumental into other, more complex, value positions introduces a range of qualities, intensities, and perspectives occluded by the functional, and centrally involves metaphor production and use.

While translation from the instrumental to higher register values can be achieved through the prism of the medical humanities, this should initially be seen as drawing out the intrinsic artistry and humanity of biomedical science and clinical and communication skills. In some cases, biomedical sciences are already delivered at higher registers beyond the instrumental, while the medical humanities may be delivered functionally. The aim is to raise and maintain value across all clinical and educational practices as increasing quality, diversity, and intensity. The medium through which this can be achieved is productive metaphor (some metaphors can be trite and unproductive), shifting registers of meaning. This is how metacognition works, embracing meta-sensing (high levels of sensibility such as close noticing), meta-affect (high levels of sensitivity and expert management of affect), and intuition (allowing imagination to flourish as the capabilities of differing kinds of creativity). This model of establishing metacognition in clinical work and medical education may be of particular interest to biomedical science and clinical faculty as it by-passes the imperative for embracing arts and humanities sensibilities that may be seen as alien, for a recovery and celebration of the intrinsic value, beauty, and humanity of bioscience. This serves our shared, cherished value of consilience.

References

Beauchamp, T.L., Childress, J.F. 1979. *The Principles of Biomedical Ethics* (1st ed.). Oxford: Oxford University Press.

Bleakley, A. 1999. From reflective practice to holistic reflexivity. *Studies in Higher Education*, 24: 315–30.

Bleakley, A. 2015. *Medical Humanities and Medical Education: How the Medical Humanities can Shape Better Doctors*. Abingdon: Routledge.

Bleakley, A. 2020. *Educating Doctors' Senses Through the Medical Humanities: "How Do I Look?"* Abingdon: Routledge.

Bleakley, A. 2021. *Medical Education, Politics and Social Justice: The Contradiction Cure*. Abingdon: Routledge.

Bleakley, A. 2023. *Medical Humanities: Ethics, Aesthetics, Politics*. London: Routledge.

Bleakley, A.A. 2024. Therapeutic intervention for an ailing medical education: The values prism model as proof of concept. *Medical Teacher*, 46: 232–38.

Bleakley, A., Neilson S. 2021. *Poetry in the Clinic: Towards a Lyrical Medicine*. Abingdon: Routledge.

Byrd, G.D., Winkelstein, P.A. 2014. Comparative analysis of moral principles and behavioral norms in eight ethical codes relevant to health sciences librarianship, medical informatics, and the health professions. *Journal Medical Library Association*, 102: 247–56.

Capra, F., Luisi, P.L. 2014. *The Systems View of Life: A Unifying Vision*. Cambridge: Cambridge University Press.

Christancho, S., Field, E., Lingard, L. 2018. What is the state of complexity science in medical education research? *Medical Education*, 53: 95–104.

Clark, A. 2016. *Surfing Uncertainty: Prediction, Action, and the Embodied Mind*. Oxford: Oxford University Press.

Dunlosky, J, Metcalfe, J. 2008. *Metacognition*. London: Sage Publications.

Dustin, M.L. 2003. The immunological synapse. *Cancer Immunology Research*, 2: 1023–33.

Engeström, Y. 2018. *Expertise in Transition: Expansive Learning in Medical Work*. Cambridge: Cambridge University Press.

Faubion, D. 2023. 7 Main Ethical Principles in Nursing + Why They're Important. *NursingProcess*. Available at: https://www.nursingprocess.org/ethical-principles-in-nursing.html Last accessed: 01 Mar 2023.
Fleming, S.M., Frith, C.D. 2014. *The Cognitive Neuroscience of Metacognition*. Dordrecht: Springer.
Fraser, S.W., Greenhalgh, T. 2001. Coping with complexity: educating for capability. *British Medical Journal*, 323: 799.
Gillon, R. 1994. Medical ethics: four principles plus attention to scope. *British Medical Journal*, 309: 184.
Heron, J. 2001. *Helping the Client: A Creative Practical Guide* (5th ed). London: Sage
Herzberg, S., Hansen, M., Schoonover, A., et al. 2019. Association between measured teamwork and medical errors: an observational study of prehospital care in the USA. *BMJ Open* 9: e025314.
Kneebone, R.L. 2016. Simulation reframed. *Advances in Simulation*, 1: 27.
Kneebone, R. 2020. *Expert: Understanding the Path to Mastery*. London: Viking.
Kulze, E. 2015. These medical models use their own bodies as teaching tools. *Vocativ*. Feb 19 2015. Available at: https://www.vocativ.com/culture/health-culture/live-model-medical-training/index.html Last accessed: 22 Feb 2023
Macklin, R. 2003. Bioethics, vulnerability, and protection. *Bioethics*, 17: 472–86.
McLachlan, J., Patten, D. 2006. Anatomy teaching: ghosts of the past, present and future. *Medical Education*, 40: 243–53.
McMenamin, P.G., McLachlan, J., Wilson, A., et al. Do we really need cadavers anymore to learn anatomy in undergraduate medicine? *Medical Teacher*. 2018; 40: 1020–29.
Metcalfe, J., Shimamura, A.P. (eds.) 1996. *Metacognition: Knowing About Knowing*. Minneapolis, MI: The MIT Press.
Moniz, T., Golafshani, M., Gaspar, C.M., et al. 2021. The prism model for integrating the arts and humanities into medical education. *Academic Medicine*, 96: 1225.
Neve, H., Hanks, S. 2016. When I say … capability. *Medical Education*, 50: 610–11.
Nussbaum, M. 2013. *Creating Capabilities: The Human Development Approach*. Cambridge, MA: Harvard University Press.
Perez, C.E. 2020. What does Peirce's Abduction reveal? *Intuition Machine*. Dec 7 2020. Available at: https://medium.com/intuitionmachine/what-does-peirces-abduction-reveal-8dccf5d3decd#:~:text=Peirce%20likely%20derived%20the%20word%20abduction%20as%20the,take%20away%2C%E2%80%9D%20and%20the%20Latin%20ducere%20%E2%80%9Cto%20lead%E2%80%9D Last accessed: 01 Mar 2023
Pinar, W. 2019. *What Is Curriculum Theory?* (3rd ed) Abingdon: Routledge.
Polanyi, M. 2009. *The Tacit Dimension*. Chicago, Ill: University of Chicago Press.
Quirk, M. 2006. *Intuition and Metacognition in Medical Education*. Dordrecht: Springer.
Reber, A.S., Allen, R. (eds.) 2022. *The Cognitive Unconscious: The First Half Century*. Oxford: Oxford University Press.
Regehr, G. 2010. It's NOT rocket science: rethinking our metaphors for research in health professions education. *Medical Education*. 44: 31–9.
Robertson, J.M., Dias, R.D., Yule, S., Smink, D.S. 2017. Operating Room Team Training with Simulation: A Systematic Review. *Journal of Laparoendoscopic & Advanced Surgical Techniques*, 27: 475–80.
Schiralkar, U. 2023. *Surgical Metacognition: Smarter Decision-making for Surgeons*. London: Surgical Psychology Publishing.
Schön, D.A. 1990. *Educating the Reflective Practitioner: Toward a New Design for Teaching and Learning in the Professions*. San Francisco, CA: Jossey-Bass.

Shtulman, A., Young, A.G. 2023. The development of cognitive reflection. *Child Development Perspectives*, 17: 59–66.

Singh, G., Goitiandia, S.W., Perry, D.. Spiers, J. 2020. *The BMJ opinion*. July 8 2020. Available at: https://blogs.bmj.com/bmj/2020/07/08/how-can-we-encourage-more-female-medical-students-to-participate-in-peer-to-peer-teaching-of-physical-exams/ Last accessed: 22 Feb 2023

Tarricone, P. 2011. *The Taxonomy of Metacognition*. Hove: Psychology Press.

Taylor, R.B. 2017. *The Amazing Language of Medicine: Understanding Medical Terms and Their Backstories*. Dordrecht: Springer

van Velzen, J. 2016. *Metacognitive Learning: Advancing Learning by Developing General Knowledge of the Learning Process*. Cham: Springer.

Vollmann, W.T. 2008. *Poor People*. New York, NY: HarperPerennial.

Wassersug, J.D. 1987. Teach humanities to doctors? Says who? *Postgraduate Medicine*, 82: 317–18.

Webb, J. 2021. *The Metacognition Handbook: A Practical Guide for Teachers and School Leaders*. Woodbridge: John Catt Educational Ltd.

Wilkinson, A. 2023. Illuminating the Brain's 'Utter Darkness'. *The New York Review of Books*. Feb 09. Available at: https://www.nybooks.com/articles/2023/02/09/illuminating-the-brains-utter-darkness-cajal-jorgensen/ Last accessed: 11 May 2023

Wohlmann, A. 2022. *Metaphor in Illness Writing: Fight and Battle Reused*. Edinburgh: University of Edinburgh Press.

Zhang, X., Yang, J., Chen, N. et al. 2019. Modeling and simulation of an anatomy teaching system. *Visual Computing for Industry, Biomedicine, and Art*, 2: 8.

3 Metacognition, meta-affect, and the clinical encounter

Language matters

Alan Bleakley

From information to meaning

Every Grammar school pupil in post-WWII Britain (at least in my own generation) studied Henry Reed's 1942 poem 'Naming of Parts'. Ostensibly, the five-stanza poem is a lecture about the parts of the Enfield rifle, the standard issue for British troops at the time:

> And this you can see is the bolt. The purpose of this
> Is to open the breech, as you see. We can slide it
> Rapidly backwards and forwards: we call this
> Easing the spring.

The tension built by sliding the bolt 'rapidly backwards and forwards' is eased by the enjambment 'Easing the spring'. As each part of the rifle is named, so it is compared with events in nature in the springtime (perhaps reflecting the wandering minds of the conscripted soldiers being taught), whence there is a pun on 'easing the spring':

> And rapidly backwards and forwards
> The early bees are assaulting and fumbling the flowers:
> They call it easing the Spring

Reed's poem is usually read as an anti-war manifesto, where the soldier's thoughts of the warm, bucolic pleasures of pastoral life are contrasted with the cold, impersonal mechanics of a war instrument. However, seemingly unbeknown to curriculum planners of the time, Reed's poem increasingly introduces sexual innuendo, unequivocal by the third and fourth stanzas.

More. The poem shifts back and forth between *information* (the rifle parts, catalogued) and *meaning* (the shift into nature, the sexual innuendo). Naming the parts of the rifle (bolt, breech, and so on) is purely information based on mechanics. Meaning is introduced where, punning on the word 'spring', the mechanical part of the rifle is contrasted with the 'assault' of the early bees on

DOI: 10.4324/9781032687339-5

the wildflowers. A simile is employed. The simile transforms into a metaphor for sex ('open the breech', 'slide it/Rapidly backwards and forwards'). The militaristic stance is then displaced by the sensual ('assault' becomes a 'fumble').

This was of course lost on myself and the other callow boys and girls in my English class in the early 1960s studying for what were then called 'O' Levels (now GCSEs), where we were required to mechanically memorise the poem through rehearsal – as information with little or no depth of meaning. The analysis offered by my English teacher at the time was superficial enough to skim over meanings, only going so far as to re-state the obvious contrast between the harsh mechanical elements of the rifle associated with war and the bucolic elements of springtime associated with peace. Education as information, the default position at the time, and perhaps one that still dominates.

Indeed, medical students today continue to learn much of their course content through a 'naming of parts'. Take anatomy, for example, where the skeleton is typically described (and therefore learned) as no more than a collection (or a naming) of parts, a hinged mechanism in which one bone connects to and articulates another. It is easy to characterise this reductionist view as a Vesalian legacy, but to do so, we must put this in the context of human anatomy in the 16th century. Vesalius was surely working within a culture of meaning rather than information, where through careful dissection (of the bodies of executed criminals) he exploded traditional Galenic anatomy and presented his new aesthetic vision by employing artists to produce exquisite drawings and engravings of his work. In this way, information took on an aesthetic dimension to raise its register to meaning. This is why I argue that it is good for medical students to not just name, but also draw, what they see.

The 'Skeleton Dance' nursery rhyme that I was taught as a child says: 'The foot bone's connected to the leg bone/The leg bone's connected to the knee bone/The knee bone's connected to the thigh bone/ … ', and so forth. Again, pure information, devoid of meaning. Mechanics. But this ditty is based on a spiritual song in which the body is etched with 'the word of the Lord'. In anatomy, there is a transformation from information to meaning when the body is seen through an aesthetic register as living and moving anatomy, a wonder of design by evolution. Information can therefore be transformed into meaning as an anatomy lecturer or demonstrator shows how an articulation allows for the knee to bend or brace, how the muscle inserts, and what happens on contraction and relaxation in the context of the movement of expert dancers or athletes or how para-athletes compensate for loss of limbs or restricted movement.

But the anatomy class needs to be reminded how a muscle contracts, and now we need the context of physics to distinguish, for example, between isotonic concentric and eccentric forms of contraction. However, we need to see this in action: where living anatomy is meaningful, dead anatomy is information. Similarly, medical students may need to know the seven steps of muscle contraction, drawing in physiology and biochemistry, from the generation of action potentials to the hydrolysing of adenosine triphosphate (ATP).

But, again, this needs to be learned as animated, meaningful material and not as dead-in-the-water information. Muscle contraction as a thing of beauty rather than just mechanics. And 'beauty' is surely a word outlawed by instrumental biomedical science, where explanation precedes (or obliterates) appreciation of a phenomenon.

All of this must be put into a bigger context, such as the body moving in space to avoid objects and the leg twisting, or the body colliding with another body, causing a knee injury. We don't want medical students to twist their knees, but we can get them to dance (helped by performance artists or a dance troupe) to show how bodies can move and expertly move around each other. In doing so, this invokes the 'medical humanities' (Bleakley 2023), and the 'naming of parts' is extended to the world of nature, to context. The medical humanities can help to shift pure information into meaning, following TS Eliot's recommendation for a life shaped by art. In his play 'The Rock', Eliot (1934) asks: 'Where is the wisdom we have lost in knowledge?/Where is the knowledge we have lost in information?' By teaching anatomy through dance and movement, medical students can both *contextualise* information to raise its register and *translate* from one medium to another as further generation of meaning. These are 'meta' ways of knowing.

Eliot may have been thinking of Socrates, who suggested that '*knowledge, when separated from justice and virtue, is seen to be cunning and not wisdom*' (Plato *Menexenus*). In other words, values-based context is vital. Information on its own is inferior to knowledge, but knowledge does not advance to meaning (and possibly to wisdom) unless it is embedded in values, again beyond the economic and functional. Meaning and wisdom might be defined as the virtuous application of knowledge, as a meta-application.

Back to anatomy: medical education can be improved when a set of bones (calcaneus, talus, navicular, cuneiform, metatarsal, phalange, and so forth) is not just named (the literal 'naming of the parts') but contextualised ('how does the body maintain an upright posture against gravity?' or 'why, mechanically can we hold our heads high – or not?'). This is our way of 'Easing the Spring', putting the body back in nature. Again, medical education must begin not in information but in meaning. What is it, for example, to learn anatomy in the context of physical disability? Is it enough to know that the navicular bone is so called because of its shape – resembling a small boat? Again, information seeking meaning (what if the boat crashes on a rock – how are its five proximal, distal, and lateral articulations affected?).

The Greek physician Anthony Papagiannis (2017) says of the poet TS Eliot's epigram:

> I first saw these well-known lines by T. S. Eliot inscribed as a motto on the flyleaf of a Greek textbook on internal medicine. I was a student then, and almost a quarter of a century passed before I pondered on their significance. We live in a world that worships information, and there is virtually no limit in our quest for broader and speedier access to it.

> In such a setting a critical approach to information would probably appear completely out of place, even bordering on heresy. Yet in medicine we need to view information in the right context and perspective. What is its relation to knowledge and wisdom? Can overgrowth of the one lead to atrophy of the other(s)?

Papagiannis defines information as 'point knowledge', referring to a fixed point in time, with a shelf life ('the lifespan of its validity'). Naked information can be false and deceitful – stripped of informing values – as well as accurate. As 'medical news', suggests Papagiannis, information shared in the public domain may be premature. He cites the popular broadsheet broadcasting the efficacy of low-dose aspirin in preventing myocardial infarction in 1988. This led to an outburst of unregulated self-medication (Relman 1988). Knowledge is the longer-term accumulation of evidence, for example from randomised controlled trials, but knowledge is also entropic; it decays. Characteristically, well over a half of what is taught to medical students now will have been forgotten or been revised in less than five years. Such knowledge is also typically ingested by medical students as gobbets of information to be regurgitated in formal examinations. Wisdom only emerges as the critical evaluation of knowledge, its selective use (e.g., according to economic and political circumstances), its ethical application, and its carefully contoured representation as sagacity (the aesthetics of knowledge), and its relation to power (the politics of knowledge). How then does a practitioner apply generalised knowledge to idiosyncratic contexts such as a specific patient's needs?

The exponential rise of information-led media has led to information overload or trivialisation (for instance as 'infotainment') and to problems of misinformation and disinformation. Physicians properly complain about 'Google-led patients' even as they subscribe to patient-centred medicine. Papagiannis (2017) bemoans,

> an asymmetrical hypertrophy of specialist knowledge without the parallel development of general education and broader critical function. One of the aims of medical education should be to teach doctors how to select out those essential morsels of information that will complement or revise existing knowledge. This requires an investment of time and effort, which can only lead to greater wisdom.

Discrimination would seem to be key here. Gary Tomlinson (2023), in a reconceptualisation of Darwinian evolutionary process and mechanisms, suggests that 'we assume that information carries meaning'. This public assumption is misguided if we read it as 'information per se is meaningful'. I think not, and Tomlinson agrees. As argued above, information can transform (e.g., as kinds of translation) into meaning and meaning can be embedded (and sometimes lost) in information. But isolated incidents of information constituting most of communication, as information scientists describe, are purely information-for-information's sake (Shannon 1948). Claude Shannon's major contribution to science was to discriminate between 'information' and 'noise', and in terms of such a contrast, information per se can be meaningful (because it is not noise) while its *content* may not carry meaning (e.g., affording aesthetic, ethical, political, or transcendental value).

For example, a gene stores, carries, and expresses information coded in combinations of nucleic acids. There is structure, but it lacks meaning. Meaning occurs later as information *creates the conditions of possibility for the emergence of meaning*. To say that 'the brain is necessary for conscious thought' is simply information. It is meaningless until we give it context, such as asking how translation occurs between perception and the processing of perception via the central nervous system, and how affect accompanies such processing via the autonomic nervous system's sympathetic and parasympathetic branches. At this point, we are still searching for more context to explain why this action occurred in this way for this person at this moment in time; and we are struggling to explain why this person spontaneously invented a strategy that brought about a novel result, or how the gap between soma and psyche is adequately grasped as a meditation on being. At each point in these examples, meaning gradually becomes more important than information, although such meaning was always implicit or embedded in information. This, of course, is the nature of evolution (Tomlinson 2023), where 'the turning of information into meaning' is surely a good definition of evolution (Haig 2020). Isn't 'the meaning of life' a recursive activity best expressed as 'the life of meaning'? We must also puzzle at why the making of meaning is not always ethical or cooperative, or contra-evolution. For example, psychopaths create meaning out of dreadful acts of violence, while narcissists create meaning purely in terms of self-interest. Meaning is not necessarily goodness and light.

The emergence of high-flying meaning from the nest of information advertises the arrival of 'meta', as in metacognition. Circling back, while information is qualitatively different from meaning, we cannot in turn label information as 'meaningless', for meaning is embedded in information and derives from it at a higher level of value, beyond the instrumental and economic to embrace other values (as illustrated in the previous chapter through the 'Values Prism'). Meaning is then birthed from information, while information is not essentially meaningless. As Tomlinson (2023) suggests, 'A coral reef, jellyfish, paramecium, or butterfly is a piece of meaningless life, but magnificently meaningless in its informational negotiations and dauntingly meaningless in our attempts to understand them'.

Metacognition

In Chapter 1, I described how the ancient Greek word 'meta', now used as prefix, literally means 'beyond'. But it also means 'after' or 'behind', as in 'afterword' and 'left behind', or 'separated from'. A modern meaning of meta is 'more comprehensive' or 'transcending'. But, imitating the fantastic ouroboric snake that eats itself by swallowing its own tail and in doing so emerges refreshed, 'meta' can mean that which is insistently self-referential, as in 'metatheory' or theorising about theory, or 'metahumour' involving joking about jokes. Tomlinson (2023) continues with a rider – that while 'Information transmission is a crucial aspect of all life-forms … information bearing meaning is rare'. Note that Tomlinson says 'bearing' and not 'birthing'. This remark can be put into context where Tomlinson is referring to all life forms. At some point in evolution, meaning, for a small number of life forms and most significantly for hominids, must have evolved from an informational nexus. Meaning is the evolutionary transcendence of the merely informational. It is ironic that, as we are now in the Anthropocene (also an Age of Information and Misinformation), so we seem to be guarding against meaning. Yet meaning, rather than information, is our primary evolutionary driver. Is the correlate of this craving of information at the expense of meaning paralleling our potential demise as a species through self-imposed climate change?

The evolution of meaning is surely what Darwin originally describes as the emergence through evolution of 'higher' or more complex life forms. In this context, it seems strange that a project such as medical education can be seen to frustrate an evolutionary impulse through a cultural effect: that of frustrating the opportunity for invention and imagination amongst medical students through persistent reduction to the insensible (Bleakley 2020) and the instrumental (Bleakley 2023) as celebration of information over meaning. This pedagogic track – bereft of complexity, beauty, and meaning – seems to me to parallel the ignorance advertised by climate change denial, albeit on a smaller scale.

Creating meaning is not restricted to humans. Other life forms do this. Bird song can serve functional or instrumental means, such as indicating territorial boundaries, but much bird song would seem to be simply for the sake of it – it is non-functional and self-expressive. But this does not make it meaningless. Bird song is largely an aesthetic expression and thus carries meaning beyond function (Taylor 2017). It is 'meta'. Similarly, the 'play' of mammals such as dolphins is expressive, beyond function such as communication of information concerning hunting or territorial behaviour (Rajalakshmi 2022). Play, of course, has a social function in dolphins as it does in humans, but this too extends beyond mere information sharing to creative meanings, as the continual re-invention of cultures and selves.

As we have seen, metacognition can be defined as 'thinking-about-thinking', or 'reflexivity' (reflecting on reflection). In considering the cognitive 'meta', we should also embrace meta-affect, as 'feeling about feeling', refining feelings, and gaining insight through – and into – catharsis, as previously discussed (Heron 1989). Meta-affect also embraces values clarification – what values primarily drive my activity, and can I – as Nietzsche encouraged – engage in the 'transvaluation of all values', or a critical relativism? Such transvaluation is, perhaps, the ultimate meta-move and is key to the establishment of authentic democracy – because it signals critical engagement with the values of others in authentic collaboration.

In terms of medical education, medical students are rarely formally taught to think about their thinking, let alone to feel about their feelings. There are singular exceptions, such as Quentin Eichbaum's work at Vanderbilt (2014, and see Chapter 1). Indeed, students are never formally taught to inquire into the nature of catharsis (the flow and release of affect, emotion, or feeling states) and how insight can be gained from catharsis – even though this is part of their being human, or 'human, all too human' in Nietzsche's 1878 aphoristic summation. Yet medicine is both high cognition and high affect, whose development depends upon the imagination and creativity of practitioners as they navigate the rapids of patients' and families' emotional fallout from suffering, illness, and loss. This shortfall in pedagogy rests at the feet of medical educators who resist meta-medicine: again, thinking-about-thinking (metacognition) and feeling-about-feeling (sensitivity) in clinical practice. This kind of reflexive education includes cultivation of the senses (sensibility), progression of medical culture through expansive imagination, the development of moral courage, recognition of aesthetic labour, the cultivation of democratic habits in collaborative work, and the making of meaning as a vocation across all fields of interest.

Nietzsche modelled this as the aphoristic life: make every gesture count, cultivate metaphor, and create impact. 'I am no man, I am dynamite'. No, not the egotistical-narcissistic (insistently self-referencing) template that is, for example, Donald Trump, but Nietzsche (1908/2005) himself – in *Ecce Homo* – referring to his possible legacy as a ground-breaking thinker blowing up habits and preconceptions through metacognition, to establish a radical relativism.

Let us not get cosy about making meaning of meaning (the transcendental effect, or the meta-shift of cognition and affect), for this process is one of creating ever-greater complexities standing at the edge of chaos through reformulations. It is dangerous work, as the practice of medicine is caught in two unavoidable binds, two paradoxes. The first is that medicine is dedicated to supporting life in the face of entropy (the inevitability of death and decay). The second is that clinical decision-making (diagnostics) seeks closure and certainty in the face of ever-present ambiguity. Medical education's task is to help medical students and junior doctors to navigate the waters between these two paradoxes, as if they were the outwitting the sea-monsters Scylla and Charybdis of Greek myth. Otherwise, the student or doctor is shipwrecked as incompetent. In the face of this challenge, a medical education must facilitate development of tolerance of ambiguity, the embrace of paradox and contradiction as opportunity and not threat, high levels of adaptability, the insistent re-invention of identity, resistance to developing cynicism and high levels of emotional insulation, capacity for enacting democratic habits such as collaboration and support of others, and psychotherapeutic acumen to manage self-care. These are tall orders, metacapabilities. And they are all enacted within multiple, intersecting, dynamic, complex adaptive systems that work at the edge of chaos. Moreover, they run against the currents of a reductive, instrumental, and linear medical education that appears to resist evolutionary thrust involving both risk (as innovation) and complexity.

In Homer's *Odyssey*, when Odysseus is faced with the dilemma of navigating the straits between Scylla and Charybdis, his ploy is to choose the lesser of the two evils, knowing that something must be sacrificed for the good of the whole crew. Judging that the whirlpool created by Charybdis will take down his raft and his whole crew, he sails close to the six-headed monster Scylla, who duly eats six of his men at one fell swoop. But the raft is recovered and the rest of the crew sail on. Medical students and junior doctors now are sacrificed to the six-headed monster that is historically conditioned, ingrained habits for medical culture such as toxic masculinity, heroic individualism, immoveable hierarchy, narcissism as a style of life, a culture of competition, and, above all, information-led training (Bleakley 2020). Scylla's victory is that of endemic burnout. However, medical education is, in patches, thankfully now progressing to become aware of its social justice responsibilities, to embrace inclusivity and democracy through a meaning-led education. But this shift must be radically accelerated as a 'meta' project, a learning-to-learn (Eichbaum 2014, Webb 2021) and a becoming-reflexive-practitioners (Bleakley 1999).

If there is one thing that we can be certain about amongst the welter of evidence that surrounds best practice in medicine and healthcare, it is the value of collaborative work – authentic inter-professional teamwork and co-inquiry with patients. Such patterns of working can improve patient care and safety and satisfaction amongst team members (Bhatt and Swick 2017). Similarly, if there is one thing that we can be certain about how medical students learn and continue to learn as doctors throughout their careers, it is that learning-to-learn trumps the cramming of facts and information focused on exams.

Both work collaboratively and learning-to-learn embraces meta-learning and other values characterising higher-order cognition and affect. On the one hand, thinking-about-thinking, and on the other, experiencing emotions to the full but being able to not be swamped by them, or maintaining a degree of 'free attention' that allows for catharsis to progress to insight (Heron 1989). Characteristically, such meta-capacities embrace ethical values ('what impact does my decision have on others?'), aesthetic values ('is my work graceful and does it engage sensibility?'), political values ('what are the power implications of what I am about to do – will my actions be democratic?'), and transcendental values ('does my work move beyond the level of putting knowledge into action to add to meaning and grace; is my work one of reformulation: creative/innovative/imaginative, and breaking new ground?').

Language and meta-language

This shift from the mundane instrumental to the meta-level of activity, inquiry, and appreciation is shaped primarily by using expressive language or linguistic tropes (figures of speech and rhetorical devices) such as metaphor, analogy, metonym, and paradox. Expressive metaphor is part and parcel of the vernacular, or everyday speech. It is also deeply embodied as non-verbal expression open to creative adaptation. Within any cultural context, we take on a variety of communication tropes, such as gesture, posture, tone of voice, gaze, and relative proximity to another, to express affect and meaning. These are everyday (but also complex) metaphorical and rhetorical activities used to convey meanings: such as persuasion, amplification, clarification, and intimacy. Quotidien embodied semiotics may be quite extraordinary but are taken for granted. In performance, drama, dance, music, sports, and other physical-expressive arts, they are raised to yet another level of meaning. In the verbal realm, the vernacular is deliberately developed as an act of metacognition, lyrical poetry perhaps being the best example of this (Bleakley and Neilson 2021). Here, innovative metaphor production is the key to the success of the art form. Indeed, poetry is not so different from medicine in that poetic composition and clinical reasoning share similar cognitive strategies, as demonstrated by Bleakley and Neilson (2021, 2024).

Patients and doctors alike inhabit the vernacular and its rich metaphoric possibilities. However, medicine (like other professions such as law) has pursued the path of developing an in-house specialist vocabulary that reduces the vernacular to technical terms. This forms an exclusive professional group of course. But such reduction is not aesthetically inclined but rather instrumental or functional. To offer a refrain from a previous chapter, the founder of the synapse – the Spanish neuroscientist, pathologist, and histologist Ramon y Cajal – first used the descriptor 'protoplasmic kisses' for the technical term 'synapse' (from the ancient Greek root *sunapsis*, meaning 'joining together'). The metaphoric/poetic 'protoplasmic kisses' trumps the instrumental, purely descriptive 'joining together' and then is more pleasing and memorable. The technical term tachypnoea (tak-ip-nee-uh) means 'panting for breath'. This term is derived from the ancient Greek roots *tachy* (swift) and *pnoe* (breathing). The word is then literalised by being moved from the vernacular ('swift breathing') to the classical ancient origin. Further vernacular translation of 'swift breathing' into 'panting for breath' more deeply embodies the metaphor, where we somatically feel the panting, the action, as we mouth the words. In the same manner, 'vomiting blood' is a deeply embodied metaphor, imaginatively enacted in the saying, where the ancient Greek term 'haematemesis' is literal and functional (from *haemato* meaning 'pertaining to the blood', plus *emesis* meaning 'vomiting') (Bleakley and Neilson 2022).

Other examples of reduction of the expressive metaphorical (in the vernacular) to the technical-medical (attached back to ancient Greek roots) include haematochezia (rectal bleeding), haematuria (blood appearing in urine), haemoptysis (coughing up blood), anuria (inability to produce urine), oedema (fluid accumulation and swelling), 'ectomy' ('removal of'), cyanosis (lack of oxygen), menorrhagia (excessively heavy periods), dyspnoea (difficulty breathing), melena (partially digested blood in the stool), pruritis (excessive itching), purulent (containing pus), rigor (abrupt attack of shivering and feeling cold), and steatorrhea (abnormal fat in faeces). Of course, as noted, such technical terms serve purposes in medical culture of brevity and concision in language and affording an identity as entry into a closed culture. But they disembody potential metaphors resulting in abstractions, and they deflect attention from the vernacular that is the cultural capital of patients. Again, common shared meanings are reduced to information (that gains meaning only as a specialist vocabulary or as an exercise in etymology).

In adopting an instrumental language that squeezes out inventive metaphor and works against a poetic imagination, we see resistance to the 'meta'. Medicine also throws a protective ring around itself that refuses admission to laypersons (patients). In abandoning the 'meta' of metaphor, the culture of medicine socialises medical students into an 'insider' professional identity. This offers exclusivity and prestige even now in the counter-current of a need for 'patient-centredness' and 'inter-professional' teamworking. In doing so, and against the spirit of the pursuit of 'meta', medical culture's historical closing of ranks can be seen as counter-productive in evolutionary terms.

To reinforce this argument, articles (e.g., https://openmd.com/guide/medical-terminology) and books about medical terminology remain at the level of description and information rather than critical reception (the 'meta' level). Where there is a basic formula to the invention of technical-medical terms (prefix + root + suffix + combining vowel), this formulaic approach of course is what reduces the inventive vernacular to the specialist lingo. This formula itself is described functionally as 'building blocks' (Bleakley and Neilson 2022) from the classical (ancient Greek or Latin) foundations. The purely lexical returns us to formulaic and instrumental thinking. Why not a return to Homer that can promote meta-reflection on insistent modern habits such as medical education's desire to educate for 'empathy', where the notion is rarely critically questioned for its roots and meanings? Homer uses the word 'pity' – now having lost its currency – to describe a more expansive notion of 'empathy' (Marshall and Bleakley 2017). Can we revisit Homeric pity for its riches and revelations?

Moreover, again a functional move, medical English has become the primary language for global communication in healthcare, as English for Medical Purposes (EMP). Reductive instrumentalism is then combined with neocolonialism, the English re-creating their Empire. Of course, this has purpose based in convenience and function, but it steamrolls cultural differences: for example, while the English poet Samuel Taylor Coleridge coined the term 'psychosomatic', it can be argued that it is French culture that has most insistently cultivated a host of irrational and efflorescent psychosomatic maladies – such as the short-lived psychotic episode *bouffée délirante* – seen particularly in new migrants or displaced persons (Johnson-Sabine et al. 1983). Here is a rich vocabulary shifting information to meaning grounded in a shared culture of malady across medicine and lay patients. Don't expect such florid terms in EMP.

Medical English then works literally and mechanically, and not poetically – from prefixes, roots, and suffixes derived from the ancient Greek and Latin. Combining vowels, usually an 'o', are added to aid in pronunciation. For example, hypothermia, one term that is now integrated into the vernacular, has the prefix hypo- ('below normal'), the root 'therm' ('heat or warmth'), and the suffix -ia (condition). Prefixes include 'macro' ('large') and 'micro' ('small'). Word roots can indicate a bodily part or condition, such as 'enceph' (brain) or 'oste' (bone). Compound words, such as cardio-pulmo-nary, reflect multiple roots (heart and lungs). Suffixes usually refer to a specialty, test, procedure, function, condition, or status, and include '-I' ('inflammation') and '-ectomy' ('removal'). A litany of functions or a 'naming of parts' as the poet Henry Reed would have it. My key point about this reductive vocabulary is its anti-poetic presence – such a corpus of technical terms remains untouched by the poetic imagination and is unlikely to stimulate a poetic approach to patient care.

Further, and taking reductive instrumentalism to its logical conclusion, the medical, healthcare, social care, and community care professions have developed a common clinical language for electronic communication, institutionalised since 2011 in the English National Health Service (NHS) as SNOMED CT (Systemized Nomenclature of Medicine – Clinical Terms) (https://www.gov.uk/government/news/common-clinical-language-for-nhs-will-help-improve-patient-care-and-safety). This is multilingual and available in more than 50 countries including the USA, Canada, Australia, Spain, Sweden, and the Netherlands. Of course, this is technically efficient, and rightly so – as 'purpose built'. But such instrumentality again masks the embrace of other value systems in medicine, healthcare, and social and community care that may be expressive, imaginative, and adaptive to the idiosyncratic patient.

On the general case of patient-friendly language in an era of strenuously promoted 'patient-centredness' in medicine and healthcare, efforts have been made in midwifery, for example, to note that '*Language matters as a way of respecting women's views and ensuring that they are empowered to make decisions*' (Mobbs et al. 2023, italics in original). Here, the thinking moves from the mundane to the 'meta' in the form of a paradox. It is sophisticated medicine that has stripped the intensely metaphoric public vernacular through promotion of technical language within a reductive biomedical register, and then concealed the former's expressiveness as the native language of 'patients'. Further, such patients themselves have been commodified, as customers, within a newly formed reductive language of medicine as business and commerce (the economic value complex forming medicine's bower, along with instrumentalism or functionalism). Here, patients are stripped of their complex and aesthetic linguistic capital – embracing metaphor and slang – that remains invested in, and controlled by, medical culture. This is an appropriation of vernacular capital, intensely felt in patients' inability to claim the fruits of their emotional labour as their own, where medical culture characteristically subverts, diverts, or inverts such emotional expression as surplus to the cognitive work of diagnosis and treatment. Patients' symptoms are entangled with their idiosyncratic verbal, non-verbal, and semiotic expressions that are often painfully squashed in the clinical encounter. Such repression of rich and potentially enabling language can amplify repressed language as symptom (self-loathing, anger at being ignored or misunderstood, and mute response in the face of arrogance).

In re-inventing poetry, shifting from high-flown and abstruse language to the vernacular, Wordsworth and Coleridge sought to talk with local labourers on their long walks in the Quantocks in Somerset at the tail end of the 18th century. Can medicine also return to the perspective of the patient's metaphoric vernacular? My illustrative example here is obstetrics, in which the patient is always a woman, yet the culture has been shaped in recent history by a masculinised surgical culture in the face of opposition by a female-inspired midwifery tradition. Specialist language then has not only been instrumentalised (stripped of metaphor), but also gendered (male). The return to everyday language contra 'medicalese' is not just political correctness, but meta-thinking – as meta-affect or acute sensitivity. This is both an ethical and aesthetic move, but it is more obviously political in resisting the objectification of mothers-to-be, where capital has been stripped from its primary producer and re-invested in another culture (again, medicine's appropriation of patients' emotional labour). I am suggesting that the return of such capital to its producers (in this case, mothers-to-be) would advertise a shift from information to meaning, or the mundane to the meta.

Mobbs and colleague (2023) suggest areas in which language can be translated from obstetrician-centred to mother-centred language. This shift does not necessarily raise the values register from the instrumental to embrace metaphor, but it does facilitate the opportunity for dialogue. Encouraging the mother-to-be to speak allows for more florid, personalised expression, but also speaks on behalf of women at large and feminine archetypes rather than stereotypes.

Respecting women as autonomous adults and decision-makers

For example, where the obstetrician habitually refers to the woman as 'good girl' during labour, this is corrected to 'you're doing really well'. The directive 'you must have' can be re-phrased as 'we suggest' or 'it is in your best interests'; 'the patient refused' is re-cast as 'the patient declined'. Returning power to the woman in this way lays the ground for allowing idiosyncratic use of language in the face of medical habit.

Respecting women as persons (rather than containers and mechanisms for producing a baby)

For example, a 'delivery' (possibly the most habitual term) becomes 'giving birth', thus losing the mechanical implications of a misplaced metaphor. In talking to colleagues, the obstetrician's habitual use of 'primigravida' (a woman pregnant for the first time) ('the primigravida in room 12') is changed to use the woman's surname or first name or both. The reclamation of the simple utterance 'it's my first baby' reclaims aesthetic linguistic capital against the instrumentalism of medical speak.

Replacing codified medical language with plain speaking

For example, instead of referring to 'SROM' ('spontaneous rupture of membranes'), the obstetrician uses the vernacular and metaphoric: 'your waters have broken'; instead of 'antepartum haemorrhage', the woman is told 'you have some bleeding'. Abstractions are replaced by physicality so that the woman is living the experience bodily and not mediated by the textbook.

Avoiding phrases that are anxiety provoking, over-dramatic, or violent

For example, 'rupture the membranes' (surgical talk) becomes 'release the waters'; 'trial of forceps' becomes 'let's see if we can help baby out using forceps'; while 'foetal distress' is translated as 'there are changes in the baby's heart rate pattern'. In each case, the surgical lingo is violent and violating, replaced by the pacific maternal.

Avoiding insensitive language

For example, the habitual 'poor maternal effort' is replaced by 'the patient is not finding it easy'; while 'failure to progress' is referred to as 'slow labour', another fine metaphor.

Meta-affect and catharsis

The experiences of new mothers will likely involve frequent moments of anticipation, fear, joy, and pain. Will this be purely expressive, or will such cathartic episodes be a source of insight and connection (e.g., to a sisterhood, or to a family nexus, or to a good or poor relationship with the father), and will the obstetrician, where involved, engage cathartically, or practice a professional 'cool reason'? There is a meta-aspect to such a question, for it engages the entanglement of myth and human culture, grounded in classical drama. The ancient Greek word *katharsis* referred to the expression of emotion as a form of purification, placing emphasis on the soothing and calming of the emotions after such expression. Here, I follow on from sections on meta-affect in previous chapters to expand the case for medical education to grapple more intently with how medical students and junior doctors might 'work with' their emotional states rather than 'against' them (through a variety of psychological defence mechanisms such as repression, rationalisation, and displacement).

In classical Greek drama, as the actors played out the tragedy, a chorus performing music, dance, poetry, and song would interact with the audience to provide commentary and interpretation. If the tragedy itself is the patient's illness or symptoms, the audience is the patient herself, distanced from that tragedy by the intervention of the physician who acts as chorus. The physician plays the roles of both diagnostician and carer, where she is instrumental in acting as facilitator of the patient's *katharsis*. Indeed, the Polish physician Andrzej Szczeklik (2005) describes medicine as, primarily, the art of managing catharsis. Medicine is necessarily meta-medicine once this perspective is adopted as it engages the ancient lineage of dramatic form. Medicine is tapping into deep-rooted aspects of human life as performance, where the discharge of emotion is deeply entangled with experiences of illness. Medical students would benefit from studying forms of drama as education into meta-affect.

While our mothers-to-be described above are rarely engaged in tragedy (some, however, will be – in the UK, one in every 225 pregnancies ends in a stillbirth, or seven babies every day), they are actresses in the theatre of clinical work, particularly during a hospital birth. So, they engage with the archetypal Greek drama scenario described above. The birthing mother represents the stage drama, the clinical team the chorus, and the birthing mother (and anyone who accompanies her) also the audience. Here, the drama of the birth process and the parallel experience of that birth by the mother coincide, with ongoing interpretation from the clinical chorus. Here, surely, is a meta-healthcare at play: obstetrics and midwifery as eliding art forms, properly staged and open to interpretation.

While issues of attention and metacognition have attracted a large literature and subsequent pedagogical innovations (such as how to educate for clinical *reasoning*), how to educate for clinical *feeling* has been overlooked. Yet meta-management of emotional states, as I have already indicated in previous chapters, is crucial to medical practice and the fact that it is poorly done is reflected in key historical symptoms of medical education's failings: characteristically poor emotional relationships with patients and fellow clinical team members, and, most importantly, failure in self-care amongst physicians leading to unacceptably high rates of anxiety, depression, burnout, and suicide ideation. Note how the 'meta' (suicide ideation) can emerge as a negative quality. For psychotherapists and counsellors in training, insight into and from catharsis is core to the education of their sensibilities and sensitivities and key to self-care (Bleakley 2021). Strangely, such cultivation of insight is again missing from medical education, where it remains the elephant in the room – for what is more emotionally disruptive than clinical work where distress, disease, and death are faced daily?

Insight into catharsis (or abreaction) – both while it is happening (reflection-in-action and reflection-as-action) and retrospectively (reflection-on-action) (see Preface) – is one of the wonders of human evolution where it forms the basis for morality. This is because human values are grounded in affect, or passions, and of course raise such passions. Doctors are humans and are invested in moral values and principles that go beyond the confines of an instrumental professionalism. But decent human conduct depends upon the gaining of insight from the exercise of passions, a meta-activity linking preverbal affect and postverbal insight. The consequent moral conscience suppresses or realigns impulses that may have dangerous, unwanted, or uncharted consequences. Psychopathy and sociopathy are defined by the consequences of lack of such moral conscience. Paradoxically, medical education's overdetermined approach to emotional insulation (keeping feelings at bay) (Kerasidou and Horn 2016) can lead to an over-detachment on the part of doctors that may appear insensitive, despite their claims to a moral conscience. Let us examine this more closely.

Aristotle's all-too-brief definition and description of catharsis (in *Poetics*) as the discharge of emotions, a purging, follows the ancient Greek theatre model discussed above, where the audience engages in catharsis through identification with the actors, as guided by the chorus. However, this view of catharsis falls short of detailing the meta-aspects, as (i) *the insight created by such discharge* and (ii) *the education into habitual seeking of insight from catharsis.*

For example, I may express anger rather than sublimate or repress it, but after purging, there may just be a hollow space. Importantly, insight should occupy that space. While catharsis has been adequately described, how might it be managed effectively, to provide the conditions for insight? This, of course, has been the basis to psychodynamic psychotherapies since Breuer and Freud, where the post-cathartic insight is generated by the analyst on behalf of the client, as an interpretation. For example, the habitual expression of a pattern of emotion does not happen in a vacuum, but is often aimed at a parental figure, where the direct link has been repressed or is disguised in sublimation, displacement, and other ego defence mechanisms.

In humanistic approaches such as co-counselling (Heron 1989), the insight is not provided by the counsellor, where the counsellor provides the conditions of support for abreaction and creates the space for the client to gain subsequent insight as a democratic gesture. The process is political at core, encouraging self-direction as an expression of power, but never at the expense of others. The ability to facilitate catharsis (and work through subsequent insights) in patients should be second nature for physicians, especially general practitioners whose caseload can be as much as 50% mental health issues. Again, a traditional medical education does not cultivate such psychotherapeutic acumen – yet it seems so clearly the best way to approach learning patient-centredness. I say this from many years of experience of working psychotherapeutically in the areas of expert clinical communication and pursuit of doctors' well-being.

The key to gaining insight from catharsis is to know and work with three kinds of attention. This applies to physicians working with both patients and colleagues, and in looking after their own mental health and psychological stability in an occupation that brings an unusual amount of emotional stress. Phenomenologists describe two kinds of attention – focused and free-floating (see Chapter 7). One can readily occlude the other. If engaged in a task occupying the senses, attention will be focused on the job at hand. But simultaneously, a surplus of 'paradoxical' attention allows us to perceive peripheral activities as we are focusing. Sometimes, this can be a distraction and sometimes of help. Perceived as a distraction, we may ratchet up our focused attention such that all 'interruptions' are closed out. However, this can be dangerous. In a well-known patient safety scenario describing the avoidable death of a patient undergoing a difficult intubation, described at length in Chapter 7, a team of surgeons and anaesthetists are so focused on the task that they fail to maintain what the patient safety culture calls 'situational awareness' (otherwise, free-floating attention). Nurses in the team, excluded from this task, notice that the patient is turning blue, where the team members working on the intubation do not. The nurses raise the alarm, but it is too late. The intubation is abandoned, and the patient is left to wake up from the anaesthetic on the recovery ward. But she has suffered from lengthy periods of poor oxygenation and fails to wake up, dying on the recovery bed (https://www.youtube.com/watch?v=JzlvgtPIof4).

This brings us to a third kind of attention beyond the focused and free-floating – extended or augmented attention, described in detail in Chapter 7. In the scenario above, the nurses in the team were providing an extended attention. Any social context can do this. Social contexts can also shut down attention, through unwanted interruptions. A self-audit study of interruptions over 25 typical shifts for a senior Emergency Medicine consultant in a UK Accident and Emergency department showed an average of six interruptions per hour (Allard et al. 2012). Around 75% of these interruptions were necessary and re-aligned current tasks, but around 25% detrimentally interrupted attention. In this kind of fluid working context, adaptability and flexibility are key, such that the two kinds of attention – focused and free-floating – are constantly being shaped by social forces such as distractions and re-alignments. We can call this an 'augmented attention'. It is key to both metacognition and meta-affect.

Augmented attention also encompasses extensions of attention provided by artefacts such as alarms and beepers, for example, in a 'crash' scenario where a patient needs to be resuscitated. Focused, free-floating (or paradoxical), and distributed attentions can all take attention into a meta-realm. For example, an interventional cardiologist shows extraordinarily focused attention in placing a stent, while allowing free-floating attention to move between screen, patient, trainee cardiologist, and nurses; a paediatrician is closely watching a child's behaviour while her peripheral attention is weighing up how an anxious mother is responding; and a surgeon, closely involved with a delicate operation, uses the simplest of instrument extensions, a clock, to monitor the pacing of her work. This brief section on forms of attention – a taster – will be fully expanded in Chapter 7.

Emotional labour

Physicians and surgeons engage in:

1 Cognitive or intellectual labour: rational thinking such as deductive and inductive problem-solving in diagnostic work and keeping up with new research and guidelines.
2 Abductive labour or 'best guess', 'best fit' intuitive reasoning, calling on creative capacities.
3 Physical labour, for physicians, mostly fine work such as debriding and stitching wounds; for surgeons, fine work such as vascular surgery and sometimes strenuous physical work such as orthopaedics.
4 Emotional labour, such as managing patient consultations, working in teams, and self-care in a stressful and demanding job embracing high-stakes outcomes.

Initial (undergraduate) medical education deals well with 1 above, and with 3 where elementary clinical skills are learned, usually in simulation. Abductive labour is rarely learned but picked up on the job. Emotional labour is learned in a patchy way with emphasis upon formulaic approaches to the consultation. Working in teams tends to focus on ideal collaborative team scenarios rather than the reality of poorly functioning teams grounded in traditional hierarchies, where medical students should be learning a set of democratic habits within a political (power) framework while this is rarely well modelled. The notion of emotional labour is neglected, so students fail to see that expert management of emotions is core to good practice. Rather, as noted previously, students are taught to repress affect, or keep it at bay, as emotional insulation (Kerasidou and Horn 2016). In distressing clinical placement settings, while a first response may be to try to comfort a patient or change the situation, medical students tend to use tactics of avoidance or repression (Doulougeri et al. 2016) as forms of emotional insulation. These include inaction (doing/saying nothing), focusing on task as displacement, denial, repression, and distancing oneself from the situation employing cognition to smother affect. Of course, such insulation serves a purpose, for over-identification with suffering can be highly distressing and emotionally taxing. But over-insulation is common, resulting in forms of insensibility and insensitivity such as lack of empathy and cynicism.

Many cultures are poor at managing affect and catharsis, particularly in the face of human vulnerability and distress. Medical education creates a contradiction where students are encouraged to be emotionally sensitive or to employ empathy, even as they are asked to emotionally insulate themselves – as noted above – so that they do not take on the inevitable distress they encounter in patients' suffering. Learning anatomy through dissection focuses this contradiction, where extreme sensitivity (as respect) and sensibility (as close noticing) are expected in dissecting a cadaver, while the very physical conditions of dissection shut down the senses just as young people are exposed to a traumatic scene, however well prepared (Bleakley 2021). Where such a contradiction has been central to socialisation into medicine, again its affective dimensions seem to have been poorly articulated and managed within medical education. Indeed, histories of the ritual of medical student dissection shows two characteristic defence mechanisms at work: first, defusing a potentially emotionally threatening situation through dark humour (often inappropriate, at the cadaver's expense); and second, intellectualising a primarily somatic-affective response to a dead body as the donor-cadaver is reduced to anatomical information (Warner and Edmonson 2009).

Indeed, histories of medical school dissection from North America show a third and sinister method of defusing emotional response: expressions of racism. Through early group 'selfie' photographic evidence, Warner and Edmonson (2009) show how white medical students at the beginning of the 20th century were provided largely with black cadavers that they openly mocked. One photograph – from the College of Physicians and Surgeons, Baltimore class of 1902 – shows a table with the black cadaver laid out and several medical students standing behind. On the table is the shocking inscription: 'all coons smell alike to us'.

Sources of potential distress are obviously multiple in medicine, but historically accrued habits have taken medical education in a direction that often fails to educate for meta-affect, or the ability to manage responses to distress as catharsis in ways that lead to insight rather than to symptoms such as poor self-care, anxiety, depression, suicidal ideation, and burnout. Such iatrogenic symptoms are deeply exacerbated by structural issues such as working long hours with under-resourcing. The latter is now the norm for medicine worldwide due largely to rising elderly populations with multiple chronic conditions in post-industrial countries, and population pressures, large infant mortality rates, and endemic poverty in developing nations.

As we have seen, John Heron (1989), writing within a co-counselling framework, argues that – regardless of the primary cause – discharge of personal distress (catharsis) properly managed leads to insight (a meta-affective capability). This embraces discharge of grief, disgust, anger, embarrassment, guilt, shame, fatigue, and boredom, commonly experienced in medical work. The medical student fears being swamped by distress and so cultivates habits of rationalising, distancing, and repressing – all facets of emotional insulation. This, rather than seeking a meta-affect context (such as therapeutic sessions, in groups or in co-counselling pair settings) in which balance of attention can be educated and cultivated, so that educated 'free attention' is available in situations of distress, rather than the exercise of repressive, distancing, or rationalising tactics, as shown in, for example, Doulougeri et al.' (2016) study.

For the practitioner – such as the medical student learning the so-called communication 'skills' on the job – gaining free attention and subsequent insight post-catharsis depends upon a subtle balance between experiencing emotion and discharge and maintaining conscious slack within the experience. (I say 'so-called' communication 'skills' because communication goes far beyond technical 'skill' as a complex capability). Insights can be multiple – identification with a patient's suffering or loss does not mean that one is swamped by distress. Rather, genuine empathy moves from low-grade sympathy to high-grade compathy (see Chapter 12), a feeling of identification without swamping. A medical student's insight may show a psychodynamic reason for feelings towards another – a genuine feeling of dislike for a patient or colleague (e.g., for the latter's perceived gender-related discrimination) may be because that person reminds the student of an overbearing parent or sibling, repressed feelings that have never been resolved or analysed. Re-evaluation of a past traumatic event may relieve such projection of affect.

However, such educational possibilities are repressed where medical students are taught to over-emotionally insulate or distance from feelings, rather than to utilise feeling states as a means of identification with patients' worlds. And later – for example, in a co-counselling, individual mentoring, or collegial Balint group therapeutic context – to work through disturbing episodes as retrospective accounting for how and why emotions were charged. In such contexts, feelings are likely to be re-stimulated and a new catharsis occurs that can be worked through for insight in a supportive therapeutic manner ('it wasn't just being in the presence of that suffering patient, I realise now that it was bringing up memories of my sister who died young, of the same illness; I hadn't realised until now how angry I was at being robbed of her presence at such a young age').

The 'meta' of clinical reasoning: language, meaning, and context

When doctors engage with patients in initial clinical consultations, the goal is usually one of making a diagnosis with a view to potential treatment or management. For experienced doctors, most diagnoses are made through Type 1 reasoning or pattern recognition, as opposed to Type 2 analytic reasoning. Pattern recognition is based on tacit, or stored, knowledge (see Chapter 11 on pattern thinking) and often draws on the use of heuristics or 'good enough' short-cuts (see Chapter 6) and aphorisms or culturally specific succinct sayings (Levine and Bleakley 2012). Quite simply, from the symptom presentation, the doctor thinks: 'I've seen many of these before, it is (x, y, or z)'. Pattern recognition can occur for multiple symptom presentations also but will be less common here, and not possible in the case of either unique presentations or those that show high ambiguity and lead to uncertainty in decision-making. Here, the doctor resorts to analytic reasoning: semantic qualifiers, and 'decision trees' or algorithms such as Bayes' theorem (Bours 2021), working rationally through possible alternatives until these are narrowed down to a differential diagnosis that may be focused much more tightly through tests or further investigations.

While Type 1 reasoning, or pattern recognition, outwardly appears straightforward, there is a complex cognitive process behind such reasoning that moves beyond the activation of memory as both recognition and recall of facts. This process draws on context, shifting ordinary cognition to extraordinary metacognition or thinking-about-thinking. Further, the catalyst for this shift is a linguistic trope or figure of speech and rhetorical device: metaphor primarily, but also metonym and paradox (Bleakley and Neilson 2021).

Context can provide the 'meta' in metacognition, meta-affect, and meta-sensing, where human activity is shaped by whatever the environment affords in each *umwelt* or ecological niche. This is reinforced (and expanded) where we include the host of material artefacts that provide extensions to thinking and sensing such as computers, mobile phones, imaging technologies, and so forth. Again, such affordance can be purely instrumental and informational (such as pharmaceutical formularies, blood samples, or radiography images) or can proffer meaning (in a psychiatric interview with a self-harming, anorexic young woman, the woman talks about family but never mentions her father; in a multidisciplinary team meeting, a patient's positive biopsy after excision of a squamous cell carcinoma leads the original surgeon to recommend further surgery, but this is judged to be too invasive by colleagues, who suggest radiotherapy, causing the surgeon to reflect on his recommendation as too hasty).

Jerome Groopman (2007) suggests that 'While modern medicine is aided by a dazzling array of technologies, like high-resolution MRI scans and pinpoint DNA analysis, language is still the bedrock of clinical practice'. Language and listening: the latter the mirror to shared words. Groopman opens his book *How Doctors Think* with a case study. 'Anne Dodge' is a woman in her thirties who since the age of fifteen had suffered from an undiagnosed condition that caused her to experience extreme stomach pains when eating. In the early stages, she found some relief from these pains by vomiting after eating. Her general practitioner suspected an eating disorder and referred her to a psychiatrist who diagnosed anorexia with bulimia. This misdiagnosis sealed Anne's fate – she was to see a string of doctors, including more psychiatrists, and nutritionists, and then psychologists, for what was now sealed as a psychiatric disorder. She was placed on antidepressant medication and weekly talk therapy. As time progressed, so symptoms accumulated, such as loss of red blood cells and platelets, osteoporosis, failure of her immune system, and a series of infections including meningitis. She spent four periods of hospitalisation in a mental health unit. Anne was further diagnosed with irritable bowel syndrome.

She reluctantly saw another doctor, who had been advised by her prior specialist to focus on Anne's supposed irritable bowel syndrome. Myron Falchuk, the new doctor, ignored this advice and pushed aside Anne's medical record to start anew, to enact, in other words, a meta-consultation. First, he gave her time and listened intently. The words and metaphors that Anne used in the consultation fed Falchuk's imagination, giving him a way of 'thinking otherwise' and 'seeing slant' (to draw on the poet Emily Dickinson's term). Part of his diagnostic breakthrough was to put on one side all previous diagnoses (that clearly had not led to successful treatments) with a hunch that perhaps from the start Anne had been misdiagnosed and this had caused a knock-on effect, locking her in to a medically imposed instrumental mindset of habitual reasoning. The chain of doctors, in other words, had their heads down on completion of task at hand – the insistence of intubation – thus losing situational awareness, in the patient safety example given earlier. Meta-reasoning had no room to breathe.

In short, Falchuk had a strong feeling that Anne's condition was not psychosomatic at all. In particular, he focused on the advice Anne had been given some years ago to eat masses of carbohydrates such as cereals and pasta. He recommended an endoscopy to look at her gut, and associated blood tests, on the basis that she had celiac disease, an allergy to gluten. Her current medically instigated diet was in fact causing her greater ruin. Falchuk's hunch was right. After appropriate treatment, Anne soon recovered body weight, energy, and mental well-being. Nausea, vomiting, cramps, and diarrhoea all disappeared.

In Groopman's account, he notes how Falchuk was meticulous in his attention to how a patient presented herself and what she said, as a good psychotherapist would be. This kind of acumen is not properly taught to medical students, as noted previously (Bleakley 2021). He engaged a meta-attention, as gentle inquirer but also attentive doubter, that would test the quality of his consultation style in real time. This style embraces reflection-on-reflection, or reflection-in-action (Schön 1983), that has also been termed 'reflection-as-action, or 'critical reflexivity' (Bleakley 1999) (see Preface). With a previous patient, Falchuk had been fooled into believing that she had intestinal malabsorption problems when she was taking a laxative and cheating the doctor – part of a psychiatric disorder. Here, with Anne, careful attention to her words and non-verbal semiotics convinced him that she was telling the truth and was utterly distraught at that truth. Falchuk had said of the patient who faked symptoms that he had a hunch that 'the picture didn't fit' – an apt metaphor. With Anne, he deliberately suspended judgement until he had fully heard her account. His metacognitive strategy was in essence simple: 'attention to detail', preceded by 'stepping out of the frame' that was constituted by Anne's prior medical encounters. Here, the 'picture would fit'. The new frame was inspired.

Falchuk is an expert in gastrointestinal absorption and so his technical prowess already provides a context of meaning beyond information. The case study further shows a meta-sensibility beyond ordinary sensory awareness – as noted, Falchuck paid close attention to Anne's bodily expressions as she recounted her symptoms and treatment histories. As reported by Groopman, Falchuk moves beyond information to meaning. The latter was provided largely by the facilitative diagnostic *umwelt* created by Falchuk – a collaborative atmosphere that embraces ethical, aesthetic, political, and transcendental values. Ethical and political because Falchuk does not abuse his power, aesthetic because his sensibility is tuned for cues and clues while he forms the shape of the clinical encounter as an act of beauty based around a metaphor ('the picture fits'), and transcendental because meaning is generated. These values describe the shaping of a therapeutic relationship, where rhetoric and persuasion are subtle.

This is far from the instrumental or functional activity of medicine that is restricted to the formalities of physical examination and testing, where the semiotic encounter is compressed or reduced to informational content. As Umberto Eco (2003, 4) suggests: 'The perfection of function is one of the requirements of an art work', or, function (the instrumental) must be raised in quality and intensity ('perfection') to qualify as 'art'. I have argued that medicine must perfect function or raise its qualities in complex acts of translation-as-negotiation, the function of which is to enrich the text – in this case, the clinical encounter. Diagnosis is often referred to as constructing a story from a plot, but here, in the case of Anne and Falchuk, the story is suspended for intense concentration on the plot. The universal plot and primary metaphor of two people falling in love is here rehearsed in the clinic as meta-variations on that theme: a doctor falls in love again with his clinical passions, while a woman regains a love of herself in a kind of rebirth, a metamorphosis.

References

Allard, J., Wyatt, J., Bleakley, A., Graham, B. 2012. "Do you really need to ask me that now?": A self-audit of interruptions to the 'shop floor' practice of a UK consultant emergency physician. *Emergency Medicine Journal*, 29: 872–76.

Bhatt, J., Swick, M. 2017. Focusing on Teamwork and Communication to Improve Patient Safety. *American Hospital Association*. Mar 15. Available at: https://www.aha.org/news/blog/2017-03-15-focusing-teamwork-and-communication-improve-patientsafety#:~:text=Patient%20safety%20experts%20agree%20that%20communication%20and%20teamwork,medical%20errors%2C%20improve%20efficiency%20and%20increase%20patient%20satisfaction Last accessed: 25 Mar 2023

Bleakley, A. 1999. From Reflective Practice to Holistic Reflexivity. *Studies in Higher Education*, 24: 315–30.

Bleakley, A. 2020. *Educating Doctors' Senses Through the Medical Humanities: "How Do I Look?"* Abingdon: Routledge.

Bleakley, A. 2021. *Medical Education, Politics and Social Justice: The Contradiction Cure*. Abingdon: Routledge.

Bleakley, A. 2023. *Medical Humanities: Ethics, Aesthetics, Politics*. London: Routledge.

Bleakley, A., Neilson, S. 2021. *Poetry in the Clinic: Towards a Lyrical Medicine*. Abingdon: Routledge.

Bleakley, A., Neilson, S. 2022. As 'synapses' become 'protoplasmic kisses': Symmetry across clinical reasoning and poetry. *Medical Education*, 57: 233–42.

Bleakley, A., Neilson, S. (eds.) 2024. *Routledge Handbook of Medicine and Poetry*. Abingdon: Routledge.

Bours, M.J.L. 2021. Bayes' rule in diagnosis. *Journal of Clinical Epidemiology*, 131: 158–60.

Doulougeri, K., Panagopoulou, E., Montgomery, A. 2016. (How) do medical students regulate their emotions?. *BMC Medical Education*, 16: 312.

Eco, U. 2003. *Mouse or Rat? Translation as Negotiation*. London: Weidenfeld & Nicolson.

Eichbaum, Q. 2014. Thinking about Thinking and Emotion: The Metacognitive Approach to the Medical Humanities that Integrates the Humanities with the Basic and Clinical Sciences. *Permanente Journal*, 18: 64–75.

Eliot, T.S. 1934. Chorus from The Rock. In: Eliot, T.S. *Selected Poems*. London: Faber & Faber, 1954.

Groopman, J. 2007. *How Doctors Think*. New York, NY: Houghton Mifflin.

Haig, D. 2020. *From Darwin to Derrida: Selfish Genes, Social Selves and the Meanings of Life*. Cambridge, MA: MIT Press.

Heron, J. 1989. *Catharsis in Human Development*. Guilford: University of Surrey. Available at: https://co-counselling.info/en/ref/catharsis-human-development Last accessed: 25 Mar 2023

Johnson-Sabine, E.C., Mann, A.H., Jacoby, R.J., et al. 1983. Bouffée délirante: an examination of its current status. *Psychological Medicine*, 13: 771–78.

Kerasidou, A., Horn, R. 2016. Making space for empathy: supporting doctors in the emotional labour of clinical care. *BMC Medical Ethics*, **17**: 8.

Levine, D., Bleakley, A. 2012. Maximising medicine through aphorisms. *Medical Education*, 46: 153–62.

Marshall R, Bleakley A. 2017. *Rejuvenating Medical Education: Seeking Help from Homer*. Newcastle: Cambridge Scholars Publications.

Mobbs, N., Williams, C., Weeks, A.D. Humanising birth: Does the language we use matter? Available at: https://blogs.bmj.com/bmj/2018/02/08/humanising-birth-does-the-language-we-use-matter/ Last accessed: 25 Mar 2023

Nietzsche, F. 1908/2005. *Ecce Homo: How One Becomes What One Is*. London: Penguin Classics.

Papagiannis, A. 2017. Eliot's triad: information, knowledge, and wisdom in medicine. Available at: https://hekint.org/2017/01/29/eliots-triad-information-knowledge-and-wisdom-in-medicine/ Last accessed: 01 Apr 2023

Plato. 2020. *Menexenus*. Cambridge, Cambridge University Press.

Rajalakshmi, N. 2022. The curious reasons why dolphins play. Mashable Voices. July 9 2022. Available at: https://mashable.com/article/why-dolphins-play-animal-behavior Last accessed: 11 Apr 2023

Reed – Naming of Parts - https://www.poetrybyheart.org.uk/poems/naming-of-parts

Relman, A.S. 1988. Reporting the aspirin study: the Journal and the media. *New England Journal of Medicine*, 318: 918–20.

Schön, D.A.. 1983. *The Reflective Practitioner: How Professionals Think in Action*. New York, NY: Basic Books.

Shannon, C.E. 1948. A Mathematical Theory of Communication. *Bell System Technical Journal*, 27: 379–423.

Szczeklik, A. 2005. *Catharsis: On the Art of Medicine*. Chicago, IL: University of Chicago Press.

Taylor, H. 2017. Birdsong has inspired humans for centuries: is it music? *The Conversation*. July 25. Available at: https://theconversation.com/birdsong-has-inspired-humans-for-centuries-is-it-music-79000 Last accessed: 06 Dec 2023

Tomlinson, G. 2023. *The Machines of Evolution and the Scope of Meaning*. Princeton, NJ: Princeton University Press.

Warner, J.H., Edmonson, J.M. 2009. *Dissection: Photographs of a Rite of Passage in American Medicine: 1880–1930*. New York, NY: Blast Books.

Webb, J. 2021. *The Metacognition Handbook: A Practical Guide for Teachers and School Leaders*. Woodbridge: John Catt Educational Ltd.

4 Knowing more than we can say

The tacit dimension and the unconscious ego

Alan Bleakley

Knowing more than we can say

Mark Quirk's (2006) *Intuition and Metacognition in Medical Education: Keys to Developing Expertise* is a ground-breaking work, not the least for its bold use of 'intuition' front and centre in an academic text (grounded largely in psychological science), for 'intuition' may seem like a dirty word to many in medicine and healthcare brought up on a diet of rationality and evidence-based approaches. Quirk's text, however, affords standard fare for cognitive psychologists where 'intuition' is a by-word for what is more commonly known as tacit knowing. Thus, as doctors gain expertise, much of what they 'know' is stored in memory and re-activated through pattern recognition of symptoms. This is like calling riding a bike 'intuitive'. Rather, it is habitual. Habits are fine until novel situations are encountered (e.g., the first time your bike's chain slips off its cog) and then thinking itself must be re-adjusted consciously (putting the chain on a few times, until this becomes automatic).

A more sophisticated account of intuition is provided by Immanuel Kant's transcendental idealism, as 'sensible intuition' (Rowlands 2003). Kant (in ibid.) points to the contradiction that supposedly abstract categories such as space and time are concrete, sense-based human constructions: 'If the subject … be removed … space and time themselves would collapse'. Intuition is then the work of the senses in the absence of metacognition. It is metacognition that allows us to make sense of sensible intuition through synthesis of such intuitions that comprises the faculty, for Kant, of 'understanding'. I have referred to this throughout as 'insight', but also as 'meaning'. Importantly, it is not the person who intuits, but what Kant called 'pure intuition' is readymade or *a priori* (prior to and independent from experience). Time and space are then conditions of possibility for the acts of sensing and experiencing. The *a priori* filters – through which we experience time and space – are abstractions such as 'substance' and 'cause and effect'. What Kant's model does is to lift us out of solipsism or self-interest, the modern taxis of looking inward for explanations of phenomena (most obviously in reduction of experience to brain mechanisms). Rather, Kant *situates* us in a shared world of metaphors, a position described as 'externalism', confounding first-person authority (ibid.). We will

DOI: 10.4324/9781032687339-6

have much to say about a sister phenomenon to externalism – 'distributed' and 'extended' cognition, models that challenge personalism and individualism, or ownership of cognition and affect.

There is a long history of formal investigation of intuitive capacity that reaches back to Aristotle's (2004) description of *phronesis* (practical reasoning). In the context of medical education, *phronesis* has been mobilised as both an exploratory and an explanatory notion for clinical judgement by one of the founders of North American narrative medicine Kathryn Montgomery (Montgomery Hunter 1991, Montgomery 2006), as well as by physician and medical ethicist Hillel Braude (2012). Both authors point to the tension between the stern, rational, scientific approach to medicine represented by epidemiological evidence-based approaches (grounded in generalised population studies) and the ambiguities presented by the unique patient, where treatment is often based on a 'best fit' approach. This tension is described by James Hillman (1986) as the differing approaches of 'egalitarian typologies' and the 'perception of the unique'. While epidemiological evidence-based practice is widely advertised as the best approach to medicine, John Gabbay and Andrée le May (2010) propose that most physicians rely more on local, specific, and contextualised 'practice-based evidence' than generalised 'evidence-based practice'. This leads to individual clinicians forming 'mindlines' from extensive patient contact that is the first port of call in a diagnosis rather than standardised clinical guidelines. 'Practice-based evidence' is 'best fit' practical reasoning around a unique patient, the latter a generalisation from evidence usually translated into protocols.

Aristotle (2004) had prefigured such a distinction where he distinguished *nous* as conscious, rational reasoning based in mind, from *phronesis* as practical reasoning based in the senses. In Book VI of *Nicomachean Ethics*, Aristotle also distinguished between *phronesis* as practical activity with an end-in-itself (closed) and *poiesis* as aesthetic production, the exercise of imagination or the creative will as an end-other-than-itself (open-ended). While Aristotle, of course, never drove a car, we can see both *nous* and *phronesis* at work in driving. On a familiar road with little distraction, we tend to go into 'automatic' driving mode where things seem to look after themselves (*phronesis*), until some new stimulus snaps us back into an attentive and alert consciousness (*nous*).

Neuroscientists such as Antonio Damasio (1999) have suggested a distinction between an 'autobiographical self' at the conscious level and a 'core self' at the visceral level. The former uses both a rational (logical) and a common-sense (sensory-intuitive) reasoning that constructs identity in real time as a conscious figurative (foregrounded) experience. The latter 'core self' is an unconscious and pre-conscious process that acts as ground, or background, to a configured life. It is the active conversation between the two levels that constitutes practical wisdom. As Aristotle first suggested, *phronesis* is sense-based (embodied and affective), where *nous* is mind-based (rational). Practical wisdom is an emergent property of the nonlinear, complex system of bodily sensing and intuiting, open to contemplation and shaping by consciousness. It is *phronesis*, or practical wisdom, that can best describe an experienced doctor's clinical reasoning (Chiavaroli and Trumble 2018). Developing my arguments from previous chapters, I would suggest that *phronesis* or practical wisdom is shaped by embodied metaphors.

Of course, this distinction between visceral background and conscious foreground is crude, as we shall see. But, as a starting point, both philosophers and experimental cognitive psychologists have posited that moment-to-moment consciousness must be extended to embrace more than we can say or what is foregrounded (Polanyi 1966, Reber 1996, Reber and Allen 2022). The background must be acknowledged as nest or container for foregrounded consciousness, a necessary incubator of meaning. The unconscious nest is neither abstract nor flimsy, but rather provides the muscle for the mind. Indeed, Sigmund Freud had promoted such robustness to unconscious life over a century ago and prefigured the mantra of postmodern cognitive psychology introduced by the philosopher Michael Polanyi (1966) that 'we know more than we can say'.

The philosopher Jacques Derrida (1974) describes this as every phenomenon carrying a 'surplus of signification', effectively an absent present, that is both intangible and unreachable. Kant had described this as unknowable yet posited *noumena* as opposed to knowable and sensed *phenomena*. Derrida brings the noumenon to earth as the ghost or shadow phenomenon, where a person's experiences are more than they can ever say. This is one of the fundamental values of writing poetry that it allows us to attempt to say the unsayable. Such surplus value can be described as 'transcendental'. Poetry might therefore be understood as the 'surplus' to science, particularly where the latter claims full explanation of a given phenomenon. Poets often describe the experience of the poem writing them and of the product as appearing strange or unfamiliar.

Expanding this line of thought concerning unaccountable surplus: what does it mean to claim that 'we know more than we can say' (Polanyi 1966)? This has been described as 'the paradox of tacit knowledge' (Dixon 2013). Michael Polanyi suggested that there are many things we do intuitively without being able to articulate the rules or procedures by which they operate, beyond automaticity or habit (such as driving a car or riding a cycle). The most obvious example is cognition or thinking itself and its articulation through language. Another is facial and voice recognition, capabilities that are key to human communication and sociability. Experimental cognitive psychologists have shown that rules can be acquired concerning, for example, the acquisition of a simple, previously unknown, rule-regulated 'language' as a cognitive strategy (Reber 1996).

Such rules can be applied in problem-solving without conscious knowledge of their structures or meanings. Here, these rules remain tacit or unconscious – or cannot be explicated – thereby serving as an 'implicate order' (Bohm 1980). Further, such rules govern behaviour that can be observed and measured even as these rules again cannot be consciously articulated. This phenomenon has been described as the exercise of a 'cognitive unconscious' by JF Kihlstrom (1987) and Arthur Reber and colleagues (Reber and Allen 2022), who described this as the acquisition of 'tacit knowledge' through 'implicit learning'. In the following section, I provide an illustrative clinical example of tacit knowing at work, where the shift from explicit to tacit knowing is marked by a change in language registers – from the plain descriptive to the more complex embodied metaphorical (Lakoff and Johnson 1999).

A nurse's intuition

Before birth, the foetus's blood gets oxygenated without going to the lungs thanks to the ductus arteriosus, a hole in the aorta, the body's main artery. In a full-term birth, the baby's blood is oxygenated in the lungs and the ductus closes. Where the ductus arteriosus is still open ('patent'), the blood will not circulate properly via the lungs. In premature births, this failure of the ductus to close is common but needs to be closely monitored.

An experienced neonatal nurse (in a North American context) reports her concerns about a premature baby in a critical situation:

> I took care of a 900-gram baby who was about 26 or 27 weeks ... who had been doing well for about two weeks. He had an open ductus that day. The difference between the way he looked at 9 a.m. and the way he looked at 11 a.m. was very dramatic. I was at that point really concerned about what was going to happen next. There are a lot of complications of the patent ductus, not just in itself, but the fact that it causes a lot of other things. I was really concerned that the baby was starting to show symptoms of all of them.
>
> (Dixon 2013)

In explaining these symptoms, the nurse says:

> The fact that the kid is more lethargic, paler, his stomach is bigger, that he is not tolerating his feedings, that his chem strip (blood test) might be a little strange. All these kinds of things ... there are clusters of things that go wrong. The baby's urine output goes down. They sound like they are in failure. This kind of stuff. Their pulses go bad, their blood pressure changes. There are a million things that go on.
>
> (Dixon 2013)

Significantly, the nurse was able to diagnose the baby's changing condition, but was unable to convince the physicians she spoke to that this was an urgent issue:

> You look at this kid because you know this kid, and you know what he looked like two hours ago. It is a dramatic difference to you, but it's hard to describe that to someone in words. You go to the resident and say: "Look, I'm really worried about X, Y, Z," and they go: "OK." Then you wait one half hour to 40 minutes, then you go to the Fellow (the teaching physician supervising the resident) and say: "You know, I am really worried about X, Y, Z." They say: "We'll talk about it on rounds."

> I talked to a nurse who had more experience and I said, "Look at this kid," and I told her my story, and she goes: "OK." Rounds started shortly after that and she walks up to the Attending [Physician in charge of patient] very quietly, sidles up and says: "You know, this kid, Jane is really worried about this kid." She told him the story, and said: "He reminds me about this kid, Jimmie, we had three weeks ago," and he said: "Oh." Everything stops. He gets out the stethoscope and listens to the kid, examines the kid and he says: "Call the surgeons".
>
> (Dixon 2013)

Suddenly there was recognition by the doctor of the urgency of the situation. Here is a refrain of the nurse's diagnosis:

> The fact that the kid is more lethargic, paler, his stomach is bigger, that he is not tolerating his feedings, that his chem strip (blood test) might be **a little strange**. All **these kinds of things** … there are **clusters of things** that go wrong. The baby's urine output goes down. They sound like they are **in failure**. **This kind of stuff**. Their **pulses go bad**, their blood pressure changes. There are **a million things that go on**.

The nurse moves between two linguistic registers: the literal and the metaphorical/hyperbolic (I have **highlighted** the latter complex register). As somebody with growing expertise in her field, the nurse was able to tick off some clinical warning signs that she describes in a mechanical or instrumental register, where the baby is reduced to symptom, and 'in-house' clinical jargon is used (such as 'tolerating his feedings', 'blood test' or 'chem strip', and 'urine output'). This literal register includes affectless, descriptive comments such *as* 'a 900-gram baby who was about 26 or 27 weeks'; 'he had an open ductus that day'; 'the kid is more lethargic, paler, his stomach is bigger … he is not tolerating his feedings'; and '[T]heir pulses go bad, their blood pressure changes'.

In contrast, there is a shift in language register from the literal to the embodied metaphorical, reflecting the nurse's deepening concerns:

- The blood test is 'a little strange' – blood tests are accurate and shown as quantitative data; here the nurse turns that into quality and intensity
- 'All these kinds of things' the phrase refers (presumably) to parallel test results, and this multiplies into the more amorphous 'clusters of things'
- 'This kind of stuff' – the biochemical certainties (test results) again become diffuse as they are enlarged or brought to the fore
- 'Pulses go bad' – clinical jargon is dropped for the vernacular, to emphasise the point
- 'A million things that go on' – now the emphasis becomes purposeful exaggeration or hyperbole, as a means of persuasion

In short, the acute shift in the baby's condition brings a parallel shift in register of language to capture what was going on in the nurse's consciousness – her cognition and feelings. She moves from descriptive to reflective mode that requires a different kind of language: as noted, a more metaphor-driven description as the baby looks worse ('You look at this kid because you know this kid, and you know what he looked like two hours ago. It is a dramatic difference to you, but it's hard to describe that to someone in words'). Her narrative offers a climax, where the doctor suddenly recognises the urgency of the situation after the second nurse has cleverly gained his attention: 'Everything stops. He gets out the stethoscope and listens to the kid, examines the kid and he says: "Call the surgeons"'. The nurse is in meta-mode, now cultivating reflection-as-action, or a critical reflexivity in praxis.

I would argue that the first nurse knew more than she could say – as if her fears for the child's well-being outstripped her specific clinical knowledge and experience, powered by an upsurge of affect. As noted at the opening of this chapter, we often call knowing more than we can say 'intuition', but this word has metaphysical overtones, and here the nurse follows her senses, in close noticing (the basis to a poetic imagination). We might say that the phenomenon and the noumenon greet each other. In terms of value shifts introduced in the previous two chapters, her clinical practice has shifted from the instrumental to embrace the transcendental. She *knew* the child was in crisis. Her attentional and observational skills had flipped the switch and now intuition or tacit knowing too had kicked in, a marked contrast to the apparent inertia of the attending doctors. She becomes super-sensitive, poetically tuned.

Our capabilities go beyond the supposed limits of our technical knowledge as a surplus of consciousness, drawing on a 'cognitive unconscious' as noted above. This is expressed in a shift from the controlled and controlling, precise, quantitative-like language of the present-known, to the qualitative territory of the future-unknown. Here, our capability seems to expand, and as the limits of technical competence are outstripped, so qualitative and metaphoric descriptors kick in, complexity is recognised, and complexity's inherent ambiguity is tolerated. Such thinking embodies recognition of the limit to closed and linear thinking, as open, nonlinear, complex, dynamic, adaptive systems thinking is adopted. The nurse provides a stable attractor in a complex system at the edge of chaos, preventing collapse into such chaos. Intuition informs the senses as a metacognition and meta-affect: described by Aristotle as the upgrading of *nous* (rational reasoning) to *phronesis* (practical reasoning with an end-in-itself), supplemented by *poiesis* (aesthetic production – or high-grade sensibility).

The use of 'intuition', particularly by professionals, can attract criticism. Carl Jung (1921) saw intuition as a valuable yet neglected asset where he discussed personality typologies (sensing, feeling, thinking, and intuitive types), but also larded intuition with mystical qualities (Pilard 2018). As an alternative term to intuition, we might consider 'meaning' as discussed in previous chapters. This, as noted in previous chapters, is based on the poet T.S. Eliot's (1934) distinction between information, knowledge, and wisdom (as 'meaning') in his 'Choruses from The Rock'. As we tacitly recognise complexity, so we shift away from the (albeit necessary, but restrictive) world of information (technical jargon and informing biomedical fact and measure) to a world of meaning (metaphor production, qualities, and intensities). Indeed, I would argue that we confront our unknown futures armed with embodied metaphor production as our primary way of sense-making.

Tacit knowing is not limited to long-term memory feeding into current thinking, but rather it involves the seemingly paradoxical notion that current thinking is informed by 'predictive processing' (Clark 2016, 2023), which is a common theme throughout this book. Here-and-now millisecond decisions are part of the loop that connects memory with prediction – an ecological awareness of what is about to happen in the immediate environment. In Andy Clark's (2016, 2023) account of this loop of consciousness, we 'surf uncertainty' in which we appear to be always just ahead of the breaking wave or living in the future-unknown on the basis that we can rapidly adapt from what we have gleaned in the known present. A split-second feedback loop is set up between prediction, forms of attention (see Chapter 7) appropriate to context, and memory that shapes activity *from the leading edge*. Effectively, intuition in another guise. As Clark explains, we live our lives in the microseconds of the near future rather than the null point of the here-and-now. What we call 'anticipation' is in fact a biological lifestyle for humans, as an evolutionary gain.

Leonard and Swap (2005), in a context of future-unknown thinking in business and management, suggest that once we have entered the territory of engaging meaning from the previous stance of working with information, we strive to continually re-create such meaning. Information-bound worlds come to irritate us because they fail to stimulate innovation, or metaphor production. Such innovation is 're-creation' – looking at the familiar from new perspectives – a form of adult play (or recreation). The psychoanalyst Donald Winnicott (1971) suggested that we are often stuck in chronic neurotic patterns of behaviour, such as fear of failure and the wish for control (typical traits of medical students), from unresolved childhood issues. Rather than replaying those childhood scenarios, as other Freudians might, Winnicott's suggestion is for the adult to engage in activities that resemble collaborative play, where chronic patterns of control might be challenged, and more democratic habits can be learned. In medical and healthcare education, this is achieved through involvement in participatory and collaborative activities such as Schwartz Rounds and the more therapeutic Balint Groups.

For a practitioner, the gaining of such meta-knowledge as the development of tacit knowing is dependent upon the relinquishing of control in the consultation such that the patient's perspective is fully inhabited. The symptom, issue, or problem experienced by the patient must be experienced by the practitioner in terms set by the patient. This means inhabiting the embodied metaphorical world of the patient as he or she explores the reason for visiting the doctor. The conversation, of course, happens at both an explicit and a tacit level. This Othering of our selves is best termed 'compathy', moving beyond sympathy and empathy to identification with – or indwelling – another's condition (see Chapter 12).

Tacit knowing and psychoanalytic strategies

What the neonatal nurse does in the earlier illustrative example, in tracking the condition of the premature baby, is to enact a psychoanalysis of context. She reads below the surface in tacit knowing, as a meta-strategy, just as a psychoanalyst reads into a client's talk, or a social situation, to shape an interpretation. As I have argued throughout this chapter, such a 'knowing more than we can say' is inherent to any kind of expert practice. Ask experts how they make decisions and how they improve their expertise, and they will probably be unable to explicate what has become implicate as tacit knowing. Making implicate order explicit is a mark of the 'meta': thinking-about-thinking at its most complex and creative. Such eversion of tacit knowing for examination is of course the central expertise of psychoanalysis and psychoanalytic psychotherapies, where the unconscious is made conscious, or available for translation through the register of 'analysis'. The language of analysis, in turn, is densely metaphoric. Indeed, I would argue it is poetic. We should remember that Freud, despite being nominated several times, failed to win a Nobel Prize for science. He did, however, win the 1930 Goethe Prize for Literature. This was, ostensibly, for the 'clarity' of his writing. But 'clarity' here conceals more than it reveals. The prize was awarded for style that includes elegant use of metaphor and innovation of psychological terms – such as 'defence mechanisms of the ego' – that 'work' because they are metaphorical, registering more complex, intense meanings that wrestle with the unknown.

One might expect that 'clarity' equates with opacity and the literal, but Freud disagreed. Again, his style is elegantly metaphorical: in *The Ego and the Id*, Freud (1962) describes patients 'clinging to the gain from illness' who paradoxically self-punish just as the analyst believes such patients are improving or making breakthroughs. In *Civilization and Its Discontents*, Freud (1939) describes falling in love as 'pathological', where '[A]t its height, the state of being in love threatens to obliterate the boundaries between ego and object', while, drawing on an aphorism by Schiller, 'hunger and love make the world go round' (1939). In *New Introductory Lectures on Psychoanalysis*, Freud (1957) describes the 'therapeutic efforts of psychoanalysis' as 'to strengthen the ego, to make it more independent of the super-ego, to widen its field of vision, and to extend its organization'. So 'where id was, there shall ego be' (one of Freud's most memorable phrases). Indeed, the whole work is one of sophisticated play on metaphor. As Freud (1957) says: 'It is reclamation work, like the draining of the ZuyderZee'. The impulsive id has drowned the reflective ego, and some 'free attention' must be reclaimed (as meta-affect) to gain insight into episodes of catharsis lest we drown in, or are overwhelmed by, our feeling states. It is a kind of detox, or purification. Is not all medical work one of such 'reclamation' as purification – the draining of pus, the draining of anxiety through anxiolytic medication, the draining of a bacterial infection through an antibiotic, the draining of pain and fever from a viral infection through painkillers and time, and the draining of pain through surgery? And, at the end of the day, the doctor too may be drained, heading for burnout – not just from overwork but also from lack of sophisticated insight through self-regulation, or meta-attention (see Chapter 7).

The notion of an 'unconscious' mind at work paralleling and shaping consciousness has a long history, which led to the widespread use of hypnosis as a therapeutic tool – from the German physician Franz Anton Mesmer (1734–1857) to the French neurologist and psychiatrist Jean Martin Charcot (1825–1893). Freud attended Charcot's clinical demonstrations of 'cure' through hypnotic trance of the so-called hysterics. Rejecting hypnosis, Freud developed psychoanalytic technique as a 'talking cure', essentially the elaboration of metaphor for therapeutic purposes. While Freud's techniques remain the cornerstone of conventional psychoanalysis, the notion of the unconscious as shaping conscious life (through imagination, dreams, and parapraxes such as slips of the tongue) has been developed in cognitive psychology as the work of a 'cognitive unconscious' as described earlier.

I see the 'meta' (or meaning) as being engaged in both medical education and clinical practice, beyond mere information-led instrumentalism, through metaphor production, tolerance of ambiguity, and related acceptance of complexity. All medical students must learn to engage consciously with the world of tacit knowing, presenting a pedagogical challenge. This can be done through gaining practical knowledge of the most basic of psychoanalytic working techniques – first, the vocabulary of transference in the clinical encounter; and second, through working knowledge of defence mechanisms of the ego. As an example of the first, it is common for doctors who have regular contact with some patients – such as general practitioners – to form a professional relationship with such patients. This can morph into a dependency on the part of the patient, where a transference effect is at play – the patient identifying with the empathy offered by the doctor primarily because such warmth was never offered by that patient's father or mother. In terms of defence mechanisms, an example is that patients can show non-compliance with taking pharmaceuticals that the doctor thinks are crucial to treatment. The non-compliance is not simply forgetfulness, but an active resistance to an authority figure.

Medical education has long failed to offer an adequate psychotherapeutic education (Bleakley 2021), despite medicine being the psychotherapeutic application of biomedical knowledge. Consultation and communication 'skills' are usually embedded in wider clinical skills and taught in formulaic ways. How a therapeutic alliance is built with patients is left largely to observation and then supervised practice on clinical placements, without learning the fundamentals of the dynamics of transference and resistance, and the defence mechanisms of the ego. Again, 'transference' describes the movement of positive or negative feelings that the patient or client has for another onto the figure of the doctor or therapist as a temporary 'stand in'. It is then the doctor's or therapist's task to help the patient or client to recover ownership of such transferred feelings and to gain insight into their meanings, possibly to resolve them. Other than psychiatrists, doctors are unlikely to worry overly about transference effects, especially if consultations are minimal or one-offs. However, with longer-term patients (e.g., in primary care), such transference effects are likely to be of greater significance.

In turn, the doctor or therapist may harbour positive or negative feelings towards the patient or client that will remain unresolved. For example, the patient reminds the doctor of a man who sexually abused her as a child; the doctor is sexually attracted to the patient and cannot shake this off through ethical 'professionalism'; unconscious bias is shown on the doctor's behalf, where, as a white person he treats black or Asian people differently from others but fails to recognise this neo-colonialism or imperialist tendency in his behaviour. This is 'countertransference' of affect.

As well as positive and negative transference and countertransference effects, resistance is a common psychodynamic element in therapeutic encounters. As noted above, the patient or client is resistant to suggestions (such as pharmaceutical prescriptions or lifestyle changes), or insights the doctor or therapist may offer. But this is irrational, based not on the quality of the suggestions or insights, but on the basis that they trigger, for example, long-supressed feelings of anger towards the patient's father, subsequently projected onto father-figures or those in authority. In turn, the doctor or therapist may, unconsciously, resist suggestions made by the patient or client about, for example, consulting style.

'Transference' and 'resistance' are tangible effects seen in behaviour shaped by values and affect, but they are also embodied metaphors. Nobody has seen an unconscious element transferred onto another, but we do see the embodied effects or outcomes of the dynamic exchange. Analysis of such dynamic is then a shaping of understanding of how a therapeutic alliance may be achieved between practitioner and patient as a metaphorical activity. We see this in the earlier example of the neonatal nurse who shifted gear from specific functional or instrumental clinical description to more complex but less specific metaphorical talk to describe the quality and intensity of her clinical judgement about a critically ill baby.

Psychoanalytic language abounds in embodied metaphors where it describes the tacit dimension to mind and body, a thinking and feeling underbelly to consciousness, or an implicate order (Bohm 1980). Given that our egos (senses of self) are fragile and easily bruised, we develop patterns of defences to prevent psychological injury, which I would liken to a myelin sheath protecting a nerve. However, such defences can be overdeveloped, and consequently we fail to gain reflexive insight into their dynamics to adjust ourselves in critical social contexts – intimacy and sexual relations, bringing up children, mixing with people who have differing values or ideologies, and professional encounters such as the clinical exchange.

Defence mechanisms, as embodied metaphors, cannot be seen, but their effects are felt. They include

- Projection and stereotyping ('the accident wasn't my fault – you know that women are notoriously bad drivers')
- Denial ('I never make mistakes')
- Sublimation (staying busy to hide fear of failure)
- Repression ('I don't remember doing that at all')
- Displacement (a simmering anger is expressed through driving erratically)
- Regression ('I just want to be comforted')
- Rationalisation ('I did it because it needed to be done')

If such defence mechanisms, again protecting fragile egos, are embodied metaphors in action, then it seems futile to disembody and literalise (or de-metaphorise) medical encounters through use of technical language. This drains medicine of its inherent poetics necessary to clinical judgement (Bleakley and Neilson 2022, 2024). Examples of systematic reduction of metaphor to the instrumental have been noted in previous chapters, to include 'synapses', originally called 'protoplasmic kisses' by Ramón y Cajal (1852–1934). Cajal describes transmission between one axon and its dendrites and another, across the synaptic gap, as 'protoplasmic kisses that appear to constitute the final ecstasy of an epic love story'. As noted previously, the derivation of synapse is from the ancient Greek *sunapsis*, meaning 'joining together' – a literal description. Regression to the literal drains the metaphor of its expression and potential. Of course, the synaptic leap of an electro-chemical transmission is not a literal 'kiss', but of course it is. This way we keep beauty in physiology and biochemistry. The leap from a mechanical, technical understanding of biomedicine to an aesthetic appreciation preceding explanation is a meta-move.

In suggesting that medical students should learn basic psychotherapeutic strategies and accompanying language, I am promoting the value of an education into the language of complexity through embodied metaphor use, fit for purpose in clinical encounters. This raises the value of practice from the instrumental to embrace other values: a practice of quality and intensity (Bleakley 2023a, 2023b). Such a meta-education formally engages the tacit dimension, so that 'we know more than we can say' is unpacked for inspection. What is the 'more'? This engagement with embodied metaphor has immediate practical value, as suggested above, such as uncovering unconscious bias. Indeed, what such an education points to is bias against the unconscious in current, frankly pedestrian, medical pedagogy.

As a rider to this section, consider that psychoanalytic approaches may be unconscious of their own biases. The most important of these is the assumption that where the ego embraces consciousness, this is ethically good as it overrides the potential of errant, affect-laden decisions. However, the ego can be seen as the most unconscious aspect of our psychological life (Hillman 1975). This is patently obvious where the ego shines strongest, for instance in masculinised heroism and narcissism. And medicine has, historically, attracted heroic types and cultivated their narcissism. This, thankfully, seems to be changing with the demographic shift towards women outnumbering men in medicine. Indeed, historically, as a largely all-male, white, and privileged environment, medicine's blind spot has been its own heroic individualism and narcissism, refusing the values of collaboration or democratic habits. The 'meta' question here has been: how shall medicine transcend its own ego, blind to its historically accumulated habits?

These habits have been touched on here and are described at length elsewhere (Bleakley 2021, 2023a). They include

- Resistance to democratic habits as investment in hierarchy, making it difficult to engage with authentic inter-professional teamwork
- Resistance to complexity and problem-stating as investment in linear, closed, problem-solving
- A miseducation into insensibility in a culture that requires deep and intensive use of the senses. This begins with learning anatomy through dissection and continues with emotional insulation, loss of empathy, and increase in cynicism
- Intolerance of ambiguity and uncertainty
- Systematic stripping away of metaphor use for the literal and mechanical, dulling ethical, aesthetic, political, and transcendental appreciation and activity
- Fear of failure
- Lack of self-care

As much as we know more than we can say and we can enjoy the fruits of tacit knowledge, we also know that these fruits are, at the same time, both delicious and poisoned. Tacit knowing is not some mechanical device or instrumental pursuit that we can just turn on and off at will. Rather, such knowing and feeling is values-laden, stacked with ethical dilemmas, aesthetic possibilities, political (power) implications, and transcendental promises (the openings to meanings and mysteries).

References

Aristotle. 2004. *The Nicomachean Ethics*. Harmondsworth: Penguin.

Bleakley A. 2021. *Medical Education, Politics and Social Justice: The Contradiction Cure*. Abingdon: Routledge.

Bleakley A. 2023a. *Medical Humanities: Ethics, Aesthetics, Politics*. London: Routledge.

Bleakley A. 2023b. A therapeutic intervention for an ailing medical education: The values prism model as proof of concept. *Medical Teacher* 46: 232–8.

Bleakley A, Neilson S. 2022. *Poetry in the Clinic: Towards a Lyrical Medicine*. Abingdon: Routledge.

Bleakley A, Neilson S (eds.). 2024. *The Routledge Handbook of Medicine and Poetry*. Abingdon: Routledge.

Bohm D. 1980. *Wholeness and the Implicate Order*. London: Routledge.
Braude H. 2012. *Intuition in Medicine: A Philosophical Defence of Clinical Reasoning*. Chicago, IL: University of Chicago Press.
Chiavaroli N, Trumble S. 2018. When I say … phronesis. *Medical Education*. 52: 1005–7.
Clark A. 2016. *Surfing Uncertainty: Prediction, Action, and the Embodied Mind*. Oxford: Oxford University Press.
Clark A. 2023. *The Experience Machine: How Our Minds Predict and Shape Reality*. Harmondsworth: Penguin/Allen Lane.
Damasio A. 1999. *The Feeling of What Happens: Body, Emotion and the Making of Consciousness*. London: Heinemann.
Derrida J. 1974. *Of Grammatology*. Baltimore, MD: John Hopkins University Press.
Dixon N. 2013. We Know More Than We Can Say: The Paradox of Tacit Knowledge – Part One. *Conversation Matters*. Aug 11 2013. Available at: https://www.nancydixonblog.com/2013/08/we-know-more-than-we-can-say-the-paradox-of-tacit-knowledge-part-ne.html#:~:text=%E2%80%9Cwe%20know%20more%20than%20we%20can%20say%E2%80%9D%20is,knowledge%2C%20rather%20than%20exclusively%20focusing%20on%20explicit%20knowledge. Last accessed: 11/05/2023. Part II: We Know More Than We Can Say: How to Use Tacit Knowledge. Oct 05 2013. Available at: https://www.nancydixonblog.com/2013/10/part-ii-we-know-more-than-we-can-say-how-to-use-tacit-knowledge.html. Last accessed 11/05/2023
Eliot TS. 1934. Chorus from *The Rock*. In: Eliot TS (ed.). *Selected Poems*. London: Faber & Faber, 1954. Available at: https://www.poetrynook.com/poem/choruses-ôç£the-rockôçø. Last accessed: 13/01/2024.
Freud S. 1939. *Civilization and its Discontents*. London: The Hogarth Press.
Freud S. 1957. *New Introductory Lectures on Psychoanalysis*. London: The Hogarth Press.
Freud S. 1962. *The Ego and the Id*. London: The Hogarth Press.
Gabbay J, le May A. 2010. *Practice-based Evidence for Healthcare: Clinical Mindlines*. London: Routledge.
Hillman J. 1975. *Re-Visioning Psychology*. New York, NY: Harper Collins.
Hillman J. 1986. *Egalitarian Typologies versus the Perception of the Unique*. Dallas, TX: Spring Publications.
Jung C. 1921. *Psychological Types*. Zurich: Raschler Verlag.
Kihlstrom JF. 1987. The cognitive unconscious. *Science* 237: 1445–52.
Lakoff G, Johnson M. 1999. *Philosophy in the Flesh: The Embodied Mind and its Challenge to Western Thought*. New York, NY: Basic Books.
Leonard D, Swap WC. 2005. *Deep Smarts: How to Cultivate and Transfer Enduring Business Wisdom*. Boston: Harvard Business Review Press.
Montgomery HK. 1991. *Doctors' Stories: The Narrative Structure of Medical Knowledge*. Princeton, NJ: Princeton University Press.
Montgomery K. 2006. *How Doctors Think: Clinical Judgment and the Practice of Medicine*. Oxford: Oxford University Press.
Pilard NCG. 2018. Jung and intuition: From the mindscape of the paranormal to the heart of psychology. *Journal of Analytical Psychology* 63: 65–84.
Polanyi M. 1966. *The Tacit Dimension*. Chicago, IL: University of Chicago Press.
Quirk M. 2006. *Intuition and Metacognition in Medical Education: Keys to Developing Expertise*. Dordrecht: Springer.
Reber A. 1996. *The Cognitive Unconscious*. Oxford: Oxford University Press.
Reber AS, Allen R (eds.) 2022. *The Cognitive Unconscious: The First Half Century*. Oxford: Oxford University Press.
Rowlands M. 2003. *Externalism: Putting Mind and World Back Together Again*. Chesham: Acumen.
Winnicott D. 1971. *Playing and Reality*. London: Tavistock Publications.

5 Thinking outside the brain

The extended mind and metahumanities

Quentin Eichbaum

Introduction

As a medical student in anatomy, and later as an academic pathologist, I have been awestruck when holding in my hand a human brain plucked from a skull and weighing but three pounds, to ponder the immensity of human thought, emotion, and endeavour that this clod of tissue once generated. The contradictory gap between its raw state and its ineffable humanistic capacities, the trillions of neurons and synaptic connections gone quiet in the darkness: how could this soft mass generate such complexity and humanistic warmth? Adding to this puzzle is my own brain pondering the brain of another, thinking outside of the brain that I hold. Metaphorically, I am Hamlet pondering Yorick's skull and musing on death. Is this not the ultimate meta-moment?

As a faculty member at Vanderbilt University School of Medicine, I later developed a medical humanities course that aimed to bridge the gulf between sciences and humanities using an approach based largely on metacognition (see Chapter 1). In this course, we considered the brain as the starting point or 'ground zero' for students' navigations of the medical world. Unless they could understand how the brain 'worked' and how it related to the world (and other brains), medical students would be unable to truly grasp essential qualities of the art of medicine (discussed in this course) such as empathy, perception, medical error, attention, cognitive bias, decision-making, and change. By committing to 'develop flexible thinkers and agile learners with the mindful capacity for cognitive and emotional monitoring and regulation', we were moreover able to justify this humanities course to the deans. We argued that 'cognitive flexibility and emotional agility' were attributes students needed to navigate the complexities of medical knowledge, the stresses of clinical work, and their own fluctuations in well-being to inoculate against potential burn-out.

While the course initially focused on metacognition in the individual mind, it became apparent that it also needed to encompass group or shared metacognition (Eichbaum 2014). Later, I came to see how cognition extends beyond mind, skin, and skull into the environment, an idea described by Andy Clark as the 'extended mind' that *thinks outside the brain* (Clark 2017, Paul 2021). In medical education, the extended mind has been discussed particularly in terms

DOI: 10.4324/9781032687339-7

of collaborative learning (Bleakley 2006), distributed clinical reasoning (Bleakley 2021), cyborg challenges to identity (Ellaway 2010), and relational empathy (Eichbaum et al. 2023).

In this chapter, I discuss cognition that goes beyond the individual mind to the group, as *shared*, and extends into the environment – as *situated, embodied*, and *distributed* cognition; and beyond that to the *extended mind* of 'active externalism', or dynamic, self-changing, participatory cognition. Throughout, I will show how *metahumanities* can be characterised as an integrated knowledge of the extended mind. Just as persons have intentionality (motive, desire, goals) so they have extentionality (persons situated in a web of other minds, of artefacts and of environmental affordances). A metahumanities perspective, as we posited in Chapter 1, implores us to 'explore alternatives that may be more accessible to those for whom traditional humanities are ineffective and counterproductive'.

In this chapter, I will further argue for metahumanities that (1) go beyond the ego-centric boundaries of skin and skull towards eco-centric spaces of environments with their artefacts, technologies, and natural and fabricated spaces; (2) are not siloed but integrate themselves with the sciences and other disciplines; (3) interweave the complexities of head (cognition), heart (emotion), and gut (intuition); and (4) go beyond just the shared and interactional towards the relational and *participatory* (from passivity to activity). More specifically, I explore group metacognition and shared/team cognition before considering situated, embodied, and distributed cognition as the trajectory towards the extended mind.

Group/shared metacognition

As noted, when I first developed a metacognitive approach to the medical humanities with Vanderbilt medical students, my focus was on individual metacognition. However, it became apparent from colloquium/group discussions (that took place in the 'communities of inquiry' in each college after my introductory talk) that a higher level of *shared* metacognition was at play in these groups (Eichbaum 2014). This was evident from student feedback showing how much they valued hearing one another's viewpoints, how significantly it impacted their own thinking, and how it convinced them to recalibrate their thinking and regulate their emotions. By now, medical education learning theory had undergone a transformation – shifting emphasis from an individual's thinking and feeling (cognitivism) to shared or collaborative learning essential to high levels of team functioning (brought to a high level of theoretical sophistication in Communities of Practice models, Actor Network Theory (ANT), and Cultural-Historical Activity Theory) (Bleakley 2006).

Metacognition consists of two components: *knowledge* and *regulation* (Schraw and Moshman 1995). *Knowledge* of cognition refers to the information and awareness that people have of their own thinking processes; where *regulation* refers to the resources needed to control the learning processes. Biasutti and Frate (2018) define group metacognition as 'the ability to reflect on the cognitive skills of the group during collaborative activities'. They further insist that 'metacognition should also be considered in a group dimension rather than only as a reflection on individual behavior, and it should be a relevant construct for understanding online collaborative processes'. The authors thus introduce artefact (computers) into extended cognition.

In considering group metacognition and its role in collaborative practice, Garrison and Akyol (2015) pose the question: 'how do we construct meaning and share understanding in a collaborative learning environment?'. They argue that the *self*-regulatory component of metacognition is insufficient and that *shared* metacognition and *co*-regulation are essential for collaborative activity: 'Simple connectivity is no guarantee of thoughtful collaboration. Metacognition is no longer simply a self-regulated activity and, therefore, must consider issues of shared metacognition and co-regulation'. Moreover, 'Collaborative learning environments must go beyond interaction with content and include interaction with others' (see also Cho and Joon 2013). So, an extended mind embodies both other fleshly minds and a range of artefacts. In expanding minds in this manner, it is imperative that values are also expanded from the purely instrumental or functional to address issues such as how expanded learning is designed (quality and aesthetic) and regulated (e.g., AI autonomy), and how power issues play out (politics) (see other chapters in this book).

Group metacognition is a first-level extension away from individualist brain-bound cognition towards the extended mind (Clark 1998, 2017; Clark and Chalmers 1998) as self-regulation morphs into co-regulation. In collaborative inquiry, participants naturally move from personal cognition and affect to metacognition and meta-affect. Such co-regulation occurs not only at the level of brain cognition but also as part of embodied cognition. Neuroscientist Lisa Feldman Barrett (2017) suggests that such coregulation is closely linked with embodied cognition (see below).

Shared and team cognition

A by-product of North American 'frontier' mentality that has led subsequently to cultures of 'self-help' is heroic individualism. Individuals think for themselves and retain knowledge as personal capital and act autonomously being responsible for those actions. In contrast, after the Soviet Revolution in 1917, Russian psychologists such as Lev Vygotsky developed models of collaborative learning and responsibility. Models of learning and attainment in the West have largely followed a model of individualism, but more recently have absorbed community and extended learning models. These have been reinforced by interest in how shared artefacts external to persons, most obviously computers, augment learning. Individualism was largely shaped by North American behaviourist and cognitive psychologists, where psychology was commonly defined as the study of the unique individual centred on personality.

Sociologists, however, studied groups and the concept of a 'group mind' was proposed in the 1930s by the father of modern sociology Émile Durkheim (1938).

Group mind was said to be comprised of mental states shared by a group but based on individual members' thoughts, perceptions, beliefs, and expectations while adding up to more than just the sum of their individual mental states. The concept regained traction decades later in the 1990s in fields such as organisational behaviour with the notion of team mental models as a path to enhancing team performance (Converse et al. 1993). Differing models of 'shared cognition' have emerged. Where Larson and Christensen (1993) define social cognition as the 'social processes that relate to the acquisition, storage, transmission, manipulation, and use of information for the purpose of creating a group level intellectual product', others view social cognition as going beyond information sharing to include sharing of beliefs, assertions, and emotions (Floyd and Wooldridge 1992, Innami 1992) – a view of relevance to humanities with its central interest in values.

More recently, and pertinent to the humanities, a cultural brain hypothesis views the dramatic evolutionary increase in human brain size and intelligence as driven by sharing of both cultural tools and ways of thinking. Here, 'our collective brains involve not just what we might normally think of as the elements of culture – tools, techniques, approaches, recipes, beliefs, and values but also how we think and what we think about ... new ways of thinking' (Henrich and Muthukrishna 2023). This view embraces thinking-about-thinking, or metacognition, extending beyond the individual to the collective.

What, then, is the relationship between shared cognition and group metacognition (a group thinking about how it thinks collectively)? If it is just passive sharing of information, it lacks the higher-order awareness and regulatory component of 'thinking-about-thinking' and then is not group metacognition. Shared metacognition aims to enhance group performance by applying a mental model that requires shared reflection on, and ensuing insight into, that performance. Such collaborative reflexivity entails a level of regulation and awareness of a higher order of cognition consistent with metacognition at a social level. This is complex behaviour that cannot be explained by linear models.

Collaboration within and across healthcare teams

Shared cognition has received considerable attention from organisational groups in health care and business management, where it is mostly viewed in terms of information sharing (Larson Jr and Christensen 1993). What has received less attention and remains controversial (in terms of both how such sharing occurs and how to access it) are cognitive attributes such as contextual knowledge, attitudes, beliefs, interpersonal knowledge, expectations, and predictions (all of relevance to the humanities). Recent work has focused on how shared cognition can enhance the performance of teams in organisations, a topic of intense interest in medical and healthcare education, particularly associated with improving patient safety. For example, Canon-Bowers et al. (2001) list three advantages of shared cognition for teams: (i) when team members share knowledge, it allows them to interpret cues from each other in similar manners, make consensus decisions, and take appropriate action; (ii) when teams share knowledge, it is easier to assess and make predictions about their effectiveness; and (iii) with shared knowledge among team members, it is easier to diagnose problems and find ways to solve them.

Team perturbation training and 'making strange' for the humanities

In an intriguing series of experiments relevant to health care teams (and, as I posit, pertinent to the humanities), Cooke and colleagues (Cooke and Shope 2004; Cooke et al. 2013) measured the performance (using validated outcome scores) of three sets of teams in simulated flying tasks of drones taking aerial photograph of reconnaissance targets. They compared the performance of teams trained using three different training approaches: *procedural, cross*, and *perturbation*. *Procedurally* trained teams followed a form of process training entailing a standard sequence of actions (a procedure) whenever presented with particular stimulus; *cross* trained teams were trained on each other's tasks, roles, and responsibilities (to produce teams with a high level of shared mental models and knowledge); *perturbation* trained teams were presented with multiple disruptions (perturbations) of standard coordination procedures during task acquisition in ways that compelled them to coordinate in adaptive ways to achieve their objectives.

Results indicated that perturbation trained teams significantly outperformed the other teams. Their training forced them to coordinate in innovative ways during task acquisition and this subsequently allowed them to generalise performance to novel conditions. Cross-trained teams demonstrated a high level of shared knowledge and performed better than procedural teams under novel task condition but not as well as perturbation teams. Procedural teams performed well on unchanging and foreseeable training tasks but were slow to adapt to changes in dynamic environments. This mirrors the well-known effect in medical education that education for tolerance of ambiguity produces more adaptable and resilient doctors (Peterkin and Bleakley 2017). The goal of perturbation training is to disrupt habituation and rigidity that are common outcomes of procedural training and cross training, and instead allow teams to acquire flexible interaction processes that they can transfer to new conditions. This notion has similarities with Bjork and Bjork's (2011) concept of 'desirable difficulties' in medical education at the individual level, but, for teams, is designed to engage 'difficulty' by introducing unpredictable and variable conditions into practice with the goal of enhancing the transfer of knowledge to new contexts (Gorman et al. 2010). Perturbation trained teams were also able to transfer knowledge to unrelated contexts. This performance was attributed to more flexible and adaptive *interactions* between team members during task acquisition.

These findings have implications for medical and health professions team training that tend to focus mainly on procedural training (for instance, through standard operating procedures) and cross training (for instance, nurse-led operating rooms in inter-professional education). The fixation and drive for certainty in medical training allows little room for anything analogous to perturbation education with its wider vision. Perturbation education (a 'meta' approach) allows teams to be flexible, agile, and adaptive when presented with uncertainty, also shifting focus from tolerance of ambiguity in individuals to the same phenomenon across teams and cultures.

A well-documented value of the arts and humanities is to generate perturbations – by creating uncertainty, ambiguity, and discomfort – that provoke critical consciousness and intense self-reflection (Nietzsche's Dionysian as opposed to Apollonian outlook). As Bleakley (2017) puts it, the arts and humanities 'create puzzlement and discomfort … ruffle feathers and upset preconceptions'. I describe the above studies to illustrate why we should more fully integrate the arts and humanities into medical education rather than leaving them at the edge of the curriculum (Eichbaum 2014). The perturbations they create can have a ripple effect through the learning process and teach students to become more adept at dealing with the discomforts and uncertainties of a dynamic learning environment in the integrated curriculum. More, the arts and humanities (as well as the qualitative social sciences) are grounded in qualities rather than quantities commonly enhanced by an extended and distributed cognition of artefacts such as computers, paint, musical instruments, and so forth.

The notion of perturbation training and its perceived outcomes has analogies with themes of disruption that the arts and humanities produce in 'making strange', the notion brought from literary criticism to medical education by Bleakley and Neilson (2023). This concept was first articulated by the Russian formalist Victor Shklovsky (1893–1984), who argued that *habituation* in thinking leads to 'automatic thinking' in which individuals, places, events, and objects lose their uniqueness to our consciousness and 'fade away'. He argued that through 'estrangement' (*ostramenie*), art distorts perceptions, renews awareness, and allows these things to be viewed afresh:

> In order to return sensation to our limbs, in order to make us feel objects, to make a stone feel stony, man has been given the tool of art. The purpose of art, then, is to lead us to knowledge of a thing through the organ of sight instead of through recognition. By 'estranging' objects and complicating form, the device of art makes perception long and laborious.
>
> (Shklovskiĭ 1991)

The notions of the arts and humanities creating *estrangement* and *perturbations* also align, at a sociopolitical level, with Megan Boler's (2017) concept of 'the pedagogy of discomfort'. Here, individuals are prompted to engage in 'witnessing' social injustices and to assume historical responsibility and agency in action. Rather than just spectating or observing and listening to social injustice while remaining unchanged,

> The aim of discomfort is for each person, myself included, to explore beliefs and value; to examine when visual "habits" and emotional selectivity have become rigid and immune to flexibility; and to identify when and how our habits harm ourselves and others.

These 'thinking outside the box' innovations constitute metahumanities. Metahumanities could be integrated into medicine and healthcare curricula at various junctures and in a range of ways (dissonant or seamless) to mitigate the traditional procedural/didactic relay of information to students and trainees. Thus, to give a somewhat simplistic example, in a basic science course where students may be using HeLa cells, there might be opportunity to introduce a 'perturbation' by talking about the injustices of how these cells were harvested from a black woman (Helen Largier, hence 'HeLa') without her consent, to be immortalised into a cancer cell line and used in thousands of laboratory experiments without her knowledge or consent. Many students will just want to learn about the biology of these cells and may be annoyed at encountering the 'perturbation' or 'discomfort' of the associated social and historical contexts. But such integrated metahumanities will ultimately also render such students more adept at 'reading the world' as Paulo Freire puts it and at the well-established educational and political notion of 'reflexivity' that teaches 'health professional students [to] interrogate their own perspectives as well as the social structures (sociocultural, historical and economic) by which their gazes, lenses, positionality, and perspectives are shaped' (Kumagai 2020).

From shared cognition to situated, distributed, and embodied cognition

'Cognition' is a catch-all word that is often used to embrace feeling as well as thinking. Where the dominant models of cognition have been derived from North American psychology, as noted earlier, they place emphasis upon the individual and what is encased in the skull. However, humans think and feel not simply through the central nervous system, but also through the autonomic nervous system with its significant division in the enteric nervous system that serves the gut. In older models of psychology, emphasis was placed also upon memory at the expense of future-thinking or speculation. As noted, collectivist models of cognition took the mind out of the skull in engaging with other persons and material artefacts, but also placed emphasis on informed speculation as the 'scaffolding' of learning, where learners take leaps into the unknown through carefully constructed pedagogical challenges set by experts.

That cognition and affect can be shared or *distributed* seems self-evident. Of course, brains do not physically join, but humans do, through language and shared artefacts. We talk and signal to each other to develop common understandings and to negotiate differences and conflicts. Cognition and affect are then context-bound or *situated* – the kind of thinking and emotional exchange that takes place in an academic brainstorming context is quite different from quiet contemplation or listening to music. We can also describe thoughts and feelings in terms of their *embodiment* – as 'thinking flesh', 'bodymind', and 'embodied metaphors' ('philosophy in the flesh' as George Lakoff and Mark Johnson put it) (Lakoff and Johnson 1999). Also, recall cradling the human brain in my hands at the start of this chapter.

The concepts of distributed, situated, and embodied cognition were developed independently of each other over a period of some decades with roots in the works of Émile Durkheim at the beginning of the 20th century. Durkheim (along with Max Weber and others) founded the academic discipline of sociology that turned interest in the psychological individual into how individuals collaborate and manage conflict in groups, communities, and societies. While Sigmund Freud did write on collective psychology, the sociological turn explicitly challenged his focus on the individual psyche. Lev Vygotsky was the pioneer of such work in the 1920s and early 1930s, focusing on how children's learning could be scaffolded by external 'minds' (both expert others and appropriate artefacts) as an extended cognition. Below, I address distributed and embodied cognition in detail, along with their significance for metahumanities.

Distributed cognition

Distributed cognition seeks to understand cognitive systems that go beyond individual brain-bound cognition 'to encompass interactions between people and resources and material in their environment' (Hutchins 2000), where 'resources and material' can be thought of as artefacts. Cannon-Bowers and colleagues (Cannon-Bowers et al. 1993) consider distributed cognition as a fourth category of cognition after (1) shared or overlapping, (2) similar or identical, and (3) complementary or compatible. *Shared or overlapping* cognition refers to situations where two or more members of a team need to have some common knowledge – such as a doctor and nurse who share overlapping but not identical knowledge. *Similar or identical* knowledge refers to the sharing of mostly similar or identical *attitudes and beliefs* that team members must hold to draw common interpretations and drive effective performance. *Complementary or compatible* knowledge refers to knowledge that can be different among team members but must be compatible or complementary to lead to similar expectations for performance – such as different multidisciplinary team members bringing specialised knowledge to a problem.

Sophisticated models of distributed cognition in the 1920s were not taken up in the West until the mid-1980s following the publication in English of Vygotsky's *Mind in Society* in 1978 and Minsky's *Society of Mind* in 1985. Michael Cole et al. (1997), after studying in Russia, brought Vygotsky's work to the West, co-editing *Mind in Society*; and Yrjö Engeström (2001) from Finland seeded the idea of 'expansive learning' in European psychology in the early 1980s as an early model of distributed cognition.

As the concept of distributed cognition took root, among the questions posed were: how could cognitive process like memory be distributed in a group of individuals; how could culture and beliefs be distributed across members of society (Schwartz 1989) or propagated over time in society, as in Dawkins' (1976, 2016) notion of 'memes' (rather than 'genes'); how could cognitive attributes of a group as a whole differ from those of its individual members; and how could artefacts in the material world impact cognition and augment human abilities (as depicted in Norman's [1993, 2014] *Things That Make Us Smart?*).

According to Edwin Hutchins (2000), a thought-leader on distributed cognition, Howard Gardner (1995) made the insightful comment that 'at some point a … more or less explicit decision was made to leave culture, history and emotion out of the early work [of cognition]'. Gardner's comment is somewhat short sighted but it does disclose that the humanities were excluded from scientific individualist psychology (focusing largely on personality, again 'strength of character'). Hutchins argues that 'attempts to reintegrate culture, context and history into this model of cognition have proved very frustrating'. He suggests that distributed cognition 'aspires to rebuild … cognitive science from the outside in … so that culture, context and history can be integrated with core concepts of cognition'. This aspiration was not attained, possibly due to the dominance of individualist experimental psychology and its failure to learn from sociology and anthropology. Metahumanities seek to fulfil that aspiration.

Clark and Chalmers (1998) have rebranded distributed cognition – or the extended mind – as 'active externalism'. This shares interests of the position of externalism in modern philosophy. Mark Rowland's (Madigan 2007) theory of externalism argues that our minds extend into, and are constantly interacting with, the environment whose artefacts become part of our cognitive processes and repositories for our memories. Most obviously, our cognition is extended by tools the most sophisticated of which is the computer. Another iterance of distributed and augmented cognition is Bruno Latour's (1996) actor-network theory that seeks to understand the construction of the social world as a network of interactions between human and non-human actors. These networks are not pre-existing structures but are fluid and constantly changing via negotiations and interactions between actors where the power and agency are distributed across the network instead of being held by a single actor. Complex social phenomena emerge from interactions between diverse actors that include non-human entities in shaping social reality.

The 'Extended Mind': a subset of distributed cognition

Ralph Waldo Emerson said 'The mind, once stretched by a new idea, never returns to its original dimensions'. Indeed, it may break dimensions, expanding beyond the skull. Clark and Chalmers' (1998) co-authored seminal article 'The Extended Mind' poses the question: 'where does the mind stop and the rest of the world begin?'. For them, the mind does not stop 'at the demarcations of skin and skull' but is 'an extended system, a coupling of biological organism and external sources'. Clark and Chalmers imagined the human mind to 'extend into the world' and suggested that 'once the hegemony of the skin and skull is usurped, we may be able to see ourselves more truly as creatures of the world'.

What is radical about their suggestion – and went beyond orthodox distributed cognition (which included the environment and shared cognition between individuals) – is the notion of 'active externalism'. Here, the mind does not just make use of material in the environment but is dynamically linked 'in a two-way interaction creating a coupled system to create a cognitive system in its own right'. This two-way interaction is composed of a cognitive loop between memory and foresight or prediction. Neither memory nor prediction is only 'in' our brains or bodies as 'muscle memory', but also 'in' the immediate environment as that provides the cues to which we respond intuitively or ahead of time. Elite tennis players can judge their shots in microseconds ahead of the ball arriving at their racquet heads. They also suggested that the evolutionary advent of language allowed humans to spread our cognitive burden into the world and that language is 'not [just] a mirror of our inner states but a complement to them' (allowing for development of devices such as metaphor, irony, and story).

Clark and Chalmers' (1998) extended mind goes beyond distributed cognition (as a form of shared cognition) in proposing that one's mental states could, moreover, be partly constituted by the states of other minds, which could also act as a repository of one's own beliefs. The extended mind implied an extended self that outstripped the boundaries of consciousness and dispositional beliefs to create a 'coupling of biological organism and external resources'. Again, and more radically, this symbiotic relationship was not one in which the human is a passive recipient of information to be processed, but rather is an active predictor of flux in the environment such that behaviour is not just responsive to environmental change, but acts, in predictive mode, to create such change.

Clark and Chambers emphasised that their concept of 'active externalism' goes beyond other forms of externalism, such as distributed cognition, in proposing an 'active role of the environment in driving cognition', where cognition changes the environment. This suggests a dynamic, bidirectional, *participatory relationship* between the mind and the world that act on, and change, each other.

In the same year that Clark co-authored *The Extended Mind*, he wrote an article on 'Embodied, situated, and distributed cognition' in which he linked the biological body with the external world, where 'Biological brains are first and foremost the control systems for biological bodies. Biological bodies move and act in rich real-world surroundings' (Clark 2017). The sensorimotor system of the body that moves in the environment filters perceptions from environment to the brain thus linking the body and environment to cognition. From a different angle, the American psychologist James J Gibson (1904–1979) (and his wife Eleanor) developed a theory of perception in which humans do not actively shape their environments, but their environments afford a series of opportunities for perception. Such 'affordances' work as feedback systems between a human perceptual apparatus where the senses would not be divided (essentially an embodied cognition) and what the immediate environment 'gives off'.

As mostly an audiovisual species, humans remain generally unaware of *other sensorimotor inputs to the mind*. In *The Meaning of Human Existence*, Edward Wilson (2017) says that

> We are chemosensory idiots by comparison with other organisms ... 99% of which rely almost exclusively on a selection of chemicals ... to communicate ... . We're like a blind man walking down a crowded New York street at night.

The realisation of our 'perceptual obliviousness' should instil in us a deep sense of humility, have a humbling impact on our approach to knowledge, on how we relate to one another, to other species, to the environment – and thus ultimately on the reach of the extended mind. Metahumanities aim to make us more aware of our perceptual obliviousness not only through scientific education but also by encouraging the arts to explore perceptual domains outside the audiovisual.

This is already happening in modern museums where visitors – instead of ambling down endless halls of paintings along the walls – are enticed to interact with a range of artefacts through touch, sound, smell, and proprioception to create a new sensorium that engages them in mixed realities outside their everyday experiences. In 2015, Tate Sensorium exhibition in London brought some of paintings alive by pairing them with non-visual senses – for example, looking at a painting by Francis Bacon, visitors were invited to taste flavours associated with charcoal, salt, and teas; and a painting by John Latham was paired with soundscape and kinesthetic sensations of using sound, light, and vibrations. Immersive experiences created through virtual reality (VR) and augmented reality (AR) offer an astounding range of other possibilities for extending the range of our sensory experiences – for instance, enabling storytellers to bring the readers as viewers more directly into their storytelling (Magsamen 2023). Given the importance of education of the senses to medical education (Bleakley 2021), it is imperative that we draw on such humanities resources.

Embodied cognition

Embodied cognition posits that cognitive processes are grounded in the whole body's interactions with the world. The mind does not work in isolation on abstract problems but requires a flesh-and-blood body as medium, situated physically in an environment. Rather than being centralised, abstract, and distinct from peripheral inputs and outputs, the mind has roots and derives its complexity through sensorimotor processing.

In *IntraConnected*, Daniel Siegel (2022) insists that the brain is both *embodied* and *relational*. He presents evidence from neuro-embryology for the derivation of the embodied brain. The human nervous system derives embryologically from the neural tube to become the spinal cord that grows to connect all the major organs in complex ways through neural networks inside the head. Ultimately, he argues, we really have three brains, or what he calls 'parallel distributed processing (PDP) networks': one around the heart, one around the gut, and one inside the head. Only the head brain developed language abilities, and this is why we conceive of it mostly as the centre of cognition. Metaphorically, we also have a 'heart brain' (emotions) and 'gut brain' (intuitions). Thus, we speak of 'heartache' to describe emotional pain (and the heart as a symbol of love and courage); and we talk of having a 'gut feeling' to describe our intuitions. Now, the metaphors are grounded in fleshly reality. Neuroscientist Antonio Damasio (2018) called the head brain the 'third brain' that operates in service of the other two brains (heart and gut) and the whole body. In *Blink—The Power of Thinking Without Thinking*, Malcolm Gladwell (2006) advocates paying more attention to our gut feelings and instincts rather than only to cerebral cognition:

> When it comes to the task of understanding ourselves and the world, I think we pay too much attention to those grand themes and too little to the particulars of those fleeting moments. But what would happen if we took our instincts seriously? … there can be as much value in the blink of an eye as in months or rational analysis.

One might conceive of a 'meta-brain' serving metahumanities to include cognition, emotions, and intuition as enfolded activities and responses to activities. When we understand that our body has neural (PDP) networks capability not just in the head's collection of neurons, we gain insight into the interaction between the body and the mind and how the body is implicated in the mind's construction of information from (broadly speaking) energy flow or cognition. From this perspective, the mind is fully embodied and is broader than the brain (or, poetically, Emily Dickinson's 'the brain is wider than the sky'). If we are to establish metahumanities to serve metahumanity (both somewhat awkward terms), then we could do this poetically through available metaphors without relying on AI to compose our poetry for us. For example, again George Lakoff and Mark Johnson (1999) speak of 'philosophy in the flesh' to describe the work of embodied metaphors.

Embodied cognition is of relevance to the humanities because it is through the senses and perceptive modalities that we bring the world into the body and the brain – to produce our uniquely human arts and humanities. Embodied cognition occurs not only through visual and auditory perception (given humans are primarily an audio-visual species) but also through other perceptive modes such as thermoception, proprioception, equilibrioception, and touch – all of which are perceptive modes through which the arts are conceived.

To further explicate the notion of embodied cognition, I will draw on Margaret Wilson's (2002) seminal article 'Six Views of Embodied Cognition'. Her approach roots itself in evolutionary biology and therefore better aligns with metahumanities (that, as explained earlier, seeks consilience between the sciences and humanities) than Steven Durning's situativity theory, introduced earlier, which is rooted mostly in medical education and clinical diagnostics. Wilson's six views of views of embodied cognition are:

1 Cognition as situated

Situated cognition posits that thinking and learning are contextually located in the physical and social environment and are in turn influenced by context. For example, a resource-rich context will support cognition better than a context that is impoverished. The focus of cognition thus shifts from the individual and information processing theory (cognitivism) to the social and cultural settings within which these activities occur (Durning and Artino 2011). The content (the 'what') of information alone is insufficient without the 'how and when' (social and physical context) to which it is applied.

Situated cognition takes place in the context of cognitive inputs and outputs that are task-relevant to environmental cues. In *The Origins of Creativity*, sociobiologist Edward O Wilson (2017) argued that the invention of fire and development of campsites were pivotal events in hominid cultural and cognitive evolution as they facilitated the development of language (developed through storytelling around these fire campsites), tool development, and art. Importantly, these are *activities* and it is activity-oriented cognition that characterises situated and extended cognition, with the 'expansion' or innovation of activities as ongoing aims. Yrjö Engeström (2018) calls such expansive cognition 'learning what is not yet there'. The evolutionary drive towards more complexity in the brain in hominids is best seen as a drive to maximise the potential for collaborative cognition, as expansive learning, or learning without boundaries. These early hominid activities present a blend of context- and task-specific 'situated' activities, and the emergence of mental activity divorced (offline) from the situated environmental contexts. Language and development of the arts and culture were responsible for the rapid enlargement of the brain – estimated at an increase of 56 billion neurons over the last 2 million years (Henrich and Muthukrishna 2023).

Margaret Wilson (2002) argues that mental activity taken in the absence of task-associated input and output is 'offline', and thus by definition not situated. Such offline non-situated cognitive abilities (that likely developed during hominid cognitive evolution as humans became increasingly sophisticated in social cooperation) embrace use of language, shaping tools that matched mental representations for use in other contexts, and producing art disconnected from environmental contexts or utility. Wilson further says that language allowed 'communication about hypotheticals, past events and other nonimmediate situations'. Key among these developments and of relevance to arts and culture (and ultimately the humanities) was the development of depictive art suggesting the ability to mentally represent what is not visible or present. While such art, as suggested above, may be seen as serving aesthetic functions (animals as objects of beauty) beyond utility (depiction of hunted animals for example), they also signal emergent metacognitive activities such as ethics (what is valued and why) and transcendental concerns (the hunted animal's spirit must be appeased so that the animals return next season) (Campbell 1983).

Situated cognition is thus the embryonic form of the extended mind. In Edward O Wilson's view, the arts and culture emerged within situated conditions but then propelled the mind forward on its exponential growth through non-situated cognitive abilities. In short, we argue throughout this book that a metacognition learned in medical education must embrace metahumanities – where humanities go beyond their traditional disciplinary boundaries to engage interdisciplinary concerns such as the expansion of an activity system, as described above. An example of this kind of metahumanistic activity is a surgical team working instrumentally (to a high level of technical skill), politically (following democratic values), ethically (concerned with patient safety), and aesthetically (where team process is fluid).

This evolutionary view of situated cognition may not fully comport with situativity theory as a model for medical education and clinical diagnostics, but it does align with metahumanities calling for consilience between humanities and evolutionary biology of the sciences.

2 Cognition as time pressured

Wilson (2002) again takes an evolutionary perspective of embodied cognition in arguing that it is 'time pressured', where 'situated agents must deal with the constraints of "real time" or "run time" … a real creature in a real environment must cope with predators, prey, and terrain as fast as that situated cognition dishes them out'. A consequence of such time-pressured cognition is that humans either 'predictably fall apart under time pressure' or it impels them towards heuristic thinking to make quick decisions. On the other hand, Wilson concedes, many situated activities of daily life are not time pressured and that once one lifts the demands of time pressure, 'some of the true power of human cognition becomes evident … . Stepping back, observing, assessing, planning, and only then taking action'.

However, studies in team-based healthcare show that time-pressured cognition need not induce a falling apart or a reliance upon heuristics but can offer a stimulus for expansion of an activity system. An illustrative example, again, would be our surgical (or any other clinical) team transcending multiprofessionalism to engage with authentic inter-professionalism. Here, democratic values are ingrained, refusing linear hierarchies of power for complex, adaptive systems that have high tolerance for ambiguity or uncertainty. Such teams operate at meta-levels even – or especially – where they do not have consistent membership but are constituted ad hoc from a clinical pool. The key factor here is that such teams, collectively, do not see systemic contradictions (such as initial disagreements over patient interventions) in a negative light, or even as a problem to be solved, but rather take such contradictions as a source for innovation and problem-stating (Engeström 2018).

The kind of non-time-pressured thinking to which Wilson refers may be akin to Kahneman's (Kahneman and Egan 2011) 'thinking slow', often a luxury for high-pressured clinical teams, but necessary for complex diagnostic reasoning, and almost certainly default for a reflective practice out of the heat of the moment or in conditions of pause. An even less time-pressured mode is the 'default mode network' of 'mind wandering' in creative thinking, or what the poet Lucy Alford (2021) calls the 'garden of unstructured time – composed of non-instrumentalized attention' or 'idled attention … toward passive reception and nonselective awareness' that undergirds creativity in poetry and other arts. (See Bleakley's chapter 7 on forms of attention, where 'idled attention' can be compared with 'paradoxical attention' and 'free-floating attention', as opposed to a vigilant or focused attention.) Embodied cognition can thus be time pressured in different ways that impact attention leading to consequences such as heuristic thinking or nonselective awareness.

A good example of cognition as both situated and time pressured is a radiologist engaging in diagnostic work when working with multiple images. Here, the extended mind can be engaged by farming out the diagnostic work to an AI programme that will achieve a result in a fraction of the time that it takes for the radiologist – who can double-check the AI programme's conclusions. This is a well-established extended cognition scenario that is validated and here to stay, as an offloading of cognitive load on to the environment – a mediating artefact.

3 Offloading cognitive work on to the environment

While we are often compelled to function 'online' (within the confines of the head brain), we also frequently run our cognitive processes 'offline'. A way of reducing cognitive workload is to use the environment strategically and leave information to be accessed as needed. A way of decreasing time pressure is to offload onto the environment rather than attempt to store and manipulate all details of a situation. There are multiple ways to offload cognitive work, including writing things down and using smartphones. In the arts, one might view the writing down of poetry from the oral narrative tradition – as in Homer – as an early form of cognitive offloading. Indeed, a history of offloading is a history of human development – from writing to the printing press to computers.

Offloading can be done to alleviate stress of both working memory and short-term memory, to avoid memorising, and to focus attention. A good example is the electronic patient record. Such offloading may be both for activities that are situated in the environment and can be stored and manipulated in the situation itself and for offloading activities that are not situated in the environment but are symbolic such as diagramming and *symbolic offloading* – for example gesturing while speaking which has been found to facilitate cognitive processes that a speaker may be trying to express. Gestures played a prominent role in early hominid communication and today are harnessed in the performing arts. While undergraduate medical education has for some time included 'communication skills' in the curriculum, such skills are often poorly taught using formulaic models, rather than, say, videotape debriefing from live clinical encounters. The medical/health humanities can facilitate the learning of non-verbal communication, for example, through medical students working collaboratively with drama coaches, actor patients, and performance studies teachers and students.

4 The environment is part of the cognitive system
As we have seen, the insight that the body and environment are linked in cognitive activity has led to the claim that cognition is not just an activity of the mind but 'distributed across the entire interacting situation, including mind, body, and environment' (Wilson 2002) (see also Clark 2017). The claim here is that forces that impel cognitive activity do not reside only in the head of the individual, but instead are distributed interactively between the situation and the individual.
5 Cognition is for action
The notion that cognition has the function of serving adaptive activity and 'has its evolutionary rationale rooted in improved motor control' comes from work on perception of memory from thinkers like Churchland and colleagues (Churchland et al. 1993). While our adaptive behaviour must have driven evolution of our cognitive architecture, it is not yet clear in what way this architecture subserves action. However, as argued above, early hominid activities leading to enlargement of the brain were a blend of context- and task-specific 'situated' activities driven largely by the emergence of language and development of the arts and culture.
6 Offline cognition is body based
In this form of cognition, Wilson suggests, we manipulate the environment to assist us in thinking about a problem. Here again, we have moved away from cognitivism and information processing theory, where cognition is brain bound, to the environment being used to assist cognition – or better, cognition is an adaptive and prospective feedback loop between brain and environment (Clark 2023). Several thinkers have argued that mental structures that evolved for perception or action were co-opted to run 'offline' uncoupled from physical inputs and outputs to assist our cognitive processes.

Conclusion

As a conclusion to this chapter, I will note the two major synthetic models of embodied metacognition that have recently emerged – the first from cognitive science and computer engineering and the second from cognitive psychology applied to medical education. Andy Clark (1998, 2023) has written about situated, distributed, and embodied cognition in terms of a 'predictive processing' mind that operates in a feedback loop with the environment. The environment prepares the body for activity just as the mind predicts what may happen next. In such predictive processing, the mind operates, as it were, out of the body. This is truly a metacognition. Clinical educators Steven Durning and others (Durning and Artino 2011, Torre et al. 2020) have proposed a 'nested rim' model (situativity theory) to show how modes of cognition relate to one another, with brain-bound cognition (dual process cognition, information processing theory, and cognitivism) at the innermost rim followed successively by embodied cognition, ecological psychology, situated cognition – and with distributed cognition on the outermost rim. The 'meta' is then achieved as an outgrowth of the personal. The metaphors each author uses are telling. Clark's main metaphor is the corrective, forward-facing feedback loop, necessarily complex, that is predictive and engages high levels of uncertainty. Durning's metaphor is the nest, one less complex system nested in another, working outwards to an environmental connection. We might read this as a conservative 'motherhood and apple pie' model, where cognition is nurtured, contained, and regulated rather than allowed to be explosive and exploratory. But –as a quote attributed the Blues singer Buddy Guy puts it – 'You can't see the whole picture when you're still inside the frame'. Clark's model in contrast posits a more radical cognition of risk as the frame is reframed as porous and adaptive.

Having established the terrain of thinking outside the brain, in Chapter 10, I proceed to show how an extended mind is *realised* through the humanities in medical education to generate metahumanities. Here, we transcend current concerns with clinical diagnostics as the primary field of extended cognition in medicine to grasp how metahumanities can enrich medicine. As the novelist Annie Dillard (1989) said in *The Writing Life*: 'If art does not make us better, then what the hell is it for?'

I began this chapter cradling a human brain in my hands. I will end with a quote from Annie Paul (2021) concerning 'augmented education':

> We often regard the brain as an organ of awesome and almost unfathomable power. But we're also apt to treat it with high handed imperiousness, expecting it to do our bidding as if it were a docile servant. Pay attention to this, we tell it, to remember that, buckle down now and get the job done. Alas, we often find that the brain is an unreliable and even impertinent attendant: fickle in its focus, porous in its memory, and inconsistent in its efforts. The problem lies in our attempt to command it. We'll elicit improved performance from the brain when we approach it with the aim, not of issuing orders, but of creating situations that draw up the desired result.

Paul asks us to create a new relationship with the brain. We outsource the brain's capacities as we collaborate with others in an extended cognition just as we feed in what others outsource, all augmented by artefacts such as stunningly sophisticated technologies. But Paul asks us to do something else, as a meta-thought. She asks us neither to bully nor boss the brain, especially where it seems to let us down, but to create situations, or contexts, in which the brain's potency may be better realised. In pedagogy, we call this 'facilitation of learning' rather than 'teaching'.

References

Alford L 2021. *Forms of Poetic Attention*. New York, NY: Columbia University Press.

Barrett LF 2017. *How Emotions Are Made: The Secret Life of the Brain*. London: Pan Macmillan.

Biasutti M, Frate S 2018. Group metacognition in online collaborative learning: Validity and. reliability of the group metacognition scale (GMS). *Educational Technology Research and Development* 66: 1321–38.

Bjork EL, Bjork RA 2011. Making things hard on yourself, but in a good way: Creating desirable difficulties to enhance learning. In: MA Gernsbacher, Pew RW, Hough LM, Pomerantz JR (eds.) *Psychology and the Real World: Essays Illustrating Fundamental Contributions to Society*. *Duffield*: Worth Publishers, 56–64.

Bleakley A 2006. Broadening conceptions of learning in medical education: The message from teamworking. *Medical Education* 40: 150–7.

Bleakley A 2017. Six fallacies that hinder development of the medical humanities in medical education. *Medical Education* 51: 126–7.

Bleakley A 2021. Re-visioning clinical reasoning, or stepping out from the skull. *Medical Teacher* 43: 456–62.

Bleakley A, Neilson S 2023. As 'synapses' become 'protoplasmic kisses': Symmetry across clinical reasoning and poetry. *Medical Education* 57: 233–42.

Boler M 2017. Pedagogies of discomfort: Inviting emotions and affect into educational change. Critical Diversity in Higher Education Research Team. Discomfort Zones: negotiating tensions and cultivating belonging in diverse college classrooms in Quebec, Quebec, Canada, May 17–18.

Campbell J 1983. *The Way of the Animal Powers*. New York, NY: Alfred Van Der Marck Editions.

Cannon-Bowers JA, Salas E, Converse S 1993. Shared mental models in expert team decision making. In: NJ Castellan Jr (ed.) *Individual and Group Decision Making: Current Issues*. Mahwah, NJ: Lawrence Erlbaum Associates, Inc., 221–46.

Cannon-Bowers JA, Salas E, Converse S 2001. Reflections on shared cognition. *Journal of Organizational Behavior: The International Journal of Industrial, Occupational and Organizational Psychology and Behavior* 22: 195–202.

Cho M-H, Joon Kim B 2013. Students' self-regulation for interaction with others in online learning environments. *The Internet and Higher Education*. 17: 69–75.

Churchland PS, Ramachandran VS, Sejnowski TJ 1993. A Critique of Pure Vision. In: C Koch, JL Davis (eds.) *Large-Scale Neuronal Theories of the Brain*. Cambridge, MA: MIT Press, 23–60.

Clark A 1998. *Being There: Putting Brain, Body, and World Together Again*. Boston, MA: MIT Press.

Clark A 2017. Embodied, situated, and distributed cognition. In: W Betchel, G Graham (eds.) *A Companion to Cognitive Science*. Oxford: Blackwell, 506–17.

Clark A 2023. *The Experience Machine: How Our Minds Predict and Shape Reality*. London: Allen Lane/Penguin.

Clark A, Chalmers D 1998. The extended mind. *Analysis* 58: 7–19.

Cole, M., Engeström, Y., Vasquez, O. A. (Eds.). (1997). *Mind, culture, and activity: Seminal papers from the Laboratory of Comparative Human Cognition*. Cambridge University Press.

Converse S, Cannon-Bowers J, Salas E 1993. Shared mental models in expert team decision making. *Individual and Group Decision Making: Current Issues* 221: 221–46.

Cooke NJ, Gorman JC, Myers CW, Duran JL 2013. Interactive team cognition. *Cognitive Science* 7: 255–85.

Cooke NJ, Shope SM 2004. Designing a synthetic task environment. In: SG Schiflett, LR Elliott, E Salas, Coovert MD (eds.) *Scaled Worlds: Development, Validation, and Application*. Tampa, FL: University of South Florida, 263–78.

Damasio A 2018. *The Strange Order of Things: Life, Feeling, and the Making of Cultures*. New York, NY: Pantheon Books.

Dawkins, R. (1976). *The selfish gene*. Oxford University Press.

Dillard A 1989. *The Writing Life*. New York, NY: HarperPerennial.

Durkheim E 1938. *Rules of Sociological Method*. New York, NY: Free Press.

Durning SJ, Artino AR 2011. Situativity theory: A perspective on how participants and the environment can interact: AMEE Guide No. 52. *Medical Teacher* 33: 188–99.

Eichbaum Q, Barbeau-Meunier C-A, White M, et al. 2023. Empathy across cultures–one size does not fit all: From the ego-logical to the eco-logical of relational empathy. *Advances in Health Sciences Education* 28: 643–57.
Eichbaum QG 2014. Thinking about thinking and emotion: The metacognitive approach to the medical humanities that integrates the humanities with the basic and clinical sciences. *Permanente Journal* 18: 64–75.
Ellaway RH 2010. OpenLabyrinth: An abstract pathway-based serious game engine for professional education. *Fifth International Conference on Digital Information Management (ICDIM).*
Engeström Y 2001. Expansive learning at work: Toward an activity-theoretical reconceptualization. *Journal of Education and Work* 14: 133–56.
Engeström Y 2018. *Expertise in Transition: Expansive Learning in Medical Work.* Cambridge: Cambridge University Press.
Floyd SW, Wooldridge W 1992. Managing strategic consensus: The foundation of effective implementation. *Academy of Management Perspectives* 6: 27–39.
Gardner H 1995. The development of competence in culturally defined domains: a preliminary framework. In: NR Goldberger (ed.) *The Culture and Psychology Reader.* New York, NY: New York University Press, 222.
Garrison DR, Akyol Z 2015. Toward the development of a metacognition construct for communities of inquiry. *The Internet and Higher Education* 24: 66–71.
Gladwell M 2006. *Blink: The Power of Thinking Without Thinking.* London: Penguin.
Gorman JC, Cooke NJ, Amazeen PG 2010. Training adaptive teams. *Human Factors* 52: 295–307.
Henrich J, Muthukrishna M 2023. What makes us smart? *Topics in Cognitive Science.* Advance online publication. https://doi.org/10.1111/tops.12656
Hutchins E 2000. Distributed cognition. *International Encyclopedia of the Social and Behavioral Sciences. Elsevier Science* 138: 1–10.
Innami I 1992. Determinants of the quality of group decisions and the effect of the consensual conflict resolution. *Academy of Management Proceedings.* Published Online: 13 Dec 2017. https://doi.org/10.5465/ambpp.1992.17515606
Kahneman D, Egan P 2011. *Thinking, Fast and Slow.* Vol. 1. New York, NY: Farrar, Straus and Giroux.
Kumagai A 2020. The cutting edge: Health humanities for equity and social justice. In: A Bleakley (ed.) *Routledge Handbook of the Medical Humanities.* Oxford: Routledge, 83–96.
Lakoff G, Johnson M 1999 (revised ed.) *Philosophy in the Flesh.* New York, NY: Basic Books.
Larson JR, Christensen C 1993. Groups as problem-solving units: Toward a new meaning of social cognition. *British Journal of Social Psychology* 32: 5–30.
Latour B 1996. On actor-network theory: A few clarifications. *Soziale welt* 47 (4): 369–81.
Madigan P 2007. Externalism: Putting mind and world back together again. By Mark Rowlands and radical externalism: Honderich's theory of consciousness discussed. Edited by Anthony Freeman. *Heythrop Journal* 48: 508–9.
Magsamen R 2023. *Your Brain on Art – how the arts transform us.* New York, NY: Random House.
Norman, D. (2014). *Things that make us smart: Defending human attributes in the age of the machine.* Diversion Books.
Paul AM 2021. *The Extended Mind: The Power of Thinking Outside the Brain.* New York, NY: Eamon Dolan Books.
Peterkin A, Bleakley A 2017. *Staying Human During the Foundation Programme and Beyond: How to Thrive After Medical School.* Baton Rouge, FLA: CRC Press.
Schraw G, Moshman D 1995. Metacognitive theories. *Educational Psychology Review* 7: 351–71.

Schwartz T 1989. The structure of national cultures. In: P Funke (ed.) *Understanding the USA: A Cross-cultural Perspective*. Berlin: Gunter Narr Verlag, 110–49.
Shklovskiĭ VB 1991. *Theory of Prose*. Champaign, IL: Dalkey Archive Press.
Siegel DJ 2022. *IntraConnected: MWe (Me+ We) as the Integration of Self, Identity, and Belonging*. New York, NY: WW Norton & Company.
Torre D, Durning SJ, Rencic J, et al. 2020. Widening the lens on teaching and assessing clinical reasoning: from “in the head” to “out in the world”. *Diagnosis* 7: 181–90.
Wilson EO 2017. *The Origins of Creativity*. New York, NY: Liveright Publishing.
Wilson M 2002. Six views of embodied cognition. *Psychonomic Bulletin & Review* 9: 625–36.

6 Heuristics and metaheuristics

Rachel Ellaway

Introduction: Giant Steps

In 1959, jazz saxophonist John Coltrane recorded a song called 'Giant Steps'. The song had no words; it was just 16 bars long, and it was played in standard 4/4 time. Despite its apparent simplicity, being able to solo over it has become a rite of passage for aspiring jazz musicians, not least because of its rapid and uneven key changes. To be clear, there are many ways to solo over 'Giant Steps'. Soloists can build on the triads of each chord (chord tones), or they can add the extensions to these chords (sevenths, ninths, thirteenths); they can play the scales of the three alternating keys or the modes of those keys, use the melody as the basis of improvisation, or use different chord substitutions. They can even improvise over the chords-free form with no plan in mind other than hoping for the best. Which approach(es) a musician uses depends on their understanding of the structure and implications of the song's melody, harmony, and rhythm; the way the problems it presents can be parsed; its opportunities realised; and the ability of the musician to think and act at great speed and to be artistic in doing so.

I am a jazz musician and have played this song many times and yet I am still finding new ways to approach it, not all of which I am happy with. To solo over 'Giant Steps' (and to solo in jazz generally) requires heuristic thinking – a 'hands on' and interactive approach to learning by trial-and-error or using loosely defined rules. For me, jazz improvisation illustrates both the conditions and the varieties of heuristic thinking, and how heuristics might be understood as a critical part of metacognition, rather than as an intrinsically flawed and undesirable mental habit. In this chapter, I extend heuristics from the world of jazz improvisation to that of improvisation in medical education and clinical practice (see Bradner et al. 2016, van Ark and Wijnen-Meijer 2019).

Heuristics and heuristic thinking

In Ancient Greece, εὑρίσκω (*heurisko*) meant to find or discover something, exemplified by Archimedes' mythic exclamation of 'eureka' when inspired while bathing to develop a theory of displacement of water by a solid body.

DOI: 10.4324/9781032687339-8

According to the *Oxford English Dictionary*, the English derivation 'heuristic' (via Latin, French, and German) means a 'process or method for problem-solving, decision-making, or discovery'. However, heuristic as a concept has more specific meanings in psychology ('decision making that is performed through intuition or common sense'), education ('learn[ing] by making discoveries'), and computing ('solv[ing] problems or mak[ing] decisions by trial and error or through empirically-derived rules').[1] It is particularly in the field of psychology that heuristics has become a contentious concept. What all these approaches share is a contemplative and processional, trial-and-error method of learning: a learning through discovery and not through using pre-set rules.

Let me, provisionally at least, define a heuristic as a particular way of solving a problem that is based on previous experience and that can be applied and its utility evaluated with relatively little effort. We do not have one heuristic; we have many that we can draw upon. Each heuristic allows us to respond to a particular kind of problem we encounter, particularly under pressure, where time and resources are limited, situations are changing rapidly, and there is uncertainty and ambiguity. Typical (and rather blunt) generic heuristics include trial and error, guessing, and weighing costs and benefits. Core to heuristic thinking is adapting what was learned from previous experience to solving problems in emerging contexts; heuristic thinking displays 'plasticity'.

The solutions that heuristics provide are not necessarily perfect or ideal, and sometimes a heuristic will not resolve a particular problem or challenge. Rather, confronted with a problem, we may select one heuristic based on its apparent applicability and utility; but, if it proves ill-suited to the challenge, then we switch to another heuristic until we find something that works, or time runs out. If we do have the necessary time and resources and we find that heuristics cannot solve the problem, then we shift to slower (and typically more effortful) analytical approaches. Drawing on Simon's (1956) concept of 'satisficing' (something that is sufficient rather than optimal), we can say that heuristics are satisficing when they provide a 'good enough' solution. If one heuristic solution does not satisfice, then a different solution needs to be sought; if a heuristic solution does satisfice, then we can move on.

Being able to draw on different heuristics allows us to act and react quickly to problems, and it allows us to be economical with our thinking and efficient in reusing our past experiences. I define 'metaheuristic thinking' as thinking that solves or otherwise responds to such challenges by using heuristics. Heuristic thinkers (most human beings) typically develop a repertoire of heuristics they can reuse in response to commonly encountered problems. Some heuristics can be applied in many different contexts (such as 'trial and error') while others are more domain and task specific (such as 'check ABC' or 'take a medical history').

The philosopher Charles Sanders Peirce (often seen as the father of Pragmatism) suggested that thinking and problem-solving do not necessarily work through gathering evidence to form a hypothesis (inductive reasoning) or testing an already formed hypothesis (deductive reasoning). Rather, we make a 'best possible guess' from what we know (such as 'the kettle is boiling, so somebody must be in the house'). The abductive nature of heuristic thinking (iteratively working towards the best available solution given the circumstances) reflects an expectation that several heuristic attempts might be necessary before a satisficing heuristic solution is found.

Although our heuristic capabilities vary, we are all heuristic thinkers; we all adapt and abduct our thinking in response to the many challenges that life and our professions place in our path. We are typically schooled in heuristic thinking (both formally and informally), and we are socialised through the expressions of heuristic thinking of others from our earliest years.

If I stopped here, you might go away thinking that collectively heuristics afford a marvellous mental ability. However, as I noted earlier, there have been many criticisms levelled at heuristic thinking. It has been criticised for its tendency to 'satisfice' and the tendency to be satisfied with 'good enough' rather than 'best possible' solutions; and for its dependence on intuition, habit, and (that most deadly sin) 'common sense'. Indeed, satisficing has been portrayed as the mark of an untrained mind, while analytics are promoted as being much less prone to such failings (Hughes et al. 2020). It might be argued that a good heuristic thinker should always be mindful that more rigorous and reliable approaches might have been taken (or might still be taken) if there were more time, resource, and certainty. Either way, we do know that clinicians tend to use heuristics daily in their diagnostic work as 'practice-based evidence' rather than 'evidence-based practice' (Gabbay and LeMay 2010).

Tversky and Kahneman (1974) described heuristics as being particularly prone to bias and error and that they should not therefore be trusted or relied on, particularly in high-stakes situations. These authors (Tversky and Kahneman 1974) and Kahneman (2011) alone (and many others) have contrasted heuristic thinking with analytical thinking, suggesting that the two are antithetical as heuristics depend on fast reactions and assumptions while analytics use rigorous methods and critical thinking. While this may be true in some circumstances or for some individuals, it is a sweeping generalisation to say that heuristics are always biased compromises or even that this is their modal state. In particular, this makes no allowance for expertise, mastery, and creativity that are not particularly analytical, but are nevertheless productive and provide valuable and reliable results. Experts are praised for thinking heuristically exactly because it leads to desirable outcomes that other forms of thinking could not achieve. Think back to my example of jazz improvisation over a melody or a set of chords, where possibilities are endless, but top-drawer players (such as Coltrane himself) produce unexpected, masterful, and sometimes mysterious turns of phrase. Masterful clinicians improvise with the same distinction.

Another critical difference between the use of heuristic and analytical thinking is the acuity of the situation. If there is plenty of time and resource available to solve a particular problem, then gathering data and being slow and analytical in your approach is not only feasible, it is also advisable, particularly if the consequences of solving the problem badly are undesirable.

However, working physicians are often not afforded much time to solve the patient problems they encounter; they must come up with solutions drawing on minimal or ambiguous knowledge of the current situation. Here, the consequences of making a wrong decision are less egregious than not acting quickly and then abducting (taking the best possible choice in the circumstance) as appropriate. Even then, expertise may afford effective heuristic solutions independent of acuity (Eva and Norman 2005). One key difference between constructing a building and making an intuitive clinical judgement is that the former deals with linear, closed, predictable systems open to engineered solutions, where the latter involves nonlinear, complex, dynamic, open, and unpredictable systems that cannot be simply engineered.

Medical thinking (and thinking in general) is not simply about guiding action under pressure, nor is it solely concerned with logics and analytics; it also requires creativity and imagination. More specifically, the craft of medicine involves thinking that is practical, adaptive, and integrative – or imaginative. Carmel (2013) defined medical craft as both skilled interaction with the material world and application of knowledge in thoughtful and insightful ways. This demands the use of metaheuristics, in part as a way of abducting and integrating different kinds and streams of thought, and in part as a way of tapping into the deep and yet tacit learning and experience that forms the core of expertise (see Chapter 4). Arguably, such thinking needs to be championed and protected in the face of the technical and administrative demands of modern medical education and medicine that can erode a physician's sense of craft and restrict opportunities to apply that craft (Oxtoby 2016).

Expert heuristics

Can and should heuristics be used deliberately? For some, heuristics are understood as intrinsically preconscious and reactive; they are our habitual rules of thumb and as such cannot be deliberate or mindful. This is reflected in Kahneman's (2011) version of dual theory of mind, such that System 1 thinking is fast and instinctive (heuristic, involving pattern recognition), while System 2 is slow and deliberate (analytic). It could be argued that any deliberate thinking, either using or about heuristics (or anything else), cannot be heuristic. To resolve this, let us return to our jazz improviser. Improvisation is the foundation of jazz, essential to its expression as an art form. Heuristics embrace aesthetics, or the making of form and beauty. It is the 'shape' (and the 'shaping') of a moment, of an arc of clinical reasoning (embracing intuition), that is realised as an aesthetic gesture. For this reason, as medical students learn clinical reasoning, it is important that they embrace aesthetics in medical practice beyond instrumentalism and that they are aware of doing so. This may be through the realisation of the intrinsic beauty, drama, and elegance of biomedicine, or through the introduction of an aesthetic counterpoint to the instrumentality of biomedicine, such as drawing on the medical humanities (Bleakley 2023).

Instead of a binary model (a modernist trope and a false dilemma if there ever was one for postmodern thinkers), we might consider a more nuanced continuum between System 1 (instinctive and biased) and System 2 (slow and deliberate) such that what we might call 'System 1.5' (heuristic metacognition) sits between them. We can understand System 1.5 thinking as employing heuristics that are developed and used deliberately (as in jazz improvisation) with the aim of becoming both faster and more expert over time. The issue therefore becomes not whether physicians should use heuristics, but what kinds of heuristic thinking are appropriate in medicine or in specific medical settings. Hall (2002) argued that purely intuitive decision-making is prone to error and worse, but her solution was not to avoid or dissuade heuristic thinking but rather to develop it. Heuristics that have been honed over time have been shown to be very effective. As Marewski and Gigerenzer (2012) argued, not only are analytic approaches that depend on more data and more complexity less able to make useful predictions than heuristic approaches, but also there are many positive aspects to the use of focused heuristic thinking in medicine, where 'features of heuristics that make them useful in health care settings … include their surprising accuracy, transparency, and wide accessibility, as well as the low costs and little time required to employ them'.

This leads us to consider the issue of whether heuristics can and should be improved, curated, and developed for and by health professionals. To some extent, whatever the views of psychologists, this is moot as medical education is not a free-for-all where students are left to figure out everything for themselves. Rather, they are taken through a complicated sequence of tasks, tests, and experiences designed to create the necessary learning opportunities and assurances for them to become capable physicians. However, such an education affords two major contradictions. First, learning to make clinical judgements must involve guided, *in vivo* work experience. Second, medical education tends to adopt closed systems thinking (problem-solving), where live clinical work involves open, dynamic, complex, adaptive systems (often at the edge of chaos and prone to spontaneous re-organisation at higher levels of complexity) with high levels of unpredictability, requiring problem-stating and problematising.

Given, then, that much of medicine involves diagnostic thinking and decision-making in clinical contexts that are pressured, ambiguous, and stressful, I would argue that medical education is (and always has been) about guiding students to be heuristic medical thinkers. They must be taught to think on their feet, to deal with ambiguity uncertainty, and pressure, and to know when to slow down or change course when things are not going as they should. The problem here is not with the paradox of implicit heuristic teaching and learning, but rather with explicit messages to students to focus on analytical thinking and avoid the use of heuristics. This may be a cause of stress and confusion, rather than something that reduces these issues. Heuristics afford a significant paradox in medical education: ubiquitous in practice and yet treated with caution in training – necessary and yet demonised.

The 'should' issue has also been debated. For instance, Detmer et al. (1978) argued against heuristics as intuitive problem-solving, urging educators to teach other approaches, while Scott (2009) argued that some heuristics are more appropriate than others and that carefully planned education and deliberate practice are needed. Indeed, it could be argued that our heuristic thinking should generally improve over time (with more experience) as we acquire new heuristics to add to our repertoire, as we refine and focus the heuristics we have, and as we become more experienced at selecting and using whatever heuristics we have or are able to use. However, we might also become lazier over time, less attentive, and more complacent about our abilities as heuristic thinkers, such that our abilities decrease. Education and assessment might address issues of backsliding, but behaviourist manipulation is far from ideal as the basis of independent professional thought. Rather, professional heuristic thinkers need to develop and maintain a deliberate focus on improving and extending their repertoire of heuristics, improving their use of the heuristics they already have, and making their heuristic skills and those of their trainees and colleagues the subject of mindful and deliberate practice. Key to this is the study of how cognition-related medical errors typically occur, for there are clear patterns and tried-and-tested tactics to challenge such patterns (Croskerry 2003, 2013).

This leads to a third issue. If heuristics can be developed and honed, then to what extent can – and should – heuristic practice be deliberate, mindful, and reflective in clinical practice as a 'metaheuristics'? One might argue that the acuity and complexity of situations that require heuristic thinking would not afford time to be mindful and reflective, and if they did, then this would also allow time for more analytical thinking. However, this would still reflect a belief that heuristics are intrinsically inferior to analytics and that thinking about heuristics would be intrinsically analytic in nature. What if that were not the case? What would that deliberate mindful practice look like?

Metaheuristics

In suggesting that heuristics do play a useful role in medical practice, McLaughlin et al. (2014) argued that heuristics are not a problem *per se*, rather that they are one interactive thought process among many, any of which can contribute to decision-making and related errors: 'Heuristics may be on the causal pathway to diagnostic error, but they are not the root cause. Instead, the result of using heuristics is largely dependent upon knowledge with confounding from task difficulty, meta-level reasoning, and luck'.

This 'meta-level' reasoning can include (depending on the model) imagining the consequences of decisions, being mindful, engaging in critical thinking, and adjusting confidence to the challenges of the situation at hand. However, it is expressed or practised; the ability to moderate and focus heuristic thinking depends largely on experience and knowledge, where 'meta-level reasoning is not invariably helpful, nor overconfidence consistently harmful, as this type of reasoning is simply another way to apply stored knowledge to a problem and its effect on diagnostic performance depends upon the quality of knowledge applied' (McLaughlin et al. 2014).

Is this meta-level thinking something in addition to analytics and heuristics or a part of them? Croskerry (2013) argued that the failures and weaknesses of System 1 intuitive heuristics can be addressed by System 2 analytics stepping in and saving the day, while Feufel and Flach (2019) argued that self-regulation is far more heuristic in nature:

> The most promising way to train (future) physicians and other health professionals in clinical decision making is not to circumvent heuristics or correct deviations from logic and probability theory but to enhance the use of heuristics by improving perspicacity, that is, by tuning the (recognition) processes that underlie the domain-specific adaptive selection of heuristics and management of ensuing errors.

However, rather than following an art versus science dialectic, what if we understand analytics as a particular kind of heuristic? After all, an analytical approach can be chosen as one amongst other heuristics, and, perhaps more importantly, if we focus on heuristic thinking as our approach to solving problems in general and not just under duress, then much of our understanding shifts from heuristics as specific problem-solving algorithms to the selection and evaluation of heuristics and the development of heuristic thinking skills from such experiences. This would require a distinction between heuristics as individual and specific problem-solving approaches and heuristic thinking as a systemic way of interacting with and reflecting on the world – a meta-level operation.

This would satisfy Occam in that all problem-solving can be understood as being heuristic in the sense of selecting approaches, appraising them, and reselecting, approximating, satisficing, and so on. Such a perspective would be more humanistic and craft-oriented and, moreover, one that rejects the dialectic of System 1 and System 2 thinking favoured by critics and proponents of heuristics alike. Let us call this a metaheuristic approach, where metaheuristics are how we iteratively and reflexively select, apply, evaluate, and refocus our problem-solving independent of whatever specific approaches we take. This is broadly anchored in the 'System 1.5' space I defined earlier within a dual theory of mind framing, but it is (or can be) so much more.

Metaheuristic and intraheuristic thinking

As McLaughlin et al. (2014) suggested, our effectiveness as heuristic thinkers depends on many factors. An individual's heuristic thinking is weak if their heuristics are weak, particularly if there is a small or underdeveloped repertoire of heuristics, if the heuristics are subject to bias or randomness, or if only one approach (such as analytics) has been applied to the exclusion of others. Such heuristic thinking might also be weak if unable or unwilling to match a heuristic to the problems faced, if there is an inability or unwillingness to identify when a heuristic is not working, or if the person is unable or unwilling to shift between heuristics or adapt them to come up with a workable problem-solving approach.

By comparison, I might argue that an effective heuristic thinker is someone who has a broad heuristic repertoire to draw on, whose heuristics are tried and tested, and who can readily and adaptively match heuristics to problems, appraise how well they are working, and change or adapt their approach as needed. A good heuristic thinker should also be open to learning and relearning new and variant techniques and to be constructively critical of personal heuristic capabilities. Not only do effective heuristic thinkers need to be adept in using their heuristics, they also need to be able to accurately assess the degree of heuristic (acting now) or analytic (slowing down) thinking required of them from one moment to the next. Effective heuristic thinkers also need to be mindful of the constraints and risks associated with both heuristic and analytic thinking. Indeed, given the need for balance, needs analysis, and adaptation, rather than calling them effective heuristic thinkers, we might be better simply calling them 'effective thinkers'.

Doing these things in mindful and deliberate ways might be a mark of an effective metaheuristic thinker, and from that, it might also be argued that effective thinking requires a significant metacognitive component. However, returning to the idea of expert heuristics being very different from lay heuristics, it is both a paradox and a requirement of expertise that the more expert one becomes, the less one is aware of, or even able to be aware of, one's thinking (Kneebone 2020). Thus, while deliberate mindfulness and reflection might play a central role in developing metaheuristic expertise, once expertise is achieved, mindfulness may be difficult to sustain, and it could become a limitation if it were sustained. A mindful metaheuristic practice might on the other hand be more sustainable if it is collaborative (such as appraising, improving, and developing others' heuristic thinking, particularly for individuals for whom you have responsibility (patients, learners, peers, and colleagues)) and where the thinking of others can constrain your own heuristic capabilities (such as through policies, structures, hierarchies, and regulations). Central to this is the metacognitive need to express and account for heuristic thought, which opens it up to critique, formalisation, and abstraction. It is from such metacognitive practices that, formally, both science and art spring.

Although some heuristics might be used algorithmically (if problem X then heuristic Y), that is a somewhat analytical framing and not the primary way in which heuristics are used. Rather, the abductive selection of heuristics is itself heuristic, one that is largely based on impressions and experience. We might select a heuristic out of habit or out of association, based on constraint and effort; or we might engage some affective or Bayesian sense of probability or risk in selecting a heuristic. This draws attention to a critical difference between thinking within a heuristic (intraheuristic) and thinking across heuristics (metaheuristic). How you think within a heuristic is of necessity shaped and constrained by the heuristic. Indeed, one might argue that heuristics work the way they do exactly because of the constraints they impose and the economies those constraints afford. However, metaheuristic thinking works across and

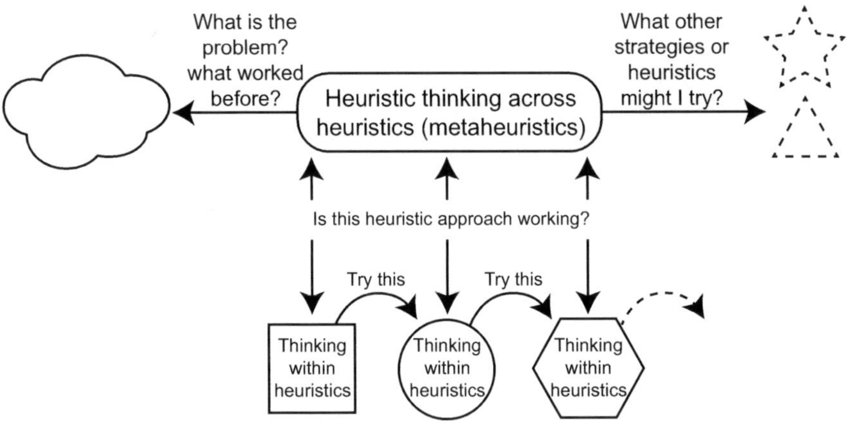

Figure 6.1 Differences and relationships between metaheuristic and intraheuristic thinking (thinking within heuristics).

between heuristics, assessing the problem or challenge, selecting. and appraising different heuristic approaches and considering alternative approaches as needed (see Figure 6.1). To this end, while intraheuristic thinking is constrained and heuristic-specific, metaheuristic thinking is of necessity abductive and expansive, and this in turn requires creativity, imagination, and improvisation in various forms and to varying extents.

Creativity, craft, imagination, and improvisation

'Creativity' can be a weasel-word. For example, Bleakley (2004) described several kinds of creativity suggesting a pluralistic approach. Creativity, like beauty, seems to be something that many people desire but few believe they have (and those that do believe they have it are often deluding themselves). Nevertheless, as Rubin (2023) argued, we are all creative in our own ways:

> 'Creativity is not a rare ability. It is not difficult to access. Creativity is a fundamental aspect of being human. It's our birthright. And it's for all of us ... to create is to bring something into existence that wasn't there before ... What you make doesn't have to be witnessed, recorded, sold, or encased in glass for it to be at work of art'.

Moreover, creativity is not random, and it is not undertaken without deliberate thought and attention. For instance, Quincy Jones (2022) described creativity in terms of left and right brain integration:

> Creativity is made up of two parts: science and soul (left and right brain). The scientific side is that which needs to be learned and practiced. But the soulful side (which is composed of emotions) is something that can't be taught – it's simply the essence of who you are as a human being

The point is well made, even if the differential left brain–right brain model has been questioned (Nielsen et al. 2013) (see Chapter 8).

Creativity in metaheuristic thinking may be expressed in many different ways. One such relates to our heuristic repertoires where existing heuristics can be adapted and elaborated, and new heuristics learned or developed. This augmentation of our heuristic repertoires may happen during problem-solving episodes or in preparation for future episodes. Metaheuristic creativity can also be about learning to use heuristics in new ways, such as combining them in parallel or in sequence, or in using a heuristic to solve a kind of problem which it has not previously been associated with.

In building an understanding of metaheuristics in medicine and medical education, we might therefore seek to distinguish creativity from craft. Craft can be understood as how we respond to anticipated typical challenges using well-honed and readily available heuristics. In medicine, there is craft in how an experienced practitioner takes patient histories, conducts physical examinations, orders tests, or works through differential diagnoses. Craft is applied where the need for adaptation is minimal and anticipated. Creativity is how we respond to problems and challenges that are novel, unexpected, and uncertain, for which we do not have readily available heuristic solutions.

Another conceptual tension we can draw on is that between script and improvisation. Script (such as a musical score) is prescriptive, while improvisation is adaptive. It might be argued that improvisation is a signature of heuristic thinking in that improvisers don't have time to come up with a carefully thought through or ideal solution; they start somewhere and then adapt and abduct as they go. Improvisation is satisficing in that whatever is done will of necessity be all there is. However, this is a somewhat deficit-focused framing as improvisation can also surprise and inspire. Indeed, improvisation can elevate performance beyond any derived or carefully curated solution as my leitmotif of John Coltrane and jazz (I hope) amply illustrates. Rather than saying that improvisation is heuristic, and that script, score, and habit are not, I would argue that they are all metaheuristic, inasmuch as they all require different kinds of problem-solving and thinking about problem-solving. Much professional practice requires metaheuristic thinking that weaves craft, creativity, habit, and improvisation together in experienced and mindful ways. From this perspective, metaheuristics are not just a matter of practical problem-solving; they are the basis of thinking both in and on action in its broadest sense.

Metaheuristics, medicine, and medical education

In exploring the implications of these concepts of metaheuristics to medicine and medical education, we might start by outlining metaheuristic capabilities that all professionals should have or should aspire to have. Earlier, I suggested that to be an effective metaheuristic thinker, an individual should have a broad and robust heuristic repertoire, a well-honed ability to match heuristics to challenges and the ability to evaluate the performance of a given heuristic approach in real time and to adapt or replace the approach as necessary. I also suggested that an effective metaheuristic thinker should be committed to continually expand and refine heuristic thinking and should seek to appraise the constraints and risks associated with such thinking. I expanded on this to suggest that an effective metaheuristic thinker should be able to weave together the metaheuristics of craft, creativity, habit, and improvisation, and that attention should be paid to the metaheuristic thinking of others as well as one's own. Whether these really are the essential or useful qualities of metaheuristics in medicine will need empirical exploration and analysis. I propose them here as a straw man to advance the thesis of this chapter.

Should we seek these metaheuristic qualities in applicants to the medical profession? Certainly, some individuals seem more metaheuristically capable than others, but where that capability comes from and how plastic it is remains unclear. For instance, it could be argued that some aspects of multiple mini-interviews in medical school admissions (Eva et al. 2004) already require an exposition of metaheuristic capabilities. If metaheuristic thinking can be developed in others, should we look for the potential for metaheuristic thinking in applicants ? If so, then do we teach these things directly or is creating the conditions for individuals to find their own way to wisdom the best we can do? Eva and Norman (2005) and Gigerenzer and Gaissmaier (2011) argued that heuristic thinking in professional contexts can be educated to be both efficient and robust through modelling, reflective practice, and creative and constructive preception. Does the development of metaheuristic capabilities follow a standard path that a whole class or cohort can follow, or is it so individual that each trainee must find their own path to it?

Should heuristic capabilities be assessed for licensure and throughout independent professional practice? At the very least, we may seek some guarantee of metaheuristic capability as a minimal standard while allowing for many idiosyncratic ways of pursuing and expressing metaheuristic expertise. It may also be that metaheuristic capabilities are, like professionalism and ethics, much more apparent in the breach than in the observance. From my own experience and in conversation with many medical teachers, they seem to notice deficits in metaheuristic thinking much more easily than they do strengths. This too deserves further empirical testing and exploration.

Are these ideal metaheuristic qualities necessary for all physicians or does the profession vary in the metaheuristic capabilities required of practitioners individually, by system, and by discipline? Are some specialties more dependent on metaheuristic thinking than others? It might be argued that primary and outpatient-focused disciplines foreground metaheuristic capabilities more than others. Certainly, my own experience has been that metaheuristics are particularly important in family medicine and emergency medicine. On the other hand, we may be better placed to anticipate and celebrate a diversity of metaheuristic expressions in trainees and practitioners without seeking to constrain them to specific specialties and subspecialties. Again, more research is needed.

We should also be attentive to the value and meaning we accord metaheuristics culturally and systemically. As I noted earlier, there are still many who are suspicious of heuristics (and by implication metaheuristics) in the profession and who would seek to shape practitioners to avoid such things and depend as much as possible on analytics. If we select applicants for their deliberate and analytical thinking, then are we not doing everyone a disservice if that is all they can do? Moreover, drilling learners to be only deliberate, analytical, and slow, and to distrust heuristics and their metaheuristic abilities is unethical and dangerous. After all, what happens when the lights go out? What happens when a physician encounters a truly new and even paradoxical situation? What becomes of their expertise if a physician lacks robust metaheuristic capabilities?

I should be clear that my argument is that the problem in medical education and practice is not the absence of metaheuristics *per se* but its arbitrariness and our inattention to its necessary qualities. That we already admit and educate many individuals who seem to have strong metaheuristic capabilities reflects a system that does not erase such thinking, but, given that we also admit and educate many individuals who seem to have weak metaheuristic capabilities, metaheuristic learning and development would seem to happen despite us rather than because of us. This reflects missed opportunities, and it potentially risks harms if practitioners who need robust metaheuristic capabilities have not been trained and assessed to make sure they meet the necessary minimum standard or who have had their heuristic capabilities inhibited by training that rejects heuristic thinking outright.

While much medical humanities work has been given over to phenomenological and existential aspects of medicine and health (Kelly 2018), embracing metaheuristics would require perspectives on problem-solving, adaptation, creativity, and improvisation. Whether Conan Doyle, John Coltrane, or Rick Rubin can or should become a part of the medical humanities canon I cannot say (although I would hope that they would). I would argue though that, whatever role the medical humanities might play in developing metaheuristic thinking, it must be more expansive than its traditional liberal arts and deficit-focused approaches. For instance, a philosophy of the medical humanities that embraces metaheuristics should also engage patterns, games, and puzzles, exploration of metacognitive habits and opportunities, and the deliberate development of combining craft, creativity, habit, and improvisation in all aspects of medical practice. That would seem to be a useful and challenging course correction to the medical humanities, but again this would need to be explored empirically as well as philosophically.

Discussion

We have articulated the essays in this volume around the concept of metahumanities as a way of challenging orthodox thinking in both medical education and the medical humanities and to explore expansive and generative perspectives on what medical education and the medical humanities might become. This is not to say that there are no deficits and weaknesses in modern medicine to be addressed; rather there is much more to medical education and the medical humanities than healing the broken souls of healthcare providers. In this chapter, I have argued that metaheuristics can contribute to metahumanities through deliberate engagement in heuristic thinking as an essential part of medical expertise. Without our heuristics, we would be unable to deal with the many uncertain, fast-moving, and emotional situations we encounter. Without metaheuristics, our heuristics are relatively weak and random and subject to the biases and errors that Tversky and Kahneman were so concerned about. Whether or not heuristics are in principle a good thing, they nevertheless feature in much physician thinking (McDonald 1996, Marewski and Gigerenzer 2012). Shifting from heuristics to metaheuristics affords perspectives to help trainees and practitioners to become expert, efficient, and adaptive heuristic thinkers.

The concept of metaheuristics intersects with many other aspects of medical education and professional development. For instance, in talking about metaheuristic thinking as a core aspect of expertise, I am in effect linking to the rich literature on expertise, including adaptive expertise (Pusic et al. 2022), novice to expert development (Dreyfus 2004, Kneebone 2020), and experiential models (Schmidt and Boshuizen 1993). I might also add the literatures on professional identity formation (Cruess et al. 2015), remediation (Kalet et al. 2017), and the role of confidence and competence (as this morphs into capability) (Gottlieb et al. 2022). Indeed, it would not be hard to make a case that all aspects of medical education relate to metaheuristics in some way or other. Similarly, much of the practices of medicine, in particular scopes of practice, career trajectories, and the maintenance of competence, the transition of competence to capability, and ongoing professional development, are all intimately tied to metaheuristic capabilities. However, other than noting these interconnections, I will leave these issues for others to consider, not least because so much of the conversation regarding heuristics and metaheuristics in medicine and medical education has been primarily framed from a psychological perspective.

This book is about both metacognition and metahumanities, and, by taking a metahumanistic perspective on metaheuristics, I would hope that the conversation can be substantially widened and rendered to be inclusive of perspectives outside those of cognitive psychology. Metaheuristic and metahumanistic perspectives can therefore serve an emancipatory function, connecting and assimilating otherwise distinct discourses and affording new and holistic directions in research and practice in the health professions. As an example, in terms of medical humanities, it might be more important to understand how artists, designers, and other creative people think, rather than what it is they are thinking about or what that thinking produces (Kneebone 2020).

This chapter proposes much but proves little. I have positioned metaheuristic thinking as something that can and should be developed as part of a physician's deliberate practice. In doing so, have I simply made a word substitution of professional heuristics for expertise? After all, I earlier criticised the concatenation of biases and heuristics. I argue that metaheuristics are useful, not because they are distinct and concrete, but because they afford ways of challenging and reorienting orthodox views in medicine and medical education; connecting erstwhile diverse conversations; and reinvigorating the medical humanities. All this notwithstanding, I will say again; more research is needed.

In closing, let me return to my opening theme of jazz. When I was learning to play in this idiom, there were two sayings that were often repeated and that have influenced me, both as a musician and as a scholar. The first was 'never the same thing once', the point being that everything is about the moment of creation, the moment of metaheuristics translating to action in the uniqueness of every moment. None of what I have argued matters in abstract; it must inform being and doing in the world. It is always here, and it is always now. The other saying was 'always be the worst musician in the band', the point being that we should always be seeking to learn from others and anticipating that others will learn from us. Metaheuristics can be transactional and social, and on the occasions when minds working together mesh into a shared groove, metaheuristics can be truly magical.

Note

1 Source: *Oxford English Dictionary*.

References

Bleakley A. 'Your creativity or mine?' A typology of creativities in higher education and the value of a pluralistic approach. *Teaching in Higher Education*. 2004; 9: 463–75.

Bleakley A. *Medical Humanities: Ethics, Aesthetics, Politics*. London: Routledge, 2023.

Bradner M, Harper DV, Ryan MH, Vanderbilt AA. 'Don't play the butter notes': jazz in medical education. *Medical Education Online*. 2016; 21: 1.

Carmel S. The craft of intensive care medicine. *Sociology of Health and Illness*. 2013; 35: 731–45.

Croskerry P. The importance of cognitive errors in diagnosis and strategies to minimize them. *Academic Medicine*. 2003; 78: 775–80.

Croskerry P. From mindless to mindful practice--cognitive bias and clinical decision making. *New England Journal of Medicine*. 2013; 368: 2445–8.

Cruess RL, Cruess SR, Boudreau JD, et al. A schematic representation of the professional identity formation and socialization of medical students and residents: a guide for medical educators. *Academic Medicine*. 2015; 90: 718–25.

Detmer DE, Fryback DG, Gassner K. Heuristics and biases in medical decision-making. *Journal of Medical Education*. 1978; 53: 682–3.

Dreyfus SE. The five-stage model of adult skill acquisition. *Bulletin of Science Technology & Society*. 2004; 24: 177.

Eva KW, Norman GR. Heuristics and biases—a biased perspective on clinical reasoning. *Medical Education*. 2005; 39: 870–2.

Eva KW, Rosenfeld J, Reiter HI, Norman GR. An admissions OSCE: the multiple mini-interview. *Medical Education*. 2004; 38: 314–26.

Feufel MA, Flach JM. Medical education should teach heuristics rather than train them away. *Medical Education*. 2019; 53: 334–44.

Gabbay J, LeMay A. *Practice-based Evidence for Healthcare: Clinical Mindlines*. Abingdon: Routledge, 2010.

Gigerenzer G, Gaissmaier W. Heuristic decision making. *Annual Review of Psychology*. 2011; 62: 451–82.

Gottlieb M, Chan TM, Zaver F, Ellaway R. Confidence-competence alignment and the role of self-confidence in medical education: a conceptual review. *Medical Education*. 2022; 56: 37–47.

Hall KH. Reviewing intuitive decision-making and uncertainty: the implications for medical education. *Medical Education*. 2002; 36: 216–24.

Hughes TM, Dossett LA, Hawley ST, Telem DA. Recognizing heuristics and bias in clinical decision-making. *Annals of Surgery*. 2020; 271: 813–4.

Jones Q. *12 Notes on Life and Creativity*. New York, NY: Abrams, 2022.

Kahneman D. *Thinking, Fast and Slow*. London: Macmillan, 2011.

Kalet A, Chou CL, Ellaway RH. To fail is human: remediating remediation in medical education. *Perspectives in Medical Education*. 2017; 6: 418–24.

Kelly M. Difficult conversations: evaluating the medical humanities. In: AD Peterkin, A Skorzewska (eds.) *Health Humanities in Postgraduate Medical Education*. New York, NY: Oxford Academic, 2018.

Kneebone R. *Expert: Understanding the Path to Mastery*. London: Viking, 2020.

Marewski JN, Gigerenzer G. Heuristic decision making in medicine. *Dialogues in Clinical Neuroscience*. 2012; 14: 77–89.

McDonald CJ. Medical heuristics: the silent adjudicators of clinical practice. *Annals of Internal Medicine*. 1996; 6: 56–62.

McLaughlin K, Eva KW, Norman GR. Reexamining our bias against heuristics. *Advances in Health Sciences Education*. 2014; 19: 457–64.

Nielsen J, Zielinski BA, Ferguson MA, et al. An evaluation of the left-brain vs. right-brain hypothesis with resting state functional connectivity magnetic resonance imaging. *PLoS ONE*. Aug 13, 2013. Available at: https://journals.plos.org/plosone/article?id=10.1371/journal.pone.0071275. Last accessed: 16 Jan 2024.

Oxtoby K. The disappearing craft of medicine. *British Medical Journal*. 2016; 352.

Pusic MV, Hall E, Billings H, et al. Educating for adaptive expertise: case examples along the medical education continuum. *Advances in Health Sciences Education*. 2022; 27: 1383–400.

Rubin R. *The Creative Act: A Way of Being*. New York, NY: Penguin, 2023.

Schmidt HG, Boshuizen HPA. On acquiring expertise in medicine. *Educational Psychology Review* 1993; 5: 205–21.
Scott IA. Errors in clinical reasoning: causes and remedial strategies. *British Medical Journal*. 2009; 338: b1860.
Simon HA. Rational choice and the structure of the environment. *Psychological Review*. 1956; 63: 129–38.
Tversky A, Kahneman D. Judgment under uncertainty: heuristics and biases. *Science*. 1974; 185 (4157): 1124–31.
Van Ark AE, Wijnen-Meijer M. "Doctor Jazz": lessons that medical professionals can learn from jazz musicians. *Medical Teacher*. 2019; 41: 201–6.

Part II

7 Forms of attention

The ground for metacognition

Alan Bleakley

Attention! Attention!

The opening sequence of Aldous Huxley's (1962: 1) novel *Island*, an optimistic counter to the earlier, dystopian *Brave New World* (1932), draws attention to the phenomenon of 'attention':

> Attention, " a voice began to call, and it was as though an oboe had suddenly become articulate. "Attention, " it repeated in the same high, nasal monotone. "Attention."
>
> ...
>
> "Attention," the voice insisted without the slightest change of tone.
>
> Leaning on one elbow, Will looked about him and saw with bewilderment, not the gray wallpaper and yellow curtains of his London bedroom, but a glade among trees and the long shadows and slanting lights of early morning in a forest. "Attention"?
>
> Why did she say, "Attention"?
>
> "Attention. Attention," the voice insisted—how strangely, how senselessly!

Huxley's late novel *Island* describes a utopian community, based on Buddhist principles, in which mynah birds are trained to say 'Attention!' and 'Karuna!' ('compassion!') at regular intervals to remind the populace to stay focused, in the here-and-now. In other words, a persistent wake-up call, a reminder to be mindful, alert, putting aside trivial distractions while parking unnecessary needs and desires. This is not, however, the harsh barking of a sergeant-major forcing attention against the will of the person and setting up resentment, but nature's reminder to wake up to what it affords as gifts in differing registers: beauty, transience, abject fear, a calming presence, and novel configurations. Yet such focused attention can swallow you whole – contrary to received opinion, its bite is worse than its bark.

Introduced briefly in Chapter 4, in a moving YouTube video, airline pilot and patient safety activist Martin Bromiley tells the tragic story of the unnecessary death of his wife Elaine at the hands of a UK surgical team

DOI: 10.4324/9781032687339-10

(https://www.youtube.com/watch?v=JzlvgtPIof4). During a difficult intubation, two experienced consultant anaesthetists, a junior anaesthetist, an experienced ENT surgeon, and three nurses attend the patient. Despite a sharp fall in oxygenation level to 40% and lower, and a falling heart rate, the doctors continue to try to intubate Elaine, even as they dismiss the nurses from the bedside. Ten minutes into the procedure, Elaine is blue – her oxygenation has been at 40% or lower for six minutes.

The three consultants continue to attempt to intubate for a further 15 minutes. They adjust oxygenation to 90%, but Elaine has been at 40% or lower for 20 minutes. At this point, they agree to abandon the procedure. However, they have not secured the airway, and they continue to stubbornly work on this for a further 10 minutes, as Elaine's oxygenation again falls to critical levels. Thirty-five minutes in, the team decide to let Elaine wake up naturally, in the recovery room. Tragically, in Martin Bromiley's own words, 'she lays there for an hour and a half and fails to wake up'.

Meanwhile, the nurses on the team had seen that Elaine had turned blue and phoned the intensive care unit – but the same nurses failed to challenge the surgical team, frozen by perceived authority and hierarchy. One of the nurses had brought in a tracheostomy set, aware that Elaine probably needed an urgent intervention, but the nurse's visible prompt was ignored by the surgical team. The nurse who phoned intensive care came in to tell the team that she had done so, but they ignored her intervention also, suggesting that she was over-reacting. This caused the nurse to contact intensive care to cancel the requested bed. While multiple factors were at work – notably a lack of leadership and poor communication within the all-male surgical team, combined with the negative effects of exercised hierarchy in the communications between doctors and nurses – our focus here is rather on forms of attention. In this case, overall awareness of the criticality of the situation was lost as the surgical team members had their heads down, concentrating on the intubation, so blinkered in a tightly focused attention that they had lost peripheral attention or situational awareness (Bleakley et al. 2013).

The philosopher Michael Polanyi (1965, 1966) differentiated between focal awareness and subsidiary awareness. In a task such as hammering a nail, focal awareness is on the nail and the fingers holding it (or it should be, to avoid an injury), while subsidiary awareness is on the hammer and the hand holding it, so that hammering becomes automatic. The surgical team would seem to have been stuck in focal awareness, losing peripheral or subsidiary awareness in terms of a sense of time, regular checking of instrumentation, and listening to the advice of the nursing team. The mynah birds had flown, attention had been lost, and so had Elaine.

Where, and how, does a doctor's or surgeon's attention fail? In the example above, I have followed the rather crude distinction between an active, focused, or *endogenous*, attention and one that is *exogenous* or free-floating. Later, I will refine this rather crude distinction as I consider non-hierarchical context-bound forms of attention adapted from the work of the literary academic Lucy

Alford (2020). While Alford's scheme was developed in the context of how differing forms of poetry come to educate differing forms of attention, this is readily adapted to address any aspect of life, as attention is the basis of all non-automatic or reflective and reflexive activity. Here, I draw on her scheme to illuminate forms of object-based attention in medical work that create differing meanings according to context. By 'object-based' attention, I mean doctors working with patients and their presenting conditions, with colleagues, and with artefacts such as instruments and test results. This analysis is readily transferable to medical education, where education of forms of attention should be core to the curriculum.

Alford also describes an 'objectless attention'. I have referred to this as free-floating, exogenous, and subsidiary. It is an awareness by nature paradoxical – in the Buddhist sense, attentive-without-attending. Both object-focused and objectless kinds of attention work in parallel, but, as we saw from the sad tale of Elaine Bromiley, sometimes focused attention blocks out peripheral, free-floating attention that would have acknowledged the nurses' concerns and been aware of the patient turning blue. Such a background attention is not merely instrumental; it can be aesthetic (it has form), ethical (it implies value judgements), political (it is implicated in power structures), and transcendental (it thinks about thinking or reflects on quality of awareness at a meta-level).

Having said that, the two kinds of attention – focused and free-floating – would seem to work in parallel, and as such we might be better to model them not as two systems but as two potentials within one feedback system between the individual embodied mind and the environment as both social collective and natural world. Again, as Andy Clark (2023) suggests, 'our minds predict and shape reality' through a forward-focusing feedback loop. 'Attention' can be thought of as 'prediction' – split-second assumptions about what will happen next based on experiences of what happened before. If the prediction turns out to be inaccurate, we rapidly adjust the forward-looking loop. Attention is of course available to introspection, but that is merely the surface element of an unconscious attention as a force for prediction. Most of this unconscious working attention is 'precision-weighting' that Clark (2023) describes as 'the predictive processing version of "attention"'. In a simple movement such as raising an arm, 'high weighting' is given to the predicted level of the raised arm, while 'actively disattending to the present state of the arm, hence damping down that sensory information'. In sophisticated movements (such as a tennis player perfecting a stroke and then innovating around that stroke), 'a cascade of prediction errors' will occur, where 'fluent, automatic corrections then deliver the stroke' (Clark 2023). Such future-focused mental rehearsal is key to expertise as it accompanies actual practices – again, attention as future-focused shaping of activity.

Clark (2023) further notes that endogenous attention 'is top-down, goal-oriented, and purposive, driven by the faculty of attention control located in the frontal cortex and basal ganglia as an executive function'. In contrast, exogenous attention 'is bottom-up, stimulus driven, powered by reflexes and receptivity networks, and sharpened by the degree of sensitivity to perceptual change' and is 'not one of directed initiative, but rather one of response' (Clark 2023). From Clark's analysis, we might again avoid splitting attention into two forms, but rather see attention as continuous and looping with memory.

In the context of Lucy Alford's (2020) analysis of attentional devices, it is again an impersonal body of literature – poetry – that is the object of contemplation rather than an anaesthetised, personal body. Nobody dies if attention to poetry is poor or not honed (although the poet and physician William Carlos Williams said that 'it is difficult to get the news from poems yet men die miserably every day for lack of what is found there'). But the principle of how forms of attention work remain the same – that the body of the poem surprises and enchants, or creates puzzlement and interrogation, not primarily for its immediate self-presentation, but for what it is not saying, saying in disguise, or hinting at. Such contextual features can be readily applied to the clinical consultation and to diagnostic work, and then to the pedagogical frameworks for learning these clinical capabilities, as we shall see.

To further illuminate differences between a focused and a free-floating attention – while bearing Clark's critique in mind that these forms may be two sides of a continuous loop (imagine a Möbius strip in which surfaces meld) – we can draw on the Gestalt notion of figure and ground, and David Bohm's (1980) distinction between an explicit and an implicate order. Key to tacit knowing in experts are embedded forms of attention. Before any other cognitive or metacognitive activity, we perceive through the senses. But before we perceive, the senses, as a complex bodily system, pay attention to whatever the environment affords in shifting contexts. Of course, these aspects of bodily being are not dis-located but act in harmony with the *umwelt* – or immediate environmental context – as a complex system. The environment shapes our perceptions just as perception attends to the environment as James Gibson (1966) sets out in affordance theory. As Gestalt psychology and phenomenology have long insisted, there is figure and ground at work in perception that are in constant movement relative to each other. Acute, focused attention dwells on, and in, the figure, while a free-ranging, free-floating, ambient, or paradoxical, attention both generates and surveys the ground out of which the figure arises.

As is the case with all educated and established capabilities, or the gaining of expertise, a highly complex set of learning – constantly being refined by ongoing circumstance – is memorised and adapted. In the process, what was previously explicit and subject to conscious contemplation gradually becomes implicit or tacit – as an 'implicate order' (Bohm 1980). David Bohm describes adding a drop of black ink to some glycerine in a tub that can be gradually churned. The ink becomes a string that eventually disappears into the glycerine ('enfolded'). However, when the churning is reversed, the string of ink reappears and is reconstituted as the blob ('unfolded'). The enfolded ink models an implicate order, paralleling tacit knowing. The beauty of Bohm's model is that it captures the continuity between implicate and explicit states. Endogenous and exogenous attentions are neither divided nor opposed, but work in parallel, intertwined.

Table 7.1 Medicine and poetry share tacit reasoning processes (isomorphic/echoic)

Poetic diction	*Clinical reasoning*
Field	Bodymind
Sensibility	Close noticing/pattern recognition
Sensitivity	Witnessing (empathy)
Rhythm	Pulse (heart) and breath
Tropes (e.g., metaphor)	Close attention to the patient's vernacular speech
Alliteration	Patient's expressive signs and symptoms
Lexical knowing	Biomedical science
Composition	Clinical guidelines
Practice/rehearsal	Use of heuristics/short cuts
Audience response	Laboratory tests

Such intertwining of figure and ground, reflected in explicit and tacit knowing, is apparent in various forms of expertise including clinical reasoning (Bleakley and Neilson 2021) (see Table 7.1).

Experts know more than they can say, for now their knowledge has become tacit or enfolded (and coded). Their reasoning process has switched from explicit Type 2 (logical, rational) to implicate Type 1 (intuitive, tacit, pattern recognition) for familiar scenarios. It will switch back to Type 2 where an unfamiliar scenario is encountered, or there is some reasonable doubt such as fear of premature closure in a critical diagnosis (Groopman 2007). Precisely because cognitive forms such as attention and decision-making are largely automatic for experts such as experienced clinicians, it is important that we maintain avenues of metacognition through which an individual can reflect upon, dissect, appreciate, and further examine their own automaticity – the realm of the 'meta'. In the realm of clinical reasoning, this reflexive work is often done after the fact by third-party commentators (Groopman 2007). Such commentators are often cognitive psychologists who, paradoxically, may fail to see their own judgement biases – for example where they site clinical reasoning in individuals' minds rather than in the social contexts of transactions (as an ecological and extended thinking). Further, examination and anatomising of clinical reasoning has been considered in relationship to other kinds of thinking common in the arts and humanities, such as both epic and lyric poetic reasoning (Bleakley and Marshall 2017; Bleakley and Neilson 2021, 2022, 2024) and forms of poetic attention, as noted (see Table 7.1).

Lucy Alford's 'forms of poetic attention'

Again, Bleakley and Neilson (2021, 2024) argue that there is correspondence, even an isomorphism, between cognitive forms of reasoning in medical decision-making and in poetic composition. This involves using a body of knowledge (biomedical/linguistic-metaphorical) to inform a set of decision-making strategies in medical work (heuristics, induction, deduction, abduction, semantic differentials, and so forth); and compositional rules and strategies in poetic work (forms, rhythm, assonance, consonance, metaphor innovation, and so forth). Common to both poetic composition and medical work (and many other forms of reasoning) is that meaning is achieved through tuning and refining attention. Attention is the gateway to cognitive effort, the portal into the cognitive and affective loop between memory and future-thinking that shapes behaviour in the here-and-now through an 'embodied mind' (Clark 2016).

Lucy Alford (2020) anatomises modes of transitive attention (directed towards objects: 'she clamped the artery') and modes of intransitive attention (expressed without objects: 'she grimaced') educated by poetry. I have noted already that we can view transitive, object-oriented attention as being focused (shifting Gestalt 'figures') and intransitive attention as being free-floating (shifting Gestalt 'grounds'). Such uses of attention can frequently be observed in medical work. For example, we might carry out an observational field study of doctors in consultations and working in teams. We will videotape them and analyse the video. From this, we can draw out differing ways in which attention is modelled under differing circumstances, such as level and nature of interruptions to a senior consultant in an emergency department setting (Allard et al. 2011). A more fulsome approach is offered by the scoping review protocol (literature review) of empirical work on attention in clinical contexts (Kissler et al. 2022), a work in progress that will hopefully provide a model of forms of attention observed in medical work that parallels Alford's exhaustive literary phenomenological analysis.

Kissler and colleagues (2022) define attention as 'a state of concentrated focus' and note its intuitive dimension. They claim that 'the practice of medicine could be thought of as a paradigmatic case of a human activity that requires attention'; however, 'medicine has had relatively little explicit discussion of attention as a whole phenomenon'. You Chen and colleagues (2022) see 'Undivided attention [as] a clinician's superpower' (also called 'deep work', 'being in the zone', and 'being in the flow'), where 'full focus and presence' is established. They cite evidence that care is safer, and 'the care process is more satisfying to patients and clinicians alike' under conditions of undivided attention. But we have seen in the case of Emily Bromley that where the surgical team had its head down and gave undivided attention to intubating the patient, free-floating or paradoxical attention was quashed, leading to error. Chen and colleagues (2022) describe the dangers of 'split attention, moments when clinicians lose focus and, as a result, risk missing important incoming data—whether a cue from the patient's body language or tone of voice, a relevant element of the past medical history, or an abnormal test result'. What these authors are referring to seems to be distraction. Focus vs distraction, however, is not the same as a meta-perception that embraces the simultaneous working of focused and paradoxical attention.

Kissler and colleagues (2021) are also interested in the way that cognitive load (reducing attention space) can be increased (as 'cognitive burdens') in clinical spaces. This is an 'ecology of attention', where empirical data are often used by organisations for utilitarian purposes – to seek efficiency and optimisation: 'As we continually try to optimize the systems in which we work, we should think ambitiously about clinical environments that optimize attention. Such thinking can improve quality, efficiency, and patient and provider satisfaction and reduce costs of care'. This instrumental approach to attention can be contrasted with that of Alford's analysis of poetry in the context of questions grounded in aesthetic values.

It is typical of medical and medical education research to reduce complex psychological phenomena, such as attention, to instrumental and formulaic representations. Ironically, this happens in the context of a workforce that is often poorly managed, under-resourced, and over-stretched. Here, attention is already so overloaded that talk of 'optimisation' of attention is hollow. The poetic imagination seeks to understand attention in less instrumental ways, grounded in the rule of 'appreciation before explanation', an aesthetic dimension.

Educating different forms of attention is what the arts and humanities do well, and this is why the medical humanities (and more so metahumanities) are important to medicine and medical education. Such education shapes the senses to be acute and receptive, forming the conditions of possibility for attention to flourish. This is vital to a medical education that seeks to refine the senses of medical students for close noticing as a prelude to clinical judgement (Bleakley 2020). To be more specific, it is embodied metaphors that tune and shape attention (Bleakley 2017). They show us not only where we should look, but how to look, as they educate attention. Alford describes how metaphor-rich poetry can act as a means of educating and shaping attention for readers in terms of the kind of attention-shaping aesthetic devices that poets draw on. In the process, she provides a manual for understanding forms of attention that bleed out from poetry into every walk of life. Again, her blueprint can readily be adapted to describe forms of attention in clinical work, and how these might be better educated based on explication of such forms. Alford's scheme allows for mapping a tacit knowing or cognitive unconscious, and then translating this into curriculum capital, or medico-pedagogical strategies (Table 7.2).

Table 7.2 Differing forms of attention discussed in this chapter

Vigilant	*Paradoxical/free-floating*	*Source*
Focused	Peripheral	Biology/ecology
Focal	Subsidiary	Michael Polanyi (philosophy)
Endogenous	Exogenous	Cognitive psychology
Object-based (transitive)	Objectless (intransitive)	Lucy Alford (literary criticism)
Figure	Ground	Gestalt psychology
Explicit order (unfolded)	Implicate order (enfolded)	David Bohm (theoretical physics)
Focused	Situational awareness	Patient safety culture

Transitive attention and the 'what' of attention

As noted above, where a verb 'accepts' one or more objects (e.g., 'Suzie enjoys a piece of music'), this reflects transitive attention. Alford points to the first principle of lyric poetry as the description of objects, in depth and often from unique angles, so that such objects of attention can be seen anew (John Keats' 1819 'Ode on a Grecian Urn' being the Ur-example). Such poetry is a work of imagination as shaped through the education of the senses. Doctors of course work daily with forms of transitive attention as they attend to patients and their presenting symptoms. Their primary work is one of close noticing (aesthetic sensibility) grounded in the senses and witnessing (ethical sensitivity) grounded in values and professionalism. Medical students largely pick up 'how to look' (and better, 'how to see') from work-based experience, but they would benefit from more formal education into forms of attention as preparatory to 'how to see', as the 'what' (rather than the 'how') of attention – the object-content rather than the process.

The nature of the object of attention

Alford distinguishes between the 'what' and the 'how' of attention. The 'what' is concerned with the object of our attention. The 'how' is the shaping of our attention by the perceived (or sometimes mis-perceived) object. This dual processing can be compared with the psychologist James Gibson's (1966) notion of 'ecological attention', where it is not primarily us who attend to the world around us, but rather what that world 'affords' that shapes our attention. Affordance is what the *umwelt* or immediate environment 'gives' and 'gives off'. We do not generally strive to attend to the world, but rather features of the world 'capture' our attention. Here, the 'what' and the 'how' of attention are collapsed into a common process, for 'what' is afforded by the environment dictates how that affordance shapes or educates an embodied attention. The notion of affordance is key to challenging the individualism of much medical education (Bleakley et al. 2011) in recovering the reality of perceptual attention – that it is embedded in context or offers 'extended cognition' (see Chapter 10).

Alford distinguishes between 'selectivity', as the resolution of the object of attention (in or out of focus); and 'spatiotemporal remove', or how the location of the object in space and time affects focus on that object. She describes the object that captures the attention of the poet as a moment of *ekphrasis* – usually described as the literary description of a visual work of art, but often widened to include verbal and written descriptions of any object of attention and close observation. In medicine, especially in diagnostic work, this can be described as 'close noticing'. It is also a form of 'witnessing' – for example of a patient's pain or suffering.

The capability of 'close noticing' is informed by both the resolution and location of the object (see Chapter 9). This is tangible and readily codified, for example, in surgical interventions, especially in minimally invasive surgery mediated by cameras; and in face-to-face consultations such as a dermatological diagnostic investigation. However, such forms of attention are less defined in diagnoses of mental health conditions. These rely more on patients' linguistic descriptions that themselves may be part of the symptom expression (e.g., continuous self-reference on the part of narcissists; leaden descriptions of depression; agitated, excited, and over-wordy descriptions of mania; dizzy, pondering, and uncertain descriptions of anxiety). Here, the object of attention may be both fuzzy and dis-located. In general, 'close noticing' – involving the resolution and location of the object – places large demands upon the medical student and junior doctor who have not yet developed specialist 'pattern recognition' for a range of presenting symptoms (see Chapter 11).

Such forms of attention can be 'hot housed', first by anatomising their elements (as above); and second through clinical learning involving structured briefing and debriefing. A paradox of the resolution of the object of attention, say with a patient's account of his or her symptoms, is that a patient's use of vernacular language can create both high texture and low resolution – fuzziness and dislocation. Vigilant attention is needed in combination with free-floating and paradoxical attention to pick up on nuances and hints. Figure and ground are entangled throughout.

Aspects of the subject of attention

As affordance theory in biology suggests, 'human–biodiversity interactions are reciprocal' (Andersson and McPhearson 2018). Attention to the object, shaped by that object as an aspect of 'affordance' or ecological perception (what the immediate context 'gives off' in terms of resolution and location of the object), is paralleled by the perceiver's 'interest' (degree of investment or motivation) and 'intentionality' (the nature of the act of attention as either active or passive) in Alford's scheme. These are self-explanatory. For Alford, poets do not recognise objects of attention fully unless the poet actively notices, selects, and is invested in the acts of perception. This is the 'how' of attention rather than the 'what'. For poets, as for medical students and doctors, there is a twist to such 'looking' and 'seeing'. One must, as the poet Emily Dickinson suggested, look 'slantwise' at objects to see them afresh or to get under their skins. The paradox of attention in medicine is that population-based rules (such as clinical guidelines) do not necessarily map onto individual patient's needs. Attention must be selective, responding to the idiosyncratic patient as the subject of attention rather than as a generalised guideline. Indeed, such a guideline may bias attention where a physician is looking for symptoms as described in a textbook rather than as they are idiosyncratically embodied in a particular patient.

Intentionality in medical work is compromised where attention is mediated by instrumentation and tests. One of the great advances in diagnostic work has been the shift from the bedside examination, facilitated by the stethoscope (using palpation, auscultation, and percussion), to greater reliance upon laboratory testing (blood, urine, and tissue samples), and imaging (ultrasound, X-ray, and MRI and CAT scans). However, while this delegation can provide more accurate diagnostic possibilities, it can also reduce the complex personal-attentional act of medicine (that embraces a range of values) to the instrumental or functional. The attentive interest and intentionality of the doctor, acting in the role of poet as creator of an artistic (imaginative and creative) relationship with their patient is quashed; or rather it is transferred to, and translated through, the diagnostic instruments of mediation. This reflects Marshall McLuhan's infamous headline that 'the medium is the message', where 'we shape our tools, and thereafter our tools shape us' (McLuhan and McLuhan 1988).

In plain terms, such translations by-pass and excise the healing potential of the 'bedside manner' or 'warm' consultation for a 'cold' diagnostic pass. In more complex terms, the aesthetic, ethical, political, and transcendental values of a medical encounter are by-passed for the instrumental, functional, or mechanical restrictions of the 'test result'. The power of medicine's poetic attentional devices is then readily undermined by the very diagnostic instruments that have improved diagnostic biomedicine. Any subsequent consultation, with test results in hand, can provide a second chance for interest and intentionality to shine, as these form the subject of attention, or the doctor's intentions shaped by interest.

Transitive (object-oriented) attention

Alford's schema of types of attention is refreshingly free from hierarchy in that there are no 'better' and 'worse' kinds of attention; rather there are good attentions/intentions, mis-intentions, thin attentions, and over-crowded attentions. I will now briefly describe the five 'dynamic coordinates' of such object-oriented attention.

i 'Interest' and 'disinterest'. Physicians are brought into conversations with patients or about patients according to how they capture their attention. Is the doctor interested in this person or is there a degree of disinterest? What interests physicians? The symptom per se, or unique and rare, or as a great illustrative example for teaching purposes? Or does the person as a whole interest them or perhaps turn them off?

ii 'Intentionality'. Do physicians home in on a particular aspect as endogenous intentionality? Or do they 'free float' as exogenous intentionality, not quite sure where to home in? Or both can be happening at once. A patient says that he drinks alcohol moderately, while his body language says that he is concealing the truth. While homing in, the physician's free-floating attention connects with memories of many other patients like this, who basically lie about their alcohol consumption despite, for example, their blood pressures remaining abnormally high, and other telling symptoms emerging.

iii 'Selectivity'. Just how wide or narrow is the physician's zone of attention? And what factors cause them to be selective about where their attention falls? Of course, they might be distracted from outside sources (as noted earlier, interruptions are common in emergency medicine, even as focus is required, and split-second decisions may need to be taken). Music played in the operating theatre has been claimed, paradoxically, to be helpful for concentration – but this is only for those who choose the music; for others, it can be a source of distraction and irritation (Bleakley 2020). The poet Wallace Stevens wrote about the stand-off between perception of the senses and the work of imagination, where 'selectivity' concerns seeing what we wish to see, or what imagination dictates. 'I've seen this before, many, many times' says the experienced physician faced with a symptom pattern, and a diagnosis is made. But there was premature closure (selectivity), and a misdiagnosis ensued, because what the physician saw was partly filled in by expectation (an imagined diagnosis), and he missed a peculiar deviance from normal presentation.

iv 'Spatio-temporal remove'. Where a stimulus is (in terms of time and space) affects how physicians perceive it (in terms of where their attention rests). Perhaps the closer the physician gets to the patient, instead of familiarity emerging, defamiliarisation sets in. 'This is not what I expected from this person. I must be mistaking them for someone else. Everything fits symptom-wise but there is something odd about it all that I cannot put my finger on'. Attention seems to roam, fails to settle in space or time, taking us for a ride.

v 'Apprehension'. Apprehension marks the limits to a focused, endogenous, vigilant attention, where the periphery of free-floating, exogenous attention begins. Just how do these attentions interact? The phenomenologist Edmund Husserl noted a distinction between noetic and noemic intentionalities. The noetic is the *how* – the act of seeing, grasping, understanding, desiring; where the noemic is the content – *what* is seen, grasped, understood, desired. Importantly, it is at the periphery of vigilant attention that the noetic gains precedence over the noemic. The act of awareness is here perhaps more important than the content, for it prefigures and flags up what might be an intentional object or content coming into being. Had the operating team in the illustrative example near the opening to this chapter mustered greater collective apprehension, they would have realised that the patient was in danger and would have taken more notice of the nurses' interventions, in particular the collective mood of these nurses – anxious, concerned, but oppressed through hierarchical constraints where the doctors' word rules.

Apprehension

There is more to be said about 'apprehension' – grasping a phenomenon through focused attention at the limits of perception. This may be where much generalist medical work sits, rather uncomfortably, as a zone high in ambiguity and uncertainty and therefore attracting higher levels of affect. Part of the issue of 'fuzzy thinking' in this zone is how to distinguish between the object and the subject of attention. An object of attention (a patient for example) is also a subject of attention as the patient's gaze is transferred back to the doctor in the consultation. The doctor pays attention to the patient as she pays attention to her own responses to the patient and his or her account. The subject's (doctor's) interest and intentionality are partly invested in the object (patient) as that patient arouses such interest and intentionality.

In the context of poetic attention, Alford describes the space between the object and subject as 'apprehension'. This is how well the object has been caught by attention. Does the poet make something of the interaction between the object she describes and her own states of attention in describing that object? This is the key 'meta' question in attending to attention. This form of (meta)attention – an attending to attention – is precisely what I am doing here with the help of Alford's scheme of forms of poetic attention. But in the heat of the moment of clinical work and decision-making, there is not the luxury of extended contemplation and analysis. As vigilant attention is exercised, so a meta-attention must be employed as a free-floating or paradoxical attention lest we find ourselves swamped by vigilant attention – too busy and all-consumed to note an objection by another team member; too focused on what to say next to note what the patient is saying now. Again, we should distinguish between *distraction* and paradoxical (free-floating) attention. The former can be destructive to the clinical encounter or intervention, where the latter is essential.

The place of metaphor

In previous chapters, I have linked metacognition, meta-affect, and meta-sensing with heightened use of embodied metaphor (specifically, innovation, intensity, and quality). What confuses the modes of transitive attention I discuss above, and why medical work must always be considered as ambiguous, even paradoxical, and sometimes contradictory, is the insistence of biomedicine to reduce patients to instrumental information. As noted throughout my chapters, this is expressed as technical jargon, in the face of vernacular language that expresses conditions through metaphor. This matters because the production of metaphor gives meaning to patient's symptoms and conditions, where reduction to technical terms reduces patients to information – the latter convenient for medicine as an intra-cultural way of exchanging information, but inconvenient for patients whose meanings are reduced to notations. Below is an illustrative case study from the *New England Journal of Medicine* (Pipito and Cascio 2023):

> A 75-year-old woman presented to the infectious diseases clinic with a 10-day history of painful lesions on the right hand and forearm. The nodules had first appeared on the back of her hand at the site of a thorn puncture she had sustained while gardening. The lesions had spread up

> the hand along a red streak and then had appeared on the forearm. Physical examination was notable for a serpentine array of firm, tender nodules on the dorsum of the right hand with overlying erythema but no drainage. On the dorsal side of the right forearm, there were two tender, erythematous nodules, with overlying ulceration of the more proximal one. Lymphadenopathy was noted in the right axilla. An aspiration of the hand lesion was performed. Bacterial culture of the aspirate grew filamentous, gram-positive, acid-fast branching rods that were subsequently identified as *Nocardia brasiliensis*. A diagnosis of sporotrichoid nodular lymphangitis was made. … After a course of trimethoprim–sulfamethoxazole, the lesions resolved.

The case study begins in the vernacular – there are no technical descriptors up to the description of the thorn puncture 'sustained while gardening'. The next sentence in the account contains a medical term – 'lesions' – that would not be used by the patient, and then a spectacular metaphor: 'along a red streak' that could readily be shared with a patient for effect. The following sentence has a beautiful metaphor – 'serpentine array' of nodules – that is specific to medical culture. After that, the descriptor (after all, it was written for physicians in a leading medical journal) becomes intensively technical, where the patient is lost to the biomedical jargon. Metaphor production is quashed. Information replaces meaning (where such information of course has meaning within technical-medical culture). We are pleased to hear that 'the lesions resolved' after treatment. We had also hoped for something humane focused on the person and not the isolated symptom (a typical objectification) like: 'the patient was cured, emerged unblemished, and felt well'. The attentional device here is specific to the genre of the 'case study' of course, focused upon symptom. But in the process, transitive attention is reduced to the instrumental. Meaning is reduced to information.

Language, particularly where metaphor operates and is used innovatively, focuses the five ways of transitive attention described above, through four main modes in Alford's scheme:

1. <u>As 'desire'</u>. This describes focused clinical work. There is an object of interest – the patient, the clinical team, a symptom, paperwork, a theory, research data, a test result, an image, a pharmaceutical – that the physician makes sense of. There is either driven interest or lack of interest.
2. <u>As 'contemplation'</u>. Here, the patient, colleague, artefacts, modes of practice, culture, and so forth become objects of contemplation, good or bad. There is nothing to be done but contemplation itself. This may result in 'desire' (above), a need to act. A surprisingly large number of physicians contemplate leaving the profession because of overwork, anxiety, and potential burnout, but numbers dwindle where this morphs into actual 'desire'. Contemplation is attentive yearning; desire is attentive doing, however destructive.

3 As 'recollection'. This is desire for a departed object – a loved one, a patient now dead, a cherished colleague who has left medicine, a burning interest now waning or extinguished. The focal object is in memory, not in the flesh.
4 As 'imagination'. Here, the object of attention is one of a wish-fulfilment, an 'as if'. This is attending to objects of the mind as fantasies. Perhaps the most common example is misdiagnosis through premature closure.

Attention must have closure

Physicians, without being conscious of the kinds of classifications that I have described based on Alford's meticulous exploration of differing kinds of poetic attention, are characterised by their transitive attention capabilities – how they focus on objects. Their work, after all, is attending to patients, being in attendance (hence 'attending physician'). They should be expert at close noticing (perception) and witnessing (ethical–professional care). Physicians also, as noted earlier, attend to their colleagues, and to artefacts such as computers, instruments, test results, and so forth. Their judgements are informed by biomedical science, to which they must always be attentive as forms of explanation. Better physicians are, arguably, meta-attentive, that means balancing expert close attention (vigilance) and free-floating attention (noticing of peripheral factors, listening to the tone of patients' stories) for accurate diagnoses, and as prophylactic against premature closure as misdiagnosis. But attention must have forms of limitation and closure, lest the physician is swamped. Knowing how to turn attention off (Alford describes this as forms of intransitive attention, objectless or object-free – rather than focused – attention) is as important as cultivating active attention. Passive attention is cultivated in relaxation and forced into being in exhaustion and burnout.

There are ironies in both the spontaneous appearance and the cultivated learning of all forms of attention. First, physicians are poor at self-attention, as a basis to self-care. While structural factors such as lack of personnel and resources are a major factor in physician exhaustion, stress, and burnout, another factor is lack of self-care. Attention to the other must include meta-attention to oneself, a fundamental rule of psychotherapeutic acumen (where supervision guarantees dedicated professional attention to this issue). As I have insisted in previous chapters, medical students should learn basic psychotherapeutic acumen early in their careers, backed up by trustworthy and durable mentorship, such as managing transference and resistance effects with patients and colleagues. Such acumen should also embrace self-care as a meta-attentive device so that catharsis does not swamp or engulf the physician, and insight can emerge from catharsis.

Physicians again must understand and be mindful of the meta-attentions of intransitive attention, or objectless attention. This is circulating attention in free play that can readily be swamped by affect to produce anxiety, panic, emotional draining, melancholia, depression, and suicidal ideation in the absence of work, or in echoic contemplation. Or it can be a radical draining of affect so that the physician feels numb, affectless, and emotionally insulated.

Physicians on the edge of burnout are at the other end of the 'meta' scale, overwhelmed such that they are numbed. Symptoms typically include lack of vigilance and resignation during flurries of activity; but excessive emotional insulation can also lead to showing apparent boredom and idleness. The scope of vigilant attention is reduced, free-floating attention floats away into apparent boredom, trivial objects of attention come into play, and time and space seem to collapse into the moment that is an affectless bubble. The person seems overly self-concerned, while, paradoxically, the self seems to have simultaneously departed. Fatigue is evident, habitual behaviour paramount – as in the Zen paradox of engaging as non-engagement.

Educating transitive attention

The conditions of possibility for educating transitive attention amongst medical students and physicians include a prior valuing of the aesthetic qualities of medical work beyond the dominant instrumental. Alford's anatomising of the 'how' of attention again forms a potential pedagogy for learning metacognition. That medical students will learn to attend to patients, to symptoms, to colleagues, and to instrumentation that mediates care and cure is not in doubt. How well this is done – the quality, intensity, depth, and range of a medical education – is another matter. Will understanding of, and insight into, forms of attention be picked up from an old-style apprenticeship of 'watch and learn', or will there be a more considered approach of a cyclical process of (a) theoretical modelling, (b) briefing, (c) work experience, (d) debriefing, and (e) reviewing and refining models?

While educating attention has critical instrumental dimensions, such as organisational efficiency and patient safety, let us also consider the ethical and aesthetic dimensions to a clinician's work. Doctors are more likely to be effective not only when they form good clinical judgements, but also when they form rewarding therapeutic alliances with patients. Both require sophisticated levels of attention that follow the contours of Alford's 'poetic attention'. This is one of the reasons why the medical humanities, as arts and humanities interventions through the media of metaphor, are worthy of inclusion in a medicine curriculum. They educate and form sensibilities as differing kinds of attention. Metaphors are attention developers and tuners.

'Meta' thinking is to think with, or through, metaphors. And spatial metaphors are the most used (Lakoff and Johnson 1980). Space and place, the key physical elements of our orientation, become linguistically enriched through metaphor use. For example, during the height of the global COVID-19 crisis, it was common to talk about 'containing' the 'spread' of the virus, in 'closing off' spaces or human contacts (Kremer and Felgenhauer 2022). In diagnosis, the doctor looks for a literal lesion (a structural change or a wound) through hands-on investigation or imaging (a physiological or biochemical change, or an interior structural change). But this becomes meta where diagnostic thinking or clinical reasoning employs metaphor: 'we'll need to take blood tests **further down the line**', 'we have no idea how quickly the cancer will **spread**', 'can you give me some idea of the **level** of pain you are suffering?' Such metaphors are common in mental health scenarios: 'is the anxiety **pressing**?', 'what is your **ideal body shape**?'; and in prescribing, where, despite exact dosage on the package, the doctor says, 'we can give you **a little something** to help with that, to **lift** your mood'.

The use of metaphor shifts cognition from the literal (known) to the abstract (unknown). The world is, as it were, constructed as we go along where we use metaphor strategies. We are already shaping sensibility and consciousness through the meta, as thinking, or imagining, more deeply. Metacognition as a *dis*placed cognition signifies an unconscious, tacit, or implicit element to cognition that provides an extra layer or supplement. This is commonly called intuition, but that has become a tainted word, implying sloppy guesswork. Intuition, however, is what experts mostly rely on in clinical reasoning – again, commonly called Type 1 reasoning in the dual processing model, where Type 2 is logical, rational, and deliberative thinking, as explored earlier.

New thinking about dual process cognition (De Neys 2022) has modified the original distinction between Type 1 (intuitive, synthetic) and Type 2 (logical, analytical, deliberative) reasoning as too definite. This mirrors suspicion in cognitive psychology circles about a clear distinction between endogenous and exogenous forms of attention. Even where an intuitive processing that may lead to a misjudgement or error occurs, deliberation is seen to occur within intuitive thinking. De Neys (2022) suggests that intuition occurs across a spectrum where one end is pure and the other is a 'logical intuition'. Further, in supposed logical, rational judgements, intuitive elements can be present, particularly where decisions are made when information presented is restricted or partial.

Such cognitive psychology models have been developed from laboratory-based decision-making scenarios. Real-life clinical decision-making is made more complex by the presence of feeling (affect), and the quality and of sensing or perception. The meta of 'sense-making' from sensory information is then tinged or biased by feelings and values that preform how and what we sense. Into this mix we must add memory (short and long term) and 'predictive processing' or judging potential outcomes of actions. As we have seen, hovering above this complex of activity is a fluid, free-floating attention that decides where focus shall rest. This acts as a metacognitive scanner. Should this attention be swamped, for example, by acute focus on an immediate issue, or an overwhelming catharsis or emotional response, then effective decision-making itself can be compromised. Attention is the net that catches all the fish of cognition and feeling. It is imperative that we give it full attention and particulate expression.

References

Alford L. 2020. *Forms of Poetic Attention*. New York, NY: Columbia University Press.

Allard J, Wyatt J, Bleakley A, Blair G. 2011. 'Do you really need to ask me that now?': a self-audit of interruptions to the 'shop floor' practice of an emergency physician. *BMJ Emergency Medicine Journal*. 29: 872–6.

Andersson E, McPhearson T. 2018. Making sense of biodiversity: The affordances of systems ecology. *Frontiers in Psychology*. 04 May 2018/*Sec. Environmental Psychology*. 9. Available at: www.frontiersin.org/articles/10.3389/fpsyg.2018.00594/full#:~:text=Affordances%20are%20defined%20in%20this,mean%20functionally%20meaningful%20whole%20situations Last accessed: 12/01/2024.

Bleakley A. 2017. *Thinking with Metaphors in Medicine: The State of the Art*. Abingdon: Routledge.

Bleakley A. 2020. *Educating Doctors' Senses Through the Medical Humanities: 'How Do I Look?'* Abingdon: Routledge.

Bleakley A, Allard J, Hobbs A. 2013. 'Achieving ensemble': communication in orthopaedic surgical teams and the development of situation awareness – an observational study using live videotaped examples. *Advances in Health Sciences Education: Theory and Practice*. 18: 33–56.

Bleakley A, Bligh J, Browne J. 2011. *Medical Education for the Future: Identity, Power and Location*. Dordrecht: Springer.

Bleakley A, Marshall RJ. 2017. *Rejuvenating Medical Education: Seeking Help from Homer*. Newcastle: Cambridge Scholars.

Bleakley A, Neilson S. 2021. *Poetry in the Clinic: Towards a Lyrical Medicine*. Abingdon: Routledge.

Bleakley A, Neilson S. 2022. As 'synapses' become 'protoplasmic kisses': Symmetry across clinical reasoning and poetry. *Medical Education*. 57: 233–42.

Bleakley A, Neilson S (eds.) 2024. *The Routledge Handbook of Medicine and Poetry*. Abingdon: Routledge.

Bohm D. 1980. *Wholeness and the Implicate Order*. London: Routledge.

Chen Y, Adler-Milstein J, Sinsky CA. 2022. Measuring and maximizing undivided attention in the context of electronic health records. *Applied Clinical Informatics*. 13: 774–7.

Clark A. 2016. *Surfing Uncertainty: Prediction, Action and The Embodied Mind*. Oxford: Oxford University Press.

Clark A. 2023. *The Experience Machine: How Our Minds Predict and Shape Reality*. Dublin: Allen Lane/Penguin.

De Neys W. 2022. Advancing theorizing about fast-and-slow thinking. *Behavioral and Brain Sciences*. 1: 68.

Gibson, JJ. 1966. *The Senses Considered as Perceptual Systems*. Boston, MA: Houghton Mifflin.

Groopman JE. 2007. *How Doctors Think*. Boston: Mass.: Houghton Mifflin.

Huxley A. 1962. *Island*. London: Chatto & Windus.

Kissler MJ, Kissler K, Burden M. 2021. Toward a medical "Ecology of Attention". *New England Journal of Medicine*. 384: 299 0150301.

Kissler MJ, Kissler K, Porter SC, et al. 2022. Concepts and metrics of clinician attention: a scoping review protocol. *BMJ Open*. 12: e052334.

Kremer D, Felgenhauer L. 2022. Reasoning COVID-19: the use of spatial metaphor in times of a crisis. *Palgrave Communications*. 9: 1–15.

Lakoff G, Johnson M. 1980. *Metaphors We Live By*. Chicago, IL: University of Chicago Press.

McLuhan M, McLuhan E. 1988. *The Laws of Media: The New Science*. Toronto: University of Toronto Press.

Polanyi M. 1965. The structure of consciousness. *Brain*. LXXXVIII: 799–810.
Polanyi M. 1966. *The Tacit Dimension*. Chicago, IL: University of Chicago Press.
Pipito L., Cascio A. 2023. Sporotrichoid Nodular Lymphangitis from Nocardia brasiliensis. *New England Journal of Medicine*. 388: 1701.

8 Perception: immaculate or illusory?

Whither then metacognition and metahumanities?

Quentin Eichbaum

Introduction

The focused uses of the senses are integral to medical practice as a basis to diagnostic work. First, one must closely notice expression of symptom whether this is perceived directly in or on the patient's body and its expressions and extrusions, or whether this is picked up indirectly through talk and non-verbal expression. Perception, however, is not contained by persons but is distributed across artefacts. Historically, the physician's sensorium affords vision, taste, smell, and touch (primarily percussion and palpation of the patient's body) that has long been extended through use of the stethoscope in auscultation (Bleakley 2020). In contemporary medicine, much of the perceptual-diagnostic work is "extended" – through laboratory testing of specimens and body scans or imaging (ultrasound, X-rays, MRI, and CT scans).

Learning to perceive, or focused education of the senses, within clinical contexts is a well-documented area in medical education. Here, I review background work on human perception that challenges the traditional ways in which medical students are socialised into clinical 'ways of seeing'. A revolution has occurred in cognition that creates an imperative for medical education to address the metacognitive, as this book soundly demonstrates. This begins with a review of perception's central place in metacognition, as an extended and situated cognition (see Chapters 5 and 10). This chapter offers a summary of recent work that demands curriculum reconceptualisation for medical students in the field of perception. The purpose of the chapter, however, is not to address the pedagogical issues in such a reconceptualisation, but to set out what needs to be known about perception prior to such educational applications.

The origin of our English 'perception' is the Latin *perceptio*, meaning 'receiving, or collecting'. This implies passivity. But perception is far from a passive process of reception. Perception is the interface between our inner and outer worlds. But just how permeable, malleable, or veridical this interface is remains uncertain. The notion of 'objective reality' has long been debated and is now mostly discredited, if not disproven. Humans perceive just a sliver of 'reality' (we can only see, hear, taste, and feel certain things) but even that sliver,

DOI: 10.4324/9781032687339-11

research now suggests, is selective. Moreover, mind and environment are in a two-way conversation: mind both 'reads' the world through perception and creates the world in the image of the perceiver – all in the interests of our biological survival, but sometimes, given the illusory/hallucinogenic ingredients of perception, creating risk for the perceiver.

In this chapter, given that humans are predominantly a visual species (Wilson 1988, 2014, 2017), I focus initially mostly on visual perception, examining the notion of 'objective reality' and the veridicality of perception, but later include also other kinds of perception and associated topics:

- How and where perceptions are processed in the brain (including predictive processing)
- The perception of self, other, and emotion
- How perceptions intersect with attention and cognitive 'traps' such as beliefs
- How perception aligns with the 'extended mind'
- The role of perception in creativity and imagination, including appreciation of beauty
- The pertinence of perception to medical education

My overarching concern is the quality of relationship between perception, reality, and consciousness that nestles at the core of our humanity. Starting from the position that perception is a participatory and predictive act and lies at the core of who we are and what we might become, the concepts I explore can provoke critical questions and conundrums that extend beyond the purview of traditional humanities and into the scope of an emerging metahumanities.

The imperfections of visual perception

Creationists see the human eye as something so perfect that it could only have been created by God, not by the unpredictable process of natural selection. Richard Dawkins (Dawkins and Ward 2006) deftly abolishes this argument by demonstrating how the human eye evolved from single photoreceptor cells in primitive organisms to viable organelles of cells with limited vision, and then to the complexities of the human eye. Moreover, as noted, the human eye is far from perfect but is a flawed organ. Light that should pass through the lens of the eye must first negotiate a gauntlet – a tangle of capillary blood vessels and interneurons – before it lands up almost by chance on distant receptors at the back of the retina. All vertebrates suffer from this structural flaw, suggesting that such an early evolutionary design investment was never corrected. Moreover, the mistake was not a 'necessary error' on the way up the evolutionary ladder because lowly cephalopods, such as the octopus and the squid, get things right with their photoreceptors situated in the front of the interneurons and blood vessels. Medical textbooks continue to erroneously depict the human eye in neat diagrams with a homunculus image of the outer world perfectly inverted on a screenlike retina, suggesting that we see the world objectively like a camera. This depiction of an exact image of the world being transmitted onto the retina is flawed and creates an erroneous understanding of human visual perception. As VS Ramachandran (2012) makes clear,

> as soon as light rays are converted into neural impulses at the back of your eye, it no longer makes sense to think of the visual information as being an image … . The brain creates symbolic descriptions … it does NOT recreate the original image.

Medical students, following their previous experience of biology, are often unsettled to learn that we do not visually perceive the world 'objectively' like a camera, particularly where it challenges the 'objectivity' of their hard-learned knowledge. But this is an important step in making them aware, with humility, of human fallibility – and, as a knock-on effect, recognising the potential for medical error. Metahumanities informed by science would dispel such views of immaculate perception as an example of a wider shift in imagination. For example, in the Vanderbilt Colloquium medical humanities course we have sessions on 'How we Perceive', 'Being Wrong', and 'How We Make Mistakes', where we discuss such imperfections of human perception as a lead-in to topics on medical error, human fallibility, and humility (Eichbaum 2014).

Are the limits of perception the limits to reality?

We may 'pity' the proverbial goldfish with its myopic water-bowl view of reality, yet in the cosmic scheme of things, the human view of reality is similarly cropped. We may think of our perceptions as objective, unconstrained, a 'perfect rendition of the raw incoming signal' (Clark 2023), but that view is flawed. There is 'no immaculate perception' (Siegel 2007). Yet we continue to believe that what we perceive is reality, not individually constrained, but the ultimate 'real reality'. The philosopher Arthur Schopenhauer (Jacquette, 2015) astutely observed that 'Each man believes that the limits of his perception are the limits of reality'.

Philosophers and scientists have struggled for centuries with the question of objective reality, and the extent to which our perceptions truthfully perceive that reality – the 'veridicality of perception' (McGilchrist 2021). If the humanities are (at least in part) about seeking truth, then perception affords a problematic base for experience and subsequent judgement if what we perceive is illusory. Stephen Palmer (1999) bluntly states that 'evolutionarily speaking, visual perception is useful only if it is reasonably accurate', while Zygmont Pizlo (2014) suggests that 'veridicality is an essential characteristic of perception and cognition. It is essential. Perception and cognition without veridicality would be like physics without the conservation laws'. Pizlo (2014) further argues that our perceptions must be veridical because evolution has shaped our sensory systems to perceive the outside world accurately to enhance our survival. Jack Loomis and colleagues (1992) agree that there are similarities between our perceptions and objective reality but insist that our perceptions can also have systematic errors, particularly regarding perceived shapes. The veridicality of visual perception is then strongly contested. Stephen Pinker (1997) contends that 'our minds evolved by natural selection to solve problems that were life and death matters to our ancestry not to commune with … correctness'.

Addressing such veridicality head on, David Marr (1982), at the time a young researcher at the Massachusetts Institute of Technology, argued that natural selection can favour a subjective perception that does not represent objective reality provided it has an adaptive advantage and that natural selection would favour veridical perception as organisms become more complex. All that may be needed 'is sufficient information … to survive'. Thus Marr (1982) argued that 'usually our perceptual processing does run correctly (it delivers a true description of what is there)'. This view of visual perception representing objective reality has, however, been contested by researchers such as Donald Hoffman and Andy Clark, as detailed below.

Donald Hoffmann: the case against reality

Donald Hoffman (2019) argues that our perceptions are 'illusory' – 'objective reality' does not 'exist' and evolution has made compromises in how and what we perceive to enhance our survival. Indeed, truth, in Hoffman's view, is fundamentality irrelevant to evolution and natural selection. He advances the Fitness-Beats-Truth (FBT) theorem that sees natural selection as favouring perceptions that disregard the 'truth' and instead score evolutionary fitness points. Hoffman's (2019) 'interface theory of perception' (ITP) argues that perception is not a direct reflection of objective reality, but rather a user interface that our brains construct to help us to navigate and to survive in the world, where, 'our perceptions are more like a simplified and useful representation of the world, rather than an accurate depiction of the objective reality'. Hoffman suggests three conceptions of veridical perception: *omniscient realism* in which we 'see all of reality as it really is'; *naive realism* in which we see 'some, but not all, of reality as it is'; and *critical realism* in which the structure of our perceptions preserves some of the structure of reality (Hoffman 2019). Of these, he suggests that *critical realism* likely best aligns with natural selection and evolution and with the FBT theorem. He further advances his model of the Perceive–Decide–Act (PDA) loop to explain how perception is linked to our actions and survival in the world. Natural selection moulds this PDA loop such that experiences steer actions that enhance survival.

The PDA loop and FBT theorem both align with the notion that perception is bidirectional and participatory in that 'each time an agent acts on the world, it changes the state of the world, and reaps a fitness reward (or punishment)'.

Andy Clark: predictive processing

Challenging passive models of perception, Andy Clark (2023) presents another, more optimistic, view on the nature of the relationship between our minds, perception, and reality – a theory he terms 'predictive processing', where

> Nothing we do or experience ... is untouched by our expectations. Instead, there's a constant give-and take in which what we experience reflects not just what the world is currently telling us, but what we – consciously or unconsciously – were expecting it to be telling us.

This is a transactional as well as predictive model of perception.

Traditional views of perception describe a 'bottom-up' process with sensations in the outer word impinging on our sensory organs and causing nerve signals to flow 'inwards' and 'upwards' to the brain where 'objective reality' is ultimately deciphered (Marr 2010). In contrast, in the 'top-down' view, perceptions do not come from outside-in and move from the bottom up to the brain, but move primarily from the top down, or inside (mind and body) to out. Our experiences are '"built as predictions", or "best guesses," about the causes of sensory signals' (Seth 2021). Sensory signals from the outer world still enter the brain but serve mostly as 'prediction errors' to be minimised or suppressed by adjusting the brain's top-down predictions (Seth 2021; Clark 2023). Predictive processing suggests that: 'what we actually perceive is a top-down, inside-out neuronal fantasy that is reined in by reality, not a transparent window onto whatever that reality may be' (Seth 2021). 'Reality' is forged from process and not 'given' as content.

This view challenges the widely accepted views of perception in the humanities, providing a challenging ground for metahumanities to consider. To be sure, modern arts, especially the visual arts, have challenged the 'bottom-up' passive view of perception and recognised a participatory role of the perceiver. Thus the 'beholder's share' view of perception popularised by Ernst Gombrich (1961) emphasises the participatory role of the 'beholder'/perceiver in 'perceiving' and ultimately 'completing' a work of art.

In contrast to Hoffman's somewhat bleak 'case against reality', Clark presents a positive aspect of predictive processing by arguing that we can 'hack the predictive mind' by changing our behaviours and practices, reframing our experiences through use of language, taking advantage of scientific advances such as the placebo effect (a consequence of expectations arising from a predictive brain) and through specific drugs (including psychedelics). The optimistic view of predictive processing re-centres language, through which humanities thrive via literature, poetry, and scholarship. Concurrently, social/behavioural science-humanities can modify and adapt behaviours and change our experience of Hoffman's illusory 'drab universe'.

Perception in the left and right hemispheres of the brain

How are perceptions processed in the brain? How do the brain hemispheres process perceptions? Understanding what 'happens' to perceptions in the left and right brain hemispheres may provide further insights into the nature of perception. Iain McGilchrist (2021, 2024) has written about respective capacities of the left and right brain hemispheres and how they contribute to perception, including the division of perception tasks between the hemispheres. The left brain/right brain divide remains a topic of some controversy centring mostly around how distinctively separate the hemispheres are in their functions, or whether they work 'seamlessly together' as Stephen Kosslyn and colleagues contend (Kosslyn and Miller 2013). McGilchrist (2021) argues that since we are not aware in our 'moment to moment' living of the 'different takes of the world that each hemisphere makes possible', the hemispheres appear to function seamlessly together from the vantage of individual experience. The connection between the hemispheres via the corpus callosum allows ready exchange of activity between them. But while they are 'massively interconnected', as McGilchrist notes, and compelled to cooperate, they also 'need to be able to function to a degree independently'. There appears to be some overlap and validity to both Kosslyn's and McGilchrist's arguments. Here, I will explore McGilchrist's substantiated views on distinctive functions of the left and right brain hemispheres as I believe they offer intriguing insights into perception.

The right brain is superior at pre-cognitive components of vision, at visual (hyper)acuity, pattern recognition, and at perceptual grouping and is superior in mental rotation and thinking in three dimensions. The right hemisphere is also superior at dealing with incomplete information as well as with ambiguity and uncertainty. The latter capacities are arguably of particular relevance to the humanities if a salient role of the arts and humanities lies in dealing with ambiguity and uncertainty – to 'create puzzlement and discomfort … ruffle feathers and upset preconceptions' (Bleakley 2017). McGilchrist (2021) also argues that

> the left hemisphere is less reliable in perceptual interpretation of experience, which goes with its being more likely to jump to conclusions, getting it right when the stimulus is predictable, but wrong when it is not; the right hemisphere is more cautious, and more reliable in the long run.

The left hemisphere is also less attuned to imagery and is more abstract and conceptual, generalised, and theoretical. According to Harvard neuroscientist Stephen Kosslyn (1987), the right hemisphere produces 'vivid, in-context, external images' whereas the left hemisphere produces primarily 'non-vivid, out-of-context, internal images'. This suggests that the right hemisphere is more deeply engaged with processing imagery input from the outer world whereas the left hemisphere has a propensity towards abstract image processing.

McGilchrist (2021, 2024) argues that our experience of the world helps to shape our brain, but our brain also shapes the world. Moreover, he suggests that the balance between the brain hemispheres even over the relatively short period of the last 500 years or so has been a swing towards the left hemisphere processing.

His claims are nuanced and are difficult to measure biologically, but align with what we now know about neuroplasticity (Doidge 2007) and the adage 'use it or lose it'. McGilchrist says the trends are culturally noticeable with shifts towards abstraction and certainty (at least in Western culture and science) and away from ambiguity and uncertainty. Metahumanities may thus serve a salutary purpose in drawing us back towards activities of the right brain that is 'more embedded in the world and its uncertainties and ambiguities' compared with left brain that is 'intrinsically abstracted from the world ... less "in touch"' (McGilchrist 2021).

McGilchrist (2021) draws attention to other differences between the left and right hemispheres regarding auditory, tactile, and global perceptions. He poses the central question: 'How veridical is the perception of either hemisphere?' How in touch with reality is each hemisphere? He asks what happens when the right hemisphere is 'no longer available to correct the left hemisphere's lack of grasp of perceptual reality?' His answer is: 'In a word, pandemonium'. Studies further show that right brain lesions more seriously alter perception with anomalies in shape, size, and three-dimensionality leading to illusions and hallucinations and a disrupted sense of reality (Cutting 2012).

Studies on brain hemispheric pathologies suggest that the boundaries of the self (Devinsky 2000) and 'coherence of the self over time' (McGilchrist 2021) are maintained predominantly by the right hemisphere. Even if both hemispheres contribute, it seems that the 'objectified self, and the self as expression of will' is dependent on the left hemisphere, whereas the 'experiential self, the self in the present moment, the self sensing what is happening in one's thoughts, feelings and body state, without purpose or goal' is more widely associated with the right hemisphere (McGilchrist 2021). Of relevance to the notion of embodied cognition (Chapters 5 and 10), the right hemisphere is also more specialised for perception of the body and has connections with the limbic system that mediates between emotions and higher cognitive functions (McGilchrist 2021).

Which of the two hemispheres better conceives the truth? McGilchrist (McGilchrist 2021) argues that the left hemisphere sees the world and the nature of truth 'as a thing, certain. fixed, and independent of interaction with it (and) ... with the consistency of a representation'. The right hemisphere in contrast sees truth and experience 'as a process, always contextual, forever coming into being through our present interaction with the world ... constantly being tested against experience'. The right hemisphere sees 'truth' as relationship, reverberation, attunement, and engagement; the left hemisphere as perfect, precise, certain, factual, and representative. For the right hemisphere, truth is evolving. Of course, regardless of substantive grounding in brain function, such descriptors of 'truth' serve as powerful metaphors.

The arts and humanities would seem to have deep (but by no means exclusive) roots in the right hemisphere whereas the left brain is more analytical, and science dominated. As individuals, we may spend our working lives predominantly in the domain of one hemisphere (possibly leading to some neglect or even atrophy in the other hemisphere). Of interest, Charles Darwin reportedly lamented that his years as a scientist destroyed his previous enjoyment of literature, while Roger Sperry said: 'One gets the suspicion that 18 or so years of formal schooling in the sciences may functionally oblate the right hemisphere' (in McGilchrist 2021). Where physicist Erwin Schrödinger (1951) argued that science may be better at imparting the knowledge to answer the question 'Who are we?', McGilchrist insists that the broader scope of the right hemisphere ultimately allows it to take stock of reality for both sides of the brain. While the extent and effects of cortical hemispheric lateralisation remain contested, these studies on the different capacities of the left and right brain provide a compelling argument for bringing the sciences and humanities into closer proximity through metahumanities. This is a central theme of my chapter contributions to this volume.

Perception of self and others

Perception involves not just sensory input from the outer world but is also about how we perceive ourselves and others – that in turn influences how we perceive the world. Perception of self and of others, in influencing how we interact with one another, thus also affects how we survive and cooperate as a species (Flannery and Marcus 2012). Perceptions of self and others also likely has deep roots in our consciousness (Seth 2021). Central to such interpersonal perceptions is regulation of emotion, for interpersonal activity is both cognitive and affective in character. Regulation of such emotions requires a bidirectional participatory loop between inner emotional perception (e.g., from the limbic system and the enteric nervous system – the 'brain in the gut') and the world. Addressing and better understanding emotional regulation is relevant to metahumanities in an increasingly divisive conflict-torn world that seems to have lost its compass for emotional regulation, relationality, and civility. Medical students are educated into emotional insulation in the face of their impending exposure to sickness and death, traditionally through the ritual of cadaver dissection, so that emotional regulation is institutionally forged (by the medical culture). In other words, students' emotions are entrained.

Drew Westen (2008) draws attention to the fallacy of the emotionally regulated 'dispassionate mind' that has pervaded Western and other cultures – noting 'the vision of the mind that has captured the imagination of philosophers, cognitive scientists, economists, and political scientists since the 18th century'. This is 'a dispassionate mind – that makes decisions by weighing the evidence and reasoning to the most valid conclusions'. However, claims Westen (2008), this 'bears no relation to how the mind and brain actually work'. It may be that our efforts to educate for emotional insulation in medical students are misguided and fail to grasp the complexity of such a task that demands an education into meta-affect or conscious regulation of the emotions (see Chapters 3 and 12).

Our capacity for emotion perception is pertinent to metahumanities in shaping how we relate to one another and the level of our relational consciousness (see Chapter 12). For instance, perceptions are at the core of empathic accuracy which relies on appropriate interpretation of the emotions and the presumed experience of an 'other' in specific contexts (Hülür et al. 2016, Zaki et al. 2008). Riess (2010; Riess and Kraft-Todd 2014) has shown that a range of body signals influence empathic accuracy. Accurate perception of emotion determines how we navigate the world and interact with other individuals and groups, how effectively we function socially, and ultimately our emotional well-being (Ruffman et al. 2016).

In medical education, a possible reason for the well-documented phenomenon of empathy decline (and growing cynicism) in later-year medical students is (mis)educating for emotional insulation. We should, instead, be trying to educate for emotional sensitivity in such students. Lisa Feldman Barrett (2017) argues that we are not at all good at understanding how others feel and reading their minds even though we think we might be:

> Anytime you think you know how someone else feels, your confidence has nothing to do with actual knowledge. You're just having a moment of affective realism. … In the classical view of emotion, the responsibility is all on the perceiver's end because emotions are supposedly displayed universally. In a construction mindset, you also bear the responsibility to be a good sender.

Perceptions and emotions are also intimately connected through interoceptive signalling, where 'Many things that seem unrelated to emotion actually have a profound effect on how you feel, because of the porous boundary between the social and the physical' (Barrett 2017).

One way of improving communication is to be more finely attuned to our emotions. Studies have shown that individuals with less granular emotion perception (which can entail not finding the right words for emotions) are less able to regulate their emotions (Barrett 2017). Marc Brackett (2019) developed the 'Mood Meter' as a tool for developing emotional awareness and regulation. Colour coding is used to teach children (and adults) to identify their emotions more specifically ('granularly') to harness and communicate feelings. It has been effectively applied in schools across the United States to teach children emotional regulation. Given that medical students are faced with the contradiction that they are plunged into emotionally charged contexts from day one (traditionally through cadaver dissection as the primary way of learning anatomy) and must regulate (suppress) such emotional flux in clinical work, some kind of 'mood meter' would surely benefit medical pedagogy.

Gross and Feldman Barrett (2017) asked: 'When does a mental state become an emotion … or some other kind of mental state?' and are emotions caused by 'distinct and specific mental states'? If so, can they be acted on by other processes? People vary in the degree to which they believe an emotion is something that can be controlled and changed; in what they infer from their perceptions of another person's behaviour; in how responsible they feel for their behaviour; and even what kind of behaviour is considered tolerable or permissible. If our perceptions concerning emotional states are often wrong or just guesses, how then do we communicate effectively with one another (see Chapter 12)? Gross and Feldman Barrett (2011) suggest that, in the face of huge variability, we communicate through the brain's predictive machinery. Emotions are guided by predictions. This chimes with Andy Clark's (2023) overarching model of cognition as predictive processing, where activity is based on a feedback loop from a predictive brain to an environment. Clark suggests that, rather than being shaped by patterns of reinforcement following actions (as behaviourism suggests), we are constantly fine-tuning our actions by moving about the world in a predictive mode and changing our behaviours according to consequences. Clark's radical view is that we live micro seconds ahead of events in a world of predictions.

Much of our emotion predictive capacity resides in language. However, language is not just a passive transmitter of thoughts and emotions. It is rather more complex, multidimensional, and organic. As Lev Vygotsky (1965) said 'A word is a microcosm of human consciousness'. Words elicit different images and may evoke different emotions. George Lakoff (2008) notes that 'Language is the surface, not the soul, of the brain'. We are interpretive beings and language shapes our interpretations of our contexts and ourselves using metaphors, frames, narratives, and emotions. If language is a major vehicle through which we mediate our emotion predictions, then the humanities (working largely through language, embracing semiotics – signs and symbols) have a critical part to play in understanding emotion. Metahumanities would re-forge these links between language, the brain's prediction machinery, and emotions, and may just provide the framework for how we inhabit Andy Clark's split-second 'near future'. Why this is important to medical education and clinical practice is that so much of medicine is about thinking on one's feet as *anticipation* – not only emergency and intensive medicine and surgery where split-second decisions can mean a life is saved, but also 'slow' medicine – such as long-term contact with patients suffering from chronic physical and mental illnesses – will invite sudden insights and revelations.

Hyperindividualism and hyperconnectedness

Thus far, I have considered perception largely from the point of view of the individual, with a caveat introduced earlier that perception always occurs in a distributed context – first in relation to objects and artefacts, or the material world; second in relation to language, particularly the semiotics of emotional life; and third, in relation to others as social and cultural effects. Such individualism is a historical product of a Western/Northern hemisphere cultural milieu. David Brooks (2020) sees a major threat to the social fabric of Western society deriving from such hyperindividualism. We need, he insists, more relationalism, laying out his arguments in a 'Relational Manifesto'. Briefly, the hyperindividualism of our age inflates the self and disparages the collective; it is founded on an 'emancipatory' narrative of the heroic self-trying to break free from the 'stifling chains of society'; and rests on egotistic drives, consumerism, tribalism, and a meritocracy conditioned on individual achievement.

Relationalism, in contrast, sees society as a 'web of connections', measuring the quality of one's life by the quality of relationships and service to others (Brooks 2020). It is a way of life rather than just a system of ideas but is not shaped by individual achievement. Rather, it is based on a moral ecology of caring and relational empathy (Eichbaum et al. 2023). Relationalism does not ignore the individual but balances the individual with the collective – or is ecological rather than ego-logical in being based on commitment to others, community, and global conditions (Eichbaum et al. 2023). There may be a neural substrate for this. The discovery of mirror neurons in the 1990s by Giacomo Rizzolatti (Rizzolatti and Sinigaglia 2008) demonstrated that we may act predominantly as cooperative agents within a social group rather than independently and individually. The potential connectivity within the brain and between brains makes individualism look like an evolutionary aberration. As Heidi Ravven (2013) says, 'We are internally connected and wired together'. But, continues Ravven, this is both 'for good and for bad'. Issues of cultural values, morality, politics, religion, and taste disturb the potential harmony of such connections. Conflict is as common as collaboration – usually a fight over identity, territory, or capital. The social and relational roots of our human agency drive and mould our responsibility as individuals, not vice versa. We are victims of social connectedness as well as benefitting from such webs. Again, evidence from mirror neuron research involving shared values (and then emotions) suggests that as 'sociality is our immediate default state', 'personal individuality is an unusual achievement' (Ravven 2013).

Medicine as an institution has, historically, followed such a hierarchical template of passive hyper-connectedness. Recently, however, three factors are shaping medical culture as a more democratic, inclusive institution: more women than men entering medicine, the transfer of patient-centred principles from client-centred psychotherapy, and the patient safety movement demanding quality inter-professional teamwork. These cultural transformations literally shape perceptions: how we see and what we see as social products.

On the positive side, intense sociality has enabled the transmission of traditions and cultures and is likely sustained largely through language. However – and herein lies the rub – our social cooperativity (and empathy) is, as already noted above, a double-edged sword as Ravven (2013) suggests:

> The central moral problem of human beings is not how to get individuals to care about each other and about the common welfare ... but rather the human tendency to fanatic belonging and loyalty to the group ... . And it's unfortunate concomitant, the disavowal of personal responsibility for the group's actions. Empathy and joint action while sounding wonderfully moral, offer a double-edged sword.

Marco Iacoboni (2009) argues that the level of activity in an individual's mirror neuron system in a specific context is an indication of that person's 'identification and affiliation with other people in that context'. Mirror neurons, Iacoboni (2009) argues, 'seemed to create some form of intimacy between self and other' that further creates our sense of belonging as affiliations with specific social groups usually more like us. Similarity and familiarity appear to create higher levels of activity in mirror neurons – or as Heidi Ravven (2013) put is: 'The "selfier" the other, the more it moves us'. Emmanuel Levinas (2000), with the Holocaust in mind, asks how we might identify with the Other who is our enemy, oppressor, or most despicable to us. Levinas suggests, uncomfortably, that it is only with respect to this Other that a self is constructed. The self is known in the mirror of the Other. For medicine, the uncomfortable Other is the patient a doctor least wishes to treat but has a professional–moral duty to do so. How then will that doctor's perception be constructed in that moment of extraordinary dilemma? This is a meta-perception, meta-affect, and metahumanities dilemma.

In summary of this section, a challenge for metahumanities may therefore lie in socially and scientifically deconstructing the countervailing forces of both hyperindividualism and hyper-connectedness to help us navigate meaningful tensive paths in our lives. Medical culture must adopt a hyper-critical, self-investigative position to examine its own perceptual constructs as these affect patient care and safety. We examine numerous such hyper-critical and reflexive positions throughout this book.

Beliefs: evidence and inference

How we learn is grounded in how we perceive, and how we act as healthcare practitioners and educators is grounded in literal and figurative perceptions. In turn, perceptions are embedded in and influenced by beliefs. I have established that we do not perceive an objective world of facts, but rather an illusory world interpreted by our perceptions (Seth 2021, Hoffman 2019). Nietzsche, a major catalyst of modern relativism, said: 'There are no facts, only interpretations'. George Lakoff (2008) argues that we are interpretive beings who see the world through cognitive frames that are a limited number of complexes of embodied metaphors (such as spatial and temporal). Such frames both filter and frame our perceptions and are among the 'cognitive structures we think with' (Lakoff 2008). We filter our experiences through interpretative frames such as favoured narratives embedded in historical and cultural frames. Cognitive frames have high emotional valence, are personally owned, and are part of how we perceive ourselves and others.

Susanna Siegel (Siegel 2016) argues that conscious visual perception includes not only complex physical properties such as shape, light, colour, and movement, but also causal characteristics like the properties of objects such as those of a bicycle – as well as desires, fears, and beliefs. She argues that our perceptual experiences can be rational or irrational and that perception is not just an input portal to rational beliefs. Further, 'if beliefs could influence your experiences, how could your experience go on to strengthen those beliefs?' (Siegel 2016). Beliefs are a major 'contaminant' of perception. Gary Marcus (2009) suggests that beliefs are products of memory, inference, and perception in interaction:

> … belief is haphazard, scarred by evolution and contaminated by emotions, moods, desires, goals, and simple self-interest – and surprisingly vulnerable to the idiosyncrasies of memory … . [E}very belief passes through the unpredictable filter of contextual memory. Either we directly recall a belief that we formed earlier, or we calculate what we believe based on whatever memories we happen to bring to mind.

Moreover, inferences are drawn from these fraught beliefs. During human evolution, beliefs and inferences became richly intertwined. Marcus (2009) sees this as a major design flaw in human cognition:

> In a system that was superlatively well-engineered, belief and the process of drawing inferences (which soon become beliefs) would be separate, with an iron wall between them; we would be able to distinguish what we had direct evidence for from what we had merely inferred.

Inversions of cognitive processes can result in cognitive dissonance or psychological discomfort when beliefs are challenged by evidence, leading to biases such as confirmation bias (when we accept evidence that confirms our beliefs).

While Marcus's point is taken, we see in contemporary life that the 'iron wall' between 'direct evidence' and inference is in fact a soft filter. (Thus, we have the strange world of 'alternative facts' introduced by the Donald Trump phenomenon and his ardent followers who also believe he is doing 'God's work' on earth and perceive him as a Christ-like figure being persecuted by Democrats. This also replays the standing debate between belief and faith vs science and evidence.) This interplay between values/beliefs and facts is central to perception in medical work, where, for instance, physicians are prone to interpret scientific evidence about best practices through the lens of their own professional values and beliefs.

Ravven (2013) suggests that 'perception follows belief rather than vice versa', and Tavris and Aronson (Tavris and Aronson 2007) more pithily insist that 'believing is seeing'. This jolts expectations that perception is immaculate or equates to an unfiltered truth. This again has important consequences for medical education. For example, dominant models and discourses of how physicians think, or models of clinical reasoning, including accounts of bias in such reasoning, are in fact biased themselves. This is because such dominant models have been developed largely within the discipline of psychology based on the behaviour of individuals. Thus, our perception of the ways that doctors reason has been shaped by belief as well as science, as such individualistic models eschew the social-collaborative and the extended mind, as discussed in the following section.

Perception and the extended mind

Moving from a passive-receptive, to an active sensation-seeking sensorium, McGilchrist (2021) says: 'Perception is the act whereby we reach out from our cage of mental constructs to taste, smell, touch, hear and see the living world'. Instead of the sense organs (or the sensorium as a system) as passive recipient of input, McGilchrist describes active seeking-out of sensation. As we think about this, though, it does not seem so strange. Piaget describes children passively assimilating the world, but also actively accommodating to it. And we have noted Andy Clark's model of cognitive extension – actively 'living into' the world, not just receiving events, but both predicting and creating them. Over 50 years ago, Eleanor Gibson (1969), the partner of James J Gibson, the father of 'ecological psychology' and champion of 'affordance theory', concluded from her observations of children's perception that 'Perceptual learning is not passive absorption, but an active process, in the sense that exploring and searching for perception itself is active. We do not just see, we look; we do not just hear, we listen'. Of course, as the Gibsons showed, perception is a social process in which assimilation and accommodation are negotiated through social and cultural exchanges. Many of these are coded as habits while others break habits to develop innovations in the way we perceive. The arts and humanities trade in such innovations, creating new 'ways of seeing' (Gibson 1969).

As I discuss in Chapters 5 and 10, cognition extends 'beyond the skin and skull' into the world (called the 'extended mind' or 'thinking outside the brain') through situated, embodied, and distributed thinking (see also Chapters 1 and 2). Embodied cognition highlights perception as mediated not just through the brain, but also through the body (and as embodied metaphor in language). Perception is not received as self-removed input from the external environment but is itself in interaction with bodily relationships. James and Eleanor Gibson, again, showed how perception is shaped by interaction with things such that we do not see objects and events *per se* but instead there are 'affordances that make possible and facilitate certain actions' (Gibson 1950). Affordances describe opportunities for action elicited by objects and events – for instance, stairs afford stepping, a door handle affords grasping, a suffering patient affords empathy. We perceive the world, according to Gibson (1950), 'through an automatic filter of affordances'.

If we cannot separate our perceptions of the world from our actions, can we assume the moral agency for understanding our actions from a removed perspective in an objective, independent, and rational manner? Perception, action, cognition, and emotion are necessarily interwoven. Our relationship to the world is that of both participant and creator. This seeming compromise of moral agency presents a conundrum for metahumanities – a challenge that can only be addressed through a multidimensional approach drawing not only on ethics, but also the social and biological sciences.

As we have seen, Andy Clark (2023) describes his idea of the predictive brain where 'experience is shaped by the flow of predictions … not just what is coming in from the outside world, but what our brain expected to be coming in'.

The predictive brain, Clark (2023) argues, presents a path towards regaining agency by allowing us 'to take control of our own experiences … to hack our predictive minds', for instance through 'self-directed language (for example in practices of self-affirmation) … engaging in talk-therapy … appreciating the power of ceremony and ritual … [and] the deliberate use of placebos'. Each of these is a meta-element that raises the tenor of everyday life into a higher register. Perception here is not naïve and passive, but educated and active. Such perceptual agency is described by Clark (2023) as 'perception-action loops'. He notes that this notion was 'left dangling' in his seminal 1990 article with David Chalmers *The Extended Mind* (Clark and Chalmers 1998). He calls this 'The Recruitment Puzzle': engaging the question of how the brain manages to recruit, activate, or exploit on the spot at the right time the right mix of problem-solving resources (internal and external) to yield 'an acceptable result with a minimum of effort' (Clark 2023). Mastery of predictive processing through pedagogic technique is Clark's (2023) own version of metacognition, meta-affect, and metahumanities,

> that explain and make possible the looping encounters that build extended minds … that constantly estimate the extent to which taking actions … will reliably reduce uncertainty in ways that help us approach our goals … by estimating which actions and policies best resolve key uncertainties and hence reduce the distance between our 'optimistic predictions'… and our current state.

The predictive brain resolves the recruitment puzzle not only through brain-bound cognition but via the extended mind that involves 'a mixture of biological and non-biological resources' that go beyond the 'barriers of skin and skull' (Clark 2023).

Jaak Panksepp (Panksepp and Panksepp 2000) stresses the entangled roles of perception and action in how the brain interacts with the world to influence such perception. This view is anticipated by Susan Hurley (1998) who argues that action is not attributable to the individual alone, but is distributed between mind, body, and world. We do not have sensory faculties that just input data from the world into the brain but rather 'we live in extended worlds' that are 'reachable' rather than 'represented' or 'depicted'. Hurley (1998) rejects the computer 'input–output' model of perception and cognition, where 'Action is no more pure output than perception is pure input'. Perception is interactive as 'environments, including linguistic environments, transform and reflect outputs from the human organism.' There are 'no sharp causal boundaries either between mind and world or between perception and action'. Linearity must give way to complexity.

But complexity does not equate with chaos (although it may operate close to chaos). Discussing Hurley's work, Heidi Ravven (2013) insists that what the human brain encounters is 'not an unstructured arena of chaotic raw data but [a world] (pre)-structured by human practices, linguistic meanings, institutions, histories, cultures, and nature itself'. Here again, metahumanities come into play.

The brain does not passively perceive 'raw data' like a camera, but experiences a structured world already filled with 'human practices, linguistic meanings, institutions, histories, cultures' (2013). The role of metahumanities is then surely to map, interpret, and then deconstruct such a 'pre-structured' world to afford innovations. This is surely the creative evolutionary path. Our biological evolution has long been superseded by cultural effects.

Perception, attention, and creativity

I have outlined how models of perception have changed from the passive to the active and interactive, and how minds shape worlds as worlds shape minds. We might think of the visual perceptual process (our focus here) as sandwiched between attention (see Chapter 7) and applied imagination or creativity (Alan Bleakley [2015, chap. 5] discusses 10 types of creativities). Our perceptions are not simply passive portals on the world but wellsprings of imagination and creativity grounded in several forms of attention (Alford 2021). Anil Seth (2021) insists that 'Perception is a generative act … an action-oriented construction, rather than a passive registration of an objective reality'. This view is echoed in Donald Hoffman's (2019) 'case against reality' and by Lisa Feldman Barrett (2017), where 'Scientific evidence shows that what we see, hear, touch, taste, and smell are largely simulations of the world, not reactions to it'. Imagination threads through perception as a major well of creativity, long since recognised by psychologically sensitive poets such as Samuel Taylor Coleridge, who first coined the term 'psychosomatic' (Nicolson 2019). Nonetheless, perception is mostly not free-floating but monitored, if not controlled, by attention (see Chapter 7) that is 'your brain's boss' according to Amishi Jha (2017). Attention controls, or is at least 'very powerful in terms of affecting perception' says Jha (2007, 2017). 'Tell me what you pay attention to and I will tell you who you are', said Ortega y Gassett (2019).

Perception is distinct from attention, but they remain intertwined. 'Perception is not the same as attention, and not at all the same as thinking. But the world we choose to attend to, indeed choose whether and how to attend to, is nothing without perception' (McGilchrist 2021). In turn, the quality and focus of attention that creativity demands varies and vacillates during the creative act. 'Divergent thinking' – a term coined by JP Guilford (1961) – is a form of dispersed generative attention that brings together non-adjacent thoughts and ideas. This contrasts with convergent thinking that relies on focused attention. McGilchrist (2021) describes the intricate relationship between perception, attention, and creativity as

> Attention is a creative act, and creation is really about the induction of a highly attentive state. It is like an ear that is listening and receptive, without actually having anything at all clear yet to hear. You've got to have some intimation of what it is that's coming, however, because otherwise it couldn't come.

Since perceptions are never 'pure' but readily distorted, filtered, and framed by interpretations, heuristics, beliefs, and other cognitive 'traps', the outcomes can be salutary, nefarious, or mixed. How we yoke our perceptions and attention as forms of creativity is a primary focus for metahumanities within medical education. Good applied biomedical science (e.g., in clinical reasoning) requires metacognition – not just the memorising and recall or recognition of information, but the associated meanings that such information can bring. This invites medical educators to educate for imagination and not just memory, where biomedical science is taught as much for its elegance as for its informational value in understanding disease. The art of biomedicine is where the medical humanities are grounded – encouraging appreciation before explanation (so that patients are not objectified) and advancing linear algorithms as well as creative thinking (to realise the potential of the mind) (Bleakley 2023).

Perception and beauty

How are beauty and perception aligned? The philosopher David Hume (2000) famously argued that beauty is in the eye of the beholder, yet the poet John Keats said: 'Beauty is truth, truth beauty' suggesting that there is a definitive marker for 'beauty'. From a selective advantage perspective, perception of beauty is likely associated with its fitness payoff which may range from perceptions of healthy food selection to viable mate selection ('could this person produce and raise viable offspring?'), to sustaining our illusions and rendering us more resilient (Magsamen 2023). Donald Hoffman (2019) examines the relationship between beauty and our illusions of perception to suggest that while beauty provides an estimate of reproductive fitness, it may also represent an example of 'exaptation in which a trait evolved for one function can co-opt a new function'. Thus, feathers in birds designed originally for temperature regulation become adapted for flying, and in turn evolve as aesthetic features in a mating ritual. Such aesthetic issues are again central to the functioning of medical culture. Exaptation is rife – stethoscopes designed for auscultation become primary markers of entry into and alignment with medical culture, affording an identity. White coats originally adopted for sterility purposes become symbols of identity along with the stethoscope. Now, white coats are found to harbour bugs and are being abandoned, but reluctantly as they carry such aesthetic cultural prestige twinned with the stethoscope (that is also being slowly abandoned as bedside examinations become less frequent where laboratory testing and imaging provide more reliable diagnostic data). Thus, perceptions change as aesthetic markers evolve.

David Brooks (2023) sums up the common 'illusory' view of perception as

> The universe is a drab, silent, colorless place. I mean this quite literally. There is no such thing as colour and sound in the universe; There's just a bunch of waves and particles. But because we have creative minds, we perceive sound and music, tastes and smells, color and beauty, all in wonder. All that stuff is here in your mind not out there in the universe.

We must modify Brooks' anthropocentrism by noting that all animal forms with sensory apparatus are somehow making sense of this 'drab, silent, colorless place' and therefore to posit such a place is aesthetically pointless as that place is universally imbued with quality through sensory experience, however the latter operates.

I have mentioned how one function of the arts and humanities is to upset perceptions, or re-arrange them, to see the world 'slant' as the poet Emily Dickinson puts it. The modern and contemporary arts have largely moved away from direct representation of objective reality and towards a constructed reality that is fraught, illusory, and ambiguous. This often captures a mood, such as Pablo Picasso's *Guernica*. Picasso said: 'Art is a lie that makes us realize the truth', while Edgar Degas said: 'Art is not what you see, but what you make others see'. Some enduring works of art seem to recapitulate not an outer objective reality but align with neurobiologic signatures or correlates in the brain, as Jonah Lehrer (2007) pointed out in *Proust Was a Neuroscientist*. Thus, Cezanne's Incognito paintings that seem abstract may indeed be the way that our brain first sees 'reality' before creating the completed gestalt of irreality. They may thus fit better with a top-down predictive processing of perception than with a bottom-up processing of sensations and perception entering the mind from the outer world. Art can then inform biomedical science by cataloguing ways of looking, or close noticing, as it also educates for witnessing and ethical positioning, as in Picasso's *Guernica*. Medical education ignores such connections at its peril.

We have arrived at the point where we can say that, thanks to cultural effects on evolution, humanity has been shaped to act as creative artists – metahumanities for all – in every perceptual act as we actively interpret rather than simply passively receive the world. McGilchrist (2021) sees our capacity for symbolic representation and language as transcending the illusory world of perceptions:

> In us something new happens: to be precise, it starts happening in the great apes. It is the ability to use symbols – tokens or representations for things. And in humans it is advanced out of all recognition by language, which gives us virtually inexhaustible way of mapping the world, to which perception is, to all intents and purposes, irrelevant – and from which it may even prove a distraction.

Anil Seth (2021), however, disagrees by insisting that the sole function of the brain is to serve evolutionary fitness and keep us alive:

> Evolution's reason for providing organisms with brains is not so they can write poetry, do crossword puzzles … pursue neuroscience … . Brains are not 'for' rational thinking, linguistic communication, or even for perceiving the world. The most fundamental reason any organism has a brain – or any kind of nervous system – is to help it stay alive.

Surely this is a bleak, functional view, countered by the physician-poet William Carlos. William's infamous dictum is that, 'It is difficult/to get the news from poems/yet men die miserably every day/for lack/of what is found there'. We have surely passed the point where evolution merely serves the function of 'survival of the fittest'. The brain has evolved beyond 'evolved' just to help us 'stay alive'; otherwise intelligent, thoughtful people would likely not engage in extreme sports, risk their lives for others, or commit suicide, for example. Rather, the brain has been evolving into more complex domains so that we 'can write poetry' which is to say that we can transcend the ordinary to engage with the 'meta'.

Perception and consciousness

Modern (quantum) physics insists that our role in the universe is not one of passive bystanders but participatory (Meijer 2015). McGilchrist (2021) links such perception to consciousness when he claims that 'Perception is not passive reception, but participation … as is all consciousness'. More radically, physicist John Wheeler averred there could be no universe until consciousness arose to perceive it (Meijer 2015). These are zingy statements – but the function and locus (if any exists) of consciousness remains unresolved and baffling. Nevertheless, there are encouraging scientific advances such as the Perturbational Complexity Index (PCI) for measuring different levels of consciousness (Massimini et al. 2005). Such approaches encapsulate what Anil Seth (2021) terms 'the real problem approach' to consciousness – an approach that accepts that consciousness exists and then asks how conscious experiences are structured, what forms they take, and how they 'relate to the properties of brains, brains that are embodied in bodies and embodied in the world'. The approach is to find correlations between brain activity patterns and different kinds of conscious experience and to develop explanations between mechanism and phenomenology that are not concocted but rather make sense.

The problem of how consciousness arises from unconsciousness (or objectivity, nothing) is captured in philosopher-neuroscientist Patricia Churchland and colleagues' (Churchland et al. 1993) poignant question (raised in Chapter 10): 'How can neurons care?' Churchland's question is aimed at how caring, empathy, and cooperativity can arise from neurons, and she answers her question with evidence from neuroendocrinology (as hormones and oxytocin). Hoffman's (2019) preoccupation is with the transition from unconsciousness to consciousness. He argues that humans will likely never understand the nature of consciousness: 'Cats can't do calculus, monkeys can't do quantum theory, so why assume that Homo sapiens can demystify consciousness?' Nonetheless, he settles with the notion of 'conscious realism' as the fundamental building block of an 'objective reality of conscious agents and their interactions' but that does not put human consciousness centre stage: 'We are prone to falsely believe that certain limitations and idiosyncrasies of our perceptions are genuine insights into objective reality'.

Hoffman (2019) argues that Galileo 'got the message' and understood the illusion of our perceptions when he said: 'I think that tastes, odors, colors, and so on … reside in consciousness. Hence if the living creature were removed, all these qualities would be wiped away and annihilated'. Thus, Galileo believed that our perceptions of objective reality were not 'real' – there are no odours, tastes, or colours in objective reality. These are illusions of our perceptions. This remains a fundamental conundrum for metahumanities. Does the illusory nature of our perceptions detract from our humanity, or from the value to us of the arts and humanities? One might legitimately ask what role the arts and metahumanities have in this drab universe?

This may be a disheartening message for the humanities. It is certainly humbling. Metahumanities should take this into account as they reassess their role in defining what human consciousness and our role in the universe is about. It might make us humbler towards other species (which also have consciousness) and more willing to share this speck of a planet with other forms of life knowing that we are not the centre of the universe. We need to stop arrogating to ourselves the Judeo-Christian notion that we sit at the pinnacle of the Great Chain of Being. Intelligence and consciousness are not the same thing, and 'consciousness has more to do with being alive than with being smart' (Seth 2021). Consciousness can exist without much intelligence. More disturbing for us as an intelligent but destructive species, intelligence can also exist without consciousness (2021). The relationships between the brain, perception, and consciousness pose deep conundrums for metahumanities.

Conclusion

The view of perception as a passive recording of an objective reality has been debunked. Perception is active, participatory, bidirectional, and predictive. Less comforting, it is also illusory, likely hallucinogenic. Perception is intimately linked to consciousness, to who we are, and to our sense of self and others. To experience anything, we must bring ourselves to relate to and bear on the world – a prospect at once filled with potential and unsettling in its responsibility. Artists in particular bear such cultural responsibility – to provide ways in which we might see the world 'otherwise' and create new ways of engagement. But the arts and humanities also have an ethical duty in the emergent Anthropocene to model a multidimensional, multidisciplinary, and consilient approach that re-conceives our place on the planet as less dominant among species, and more integrated and relational – an approach encompassed in a reconstructive metahumanities shaping productive perceptions.

References

Alford L. 2021. *Forms of Poetic Attention*. New York, NY: Columbia University Press.

Barrett, L.F., 2017. *How Emotions are Made: The Secret Life of the Brain*. Pan Macmillan.

Bleakley A. 2017. Six fallacies that hinder development of the medical humanities in medical education. *Medical Education*. 51: 126–7.

Bleakley A. 2020. *Educating Doctors' Senses Through the Medical Humanities: 'How Do I Look?'*. Abingdon: Routledge.

Bleakley, A., 2023. *Medical Humanities: Ethics, Aesthetics, Politics*. London: Routledge.

Brackett, M. (2019). *Permission to Feel: Unlocking the Power of Emotions to Help Our Kids, Ourselves, and Our Society Thrive*. Celadon Books.

Brooks D 2020. *The Second Mountain: The Quest for a Moral Life*. New York, NY: Random House Trade Paperbacks.

Brooks, D. (2023). *How to Know a Person: The Art of Seeing Others Deeply and Being Deeply Seen*. Random House.

Churchland PS, Ramachandran VS, Sejnowski TJ. 1993. *A Critique of Pure Vision: Large-Scale Neuronal Theories of the Brain*. Cambridge MA: MIT Press.

Clark A. 2023. *The Experience Machine: How our Minds Predict and Shape Reality*. New York, NY: Pantheon Books.

Clark A, Chalmers D. 1998. The extended mind. *Analysis*. 58: 7–19.

Cutting JC. 2012. *A Critique of Psychopathology*. Berlin: Parados.

Dawkins R, Ward L. 2006. *The God Delusion*. Boston, MA: Houghton Mifflin Company.

Devinsky O. 2000. Right cerebral hemisphere dominance for a sense of corporeal and emotional self. *Epilepsy & Behavior*. 1: 60–73.

Doidge N. 2007. *The Brain that Changes Itself*. New York, NY: Penguin Books.

Eichbaum, Q., Barbeau-Meunier, C. A., White, M., Ravi, R., Grant, E., Riess, H., Bleakley, A. (2023). Empathy across cultures–one size does not fit all: from the ego-logical to the eco-logical of relational empathy. *Advances in Health Sciences Education*, *28*(2), 643–657.

Eichbaum QG. 2014. Thinking about thinking and emotion: the metacognitive approach to the medical humanities that integrates the humanities with the basic and clinical sciences. *Permanente Journal*. 18: 64–75.

Flannery K, Marcus J. 2012. *The Creation of Inequality*. Cambridge, MA: Harvard University Press.

Gibson EJ. 1969. *Principles of Perceptual Learning and Development*. USA: Appleton-Century-Crofts.

Gibson JJ. 1950. *The Perception of the Visual World*. Boston, MA: Houghton Mifflin.

Gombrich EH. 1961. *Art and Illusion*. New York, NY: Pantheon Books.

Gross JJ, Barrett LF. 2011. Emotion Generation and Emotion Regulation: One or Two Depends on Your Point of View. *Emot Rev*. Jan;3(1):8–16.

Guilford JP. 1961. Three faces of intellect. In: JJ Jenkins, DJ Pederson (eds.) *Studies in Individual Differences: The Search for Intelligence*. New York, NY: Appleton-Century-Crofts.

Hoffman D. 2019. *The Case Against Reality: Why Evolution Hid the Truth From Our Eyes*. New York, NY: WW Norton & Company.

Hülür G, Hoppmann CA, Rauers A, et al. 2016. Empathic accuracy for happiness in the daily lives of older couples: Fluid cognitive performance predicts pattern accuracy among men. *Psychology and Ageing*. 31: 545.

Hume, D. (2000). *A treatise of Human Nature*. Oxford University Press.

Hurley SL. 1998. *Consciousness in Action*. Cambridge, MA: Harvard University Press.

Jacquette, D. (2015). *The Philosophy of Schopenhauer*. Routledge.

Jha A. 2017. The science of training the wandering mind. Available at: https://www.mindful.org/taming-the-wandering-mind/. Last accessed: 16/01/2024.

Kosslyn S, Miller G. 2013. There is no left brain/right brain divide. *Time*. Nov 29.

Kosslyn, S. M. (1987). Seeing and imagining in the cerebral hemispheres: a computational approach. *Psychological review*, *94*(2), 148.

Jha, AP, Krompinger J, Baime MJ. 2007. Mindfulness training modifies subsystems of attention. *Cognitive, Affective, & Behavioral Neuroscience*. 7: 109–19.

Lakoff, G., Johnson, M. (2008). *Metaphors We Live By*. University of Chicago press.

Lehrer, J. (2007). *Proust was a Neuroscientist*. Houghton Mifflin Harcourt.
Magsamen R 2023. *Your Brain on Art - How the Arts Transform Us*. New York, NY: Random House.
Marr D. 2010. *Vision: A Computational Investigation Into the Human Representation and Processing of Visual Information*. Cambridge, MA: MIT Press.
Massimini M, Ferrarelli F, Huber R, et al. 2005. Breakdown of cortical effective connectivity during sleep. *Science*. 309: 2228–32.
McGilchrist I. 2021. *The Matter with Things: Our Brains, our Delusions, and the Unmaking of the World*. London: Perspectiva Press.
Meijer DKF. 2015. The universe as a cyclic organized information system: John Wheeler's world revisited. *NeuroQuantology*. 13: 57–78.
Nicolson A. 2019. *The Making of Poetry: Coleridge, the Wordsworths and Their Year of Marvels*. London: William Collins.
Ortega y Gasset J. 2019. *The Dehumanization of Art and Other Essays on Art, Culture, and Literature*. Princeton, NJ: Princeton University Press.
Palmer SE. 1999. *Vision Science: Photons to Phenomenology*. Boston, MA: MIT Press.
Panksepp J, Panksepp JB. 2000. The seven sins of evolutionary psychology. *Evolution and Cognition*. 6: 108–31.
Pinker, S. (1997). Words and rules in the human brain. *Nature*, *387*(6633), 547–548.
Pizlo, Z. (2014). *Making a Machine That Sees Like Us*. Oxford University Press, USA.
Ramachandran, V. S. (2012). *The Tell-tale Brain: A Neuroscientist's Quest for What Makes us Human*. WW Norton & Company.
Ravven H. 2013. *The Self Beyond Itself: An Alternative History of Ethics, the New Brain Sciences, and the Myth of Free Will*. New York, NY: The New Press.
Riess, H. (2010). Empathy in medicine—A neurobiological perspective. *Jama*, *304*(14), 1604–1605.
Riess, H., Kraft-Todd, G., 2014. EMPATHY: a tool to enhance nonverbal communication between clinicians and their patients. *Academic Medicine*, *89*(8), 1108–1112.
Rizzolatti G, Sinigaglia C. 2008. *Mirrors in the Brain: How Our Minds Share Actions and Emotions*. Oxford: Oxford University Press.
Ruffman T, Zhang J, Taumoepeau M, Skeaff S. 2016. Your way to a better theory of mind: A healthy diet relates to better faux pas recognition in older adults. *Experimental Aging Research*. 42: 279–88.
Schrödinger, E. (1951). *Science and Humanism: Physics in Our Time*. Cambridge University Press.
Seth A. 2021. *Being You: A New Science of Consciousness*. London: Penguin.
Siegel DJ. 2007. *The Mindful Brain: Reflection and Attunement in the Cultivation of Well-being*. New York, NY: WW Norton & Company.
Siegel S. 2016. *The Rationality of Perception*. Oxford: Oxford University Press.
Tavris C, Aronson E. 2007. *Mistakes Were Made (But Not by Me): Why We Justify Foolish Beliefs, Bad Decisions, and Hurtful Acts*. New York, NY: Harcourt.
Vygotsky LS. 1965. *Thought and Language*, MIT Press.
Westen, D. (2008). *The Political Brain: The Role of Emotion in Deciding the Fate of the Nation*. PublicAffairs.
Wilson EO. 1988. *On Human Nature*. Boston, MA: Harvard University Press.
Wilson EO. 2014. *The Meaning of Human Existence*. New York, NY: WW Norton & Company.
Wilson EO. 2017. *The Origins of Creativity*. New York, NY: Liveright Publishing.
Zaki J, Bolger N, Ochsner K. 2008. It takes two: The interpersonal nature of empathic accuracy. *Psychological Science*. 19: 399–404.

9 Capability, augmentation, and metacognition

Rachel Ellaway

Introduction

As humans, we can do lots of things, we can be lots of things, and we have the potential to do and be much more than we are. Our potential can be put down to either our intrinsic abilities or to those abilities we can develop in ourselves or in each other. Our physical abilities may vary in terms of stature, strength, endurance, suppleness, agility, and precision, while our mental abilities may vary in terms of our knowledge, recall, critical and analytical thought, discipline, creativity, and so on. Whatever our abilities are, they shape our lives in profound ways. The concept of 'disability' demonstrates that ability can be limiting as well as liberating, and it suggests that using our abilities is contingent on circumstance as well as on intrinsic facility.

This circumstantial sense of ability is clearly reflected in situations where individuals' opportunities to use their abilities are constrained (for instance through social stigma or control) or they have insufficient or mismatched abilities (for instance a lack of resources or knowledge). For instance, one individual's privilege may provide them with better access to medical education than an individual from a less privileged background even if the individual with less opportunity has superior abilities to perform as a physician. Rather than considering ability or opportunity as independent constructs, we can understand them as being woven together in the construct of 'capability'.

Amartya Sen (1992) defined capability as being dependent on various freedoms, with an individual's capabilities being expressed in combinations of beings (what someone can be) and doings (what someone can do). Martha Nussbaum (2011), who had originally worked with Sen, later defined capability as the product of an individual's abilities and their opportunities to use them. In advancing her 'human capabilities approach', Nussbaum outlined a series of essential capabilities that all humans should have – see Table 9.1.[1]

The human capabilities approach not only challenges us to consider whether an individual has the opportunity to use abilities or not (although it is certainly a valid question), it also requires us to ask how ability is constructed, deconstructed, or otherwise altered by the contexts individuals find themselves in (or have previously been in), and the social construction of capability in

DOI: 10.4324/9781032687339-12

Table 9.1 Summary of Martha Nussbaum's core human capabilities

Capability	*All humans should have the capability to …*
Life	Have a full human lifetime that is worth living
Health	Be healthy, nourished, able to reproduce, and have shelter
Bodily Integrity	Have freedom of movement, freedom from violence, and choice in matters of sex and reproduction
Senses	Be educated to be able to engage in imagination, thinking, reasoning, and creativity; to have freedom of creative and religious expression; and be able to seek pleasure
Emotions	Be free to create attachments; to experience love, grief, longing, gratitude, anger, and not be blighted by fear and anxiety
Reason	Be free to distinguish between good and bad and be able to plan and direct their lives
Affiliation	Be free to interact with others, to show concern, to retain self-respect, and to not be discriminated against
Other species	Be able to relate to animals, plants, and the world of nature
Play	Be able to enjoy things and activities
Environment	Be able to engage in politics, to hold property and goods, to seek employment, and to be free from unwarranted search, seizure, or imprisonment

terms of cultures, systems, and ideologies. For instance, it may be that an individual's opportunities were not engaged consciously or willingly, such as those afforded by material wealth or poverty, but they will nevertheless have shaped that individual's path through life. Indeed, it might be argued that the capabilities of systemically disadvantaged peoples are, by definition, broadly diminished independent of their talents (abilities) or capacities (the potential of their abilities), while the capabilities of systemically advantaged peoples are, by definition, broadly enhanced or extended independent of their abilities.

Applications of the human capabilities approach have tended to be focused on the relative capabilities of individuals and societies, in particular what capabilities are available to some but not to others, and what capabilities should be available to all (Robeyns 2017). To that end, the human capabilities approach posits a social construction of capability based on cultures, systems, and ideologies, as well as according to individual circumstances. Reflecting this, much of the work around human capabilities has explored the ways in which abilities might be constrained and the ways in which certain abilities are afforded to some while being denied to others (Robeyns 2017). Think for instance of the concept of 'social determinants of health' where health and disease are understood as being socially constructed such that access to care and the ability to benefit from it are shaped by circumstantial capabilities (Ruger 2004).

Not only can the human capabilities approach be applied to broad social and policy-related domains, but it can also be used to explore interactions of abilities and opportunities in the construction of individual capabilities, and from this it can afford opportunities to consider factors such as needs, wishes, and expectations, as well as individual agency as shaping an individual's capabilities.

This in turn affords useful and often neglected metacognitive perspectives both on how an individual's capabilities vary according to circumstance and on how that individual's opportunities to change their capabilities are also circumstantial. For instance, although its origins were in international development and human rights, by relating capability to what it means to live a meaningful and fulfilling life, the human capabilities approach can provide a foundation for reflection on one's own capabilities as well as that of others, such as peers, patients, and trainees.

From a metahumanistic perspective, the human capabilities approach could also be used to reappraise the medical humanities, particularly those that focus on medium and idiom rather than on ability and opportunity. Indeed, much of the thinking that underlies medical humanities would seem to be based on the same postsecondary 'sorting hat' that has long separated the academy into the sciences (nowadays more typically identified as STEM (science, technology, engineering, mathematics)) and the humanities. From this perspective, the medical humanities have often been portrayed or pursued as a way of restoring balance in the face of scientific domination in medicine and medical education, and as such is based on addressing assumed deficits (Katz 2014). A capability-based medical metahumanism could be used to explore whether such dialectical thinking has been as productive as intended and what alternative perspectives might offer. For example, we might consider which of Nussbaum's core capabilities are inhibited or underdeveloped in medicine and medical education, and what we might do to disinhibit or develop them. Whether or not that involves the use of theatre or reading and writing poetry becomes secondary to the capability change(s) we might seek to realise.

Human capabilities in medicine and medical education

As much as a capabilities approach has many possible intersections with medicine and medical education (both theoretical and practical), it has not so far featured in mainstream discussion and debate (Teunissen et al. 2021). For instance, in assessing who is admitted to medical school, much attention has been paid to candidates' abilities (Albanese et al. 2003) but rather less to their opportunities, although the growing attention to socioeconomic disparities in admissions reflects a shifting balance in this regard (Ellaway et al. 2019, Thomas and Dockter 2019). For those admitted to the profession, abilities continue to be a central concern in monitoring trainees' progress (particularly through the battery of assessments this involves). Ability is also closely linked to medical career choices and trajectories, to licensing and maintenance of competence, and to scopes of practice, accountability, and remediation.

Opportunity certainly is a matter of concern in medical education, but it is almost always framed as the responsibility of those providing the training rather than of those who are receiving it. Educators are tasked with providing their trainees with the necessary opportunities (however they are defined) to develop the required competencies for a particular specialty or scope of practice, and they are required to do so fairly and equitably. For instance, there has been growing attention to relative privilege and (dis)advantage in providing accommodations for learners with certain learning disabilities or needs (Zazove et al. 2016). Opportunity-related issues can also be found in medical syllabi, particularly where patient health, suffering, harm, and competence are linked to socioeconomic opportunities. These indicators notwithstanding, a dominant concept in medical education is (at the time of writing) that of 'competency', a construct that is usually linked to ability (Frank et al. 2015) but rarely to opportunity or capability. As a result, ability, opportunity, and their confluence in capability are often not connected or associated, nor are ability or capability well-theorised or situated within current discourses of medical education.

This is a significant missed opportunity. If, from a medical humanities perspective, we were concerned with all of a person's human capabilities then a capabilities approach to the humanities could include developing individuals' capabilities to use their imagination, thinking, reasoning, and creativity. Indeed, a capabilities approach could also encompass developing learners' physiological capabilities through exercise, nutrition, and other wellness approaches, while changing capabilities related to emotions might include attending more to learners' fears, anxieties, and experiences of moral injury. From a capability perspective, much, if not all, of existing curricula could therefore fall under a metahumanities umbrella. For instance, ethics and professionalism might be expanded to consider politics, pay, contracts, and autonomy in medical practice, and therapeutic options might be understood in terms of changes to patients' and providers' abilities and opportunities. A capability perspective focused on one's colleagues and trainees in healthcare might consider their apparent strengths and weaknesses as the product of their intersecting and interacting capabilities. Similar perspectives could be applied at different scales, for instance to the medical profession, to healthcare systems, and more broadly to society. Taking a capabilities approach arguably dissolves the 'medical humanities' into a more embracing and holistic sense of medical education and practice than has been afforded by oppositional deficit-focused approaches.

In summary, a capability approach (whether or not it is based on the human capabilities approach or something similar) can provide a particularly compelling and useful model to advance understanding in medicine, one moreover that has more depth than many other models (such as those of competence or of ability) and one that can be used to challenge orthodox thinking in the medical humanities. Indeed, a capability approach has the potential to expand metahumanities as a frame of reference to include and integrate much more of medical education thinking and practice than might otherwise be the case. I use the rest of this chapter to explore this proposition.

Capability and metacapability

A capability perspective can allow for reflection on one's own capabilities, on the capabilities of those people one interacts with (colleagues, patients, and learners), and on how all of these capabilities interact. Consider as an example how you might adapt your practice when a learner or colleague is underperforming to the point that your capabilities are also reduced (such as lost confidence or trust in them and the time it takes to identify and fix their mistakes). As a result, you may seek to alter their capabilities (such as reducing their opportunities to hinder you or by increasing their opportunities to remediate their shortcomings) as a way of restoring or protecting your own capabilities. Similarly, your capabilities might be impacted by the strength or complementarity of the capabilities of those you interact with. For instance, having a colleague with particularly strong statistical or surgical skills might extend what you can do as an individual and as a member of a team. It is interesting to note that, while this entanglement of capabilities is suggested in concepts of patient competency and capacity (Leo 1999), it has yet to be picked up in the context of professional development and professional identity formation.

A capability perspective would also suggest that our cognitive capabilities are a product of our cognitive abilities and opportunities. Consider a trainee who has great potential for reflection and mindfulness but whose relentless clinical schedule gives them little opportunity to make use of these abilities. In thinking about professional identity formation, a capabilities lens could allow a learner to reflect on how their individual abilities and opportunities have made them the kind of professional they are or are becoming. A learner might also consider productively reflect on how much of their growing professional identity they shaped and how much was shaped for them.

A second issue is something I will call 'capability affordance', which relates to an individual's capability to pursue metacognitive opportunities. This is not just a matter of what capabilities might be developed; it also projects a normative sense of what kinds and levels of metacognition an individual should be able to engage in, what kinds and levels of metacognition might be expected of them, and how much agency and autonomy they have in engaging in metacognition. We might therefore ask questions such as:

- What abilities and opportunities do you (and everyone else) have or need to become metacognitive?
- If metacognition requires time and focus, then do you have the time and can you maintain focus?
- If metacognition requires frameworks and tools, then do you have these available to you and are you able to make use of them?
- If metacognition requires legitimacy and rigour, then do you and those around you believe that metacognition is a legitimate part of medical education and practice?
- Do you have the ability and opportunity to be rigorous in your metacognitive activities?

Let us consider 'metacapability' as the capability to have capabilities, which allows us to consider many issues that have otherwise found little traction in medicine and medical education. For instance, rather than limiting ourselves to the somewhat simplistic question of what capabilities a generic physician or surgeon needs, we might ask what capabilities they might choose to have (and to not have), or what unanticipated or tacit capabilities they develop over time. Rather than simply asking as part of medical school admissions whether applicants have the capability to perform as medical learners, we might instead consider what capabilities applicants already have and what their capabilities to develop other capabilities are. This approach presents a direct challenge to reductive models of selection, training, and assessment based on limited generic competencies. Can we not embrace a more fulsome and holistic capability approach in medical education to focus on potential as the development of metacapabilities?

A metacapability lens also allows us to ask what the necessary capabilities for patients, colleagues, and students are, and whether those performing these roles have the metacapability to express or develop the necessary capabilities. For instance, if we were to commit to the capability for everyone to access healthcare whenever they need it, then how might that change providers' roles, responsibilities, and scopes of practice? If learners need to demonstrate particular capabilities in performing essential mental tasks, then how can we vary their opportunities to develop these capabilities so as to optimise the abilities they do have and compensate for those they do not? Or do we instead place the onus on learners such that they all get the same learning opportunities and only those who can demonstrate the necessary capabilities are allowed to continue into practice? Such questions are the foundation of debates over accommodation practices in medical education (Clarke 2023) but have, I would argue, previously lacked theoretical depth.

Metacapability might also be concerned with an individual's opportunity to use their abilities, and their ability to use their opportunities. More specifically, an individual's ability to use or develop their abilities might depend on a realistic understanding of what those abilities are, the motivation and will to use or change them, and the enabling abilities required to use or change other abilities. We might also seek to better understand the opportunities individual learners have to use or develop their abilities, and how these opportunities might be constrained or enabled by rules and regulations, by social conventions, by wealth and privilege, or by other factors.

Of course, the ability to use or develop one's opportunities would still depend to an extent on what is meant by 'opportunity'. If opportunity means 'available', then there may still be limitations to accessing or using it based on ability. To access a particular opportunity (such as getting into medical school) may require stature, strength, visual acuity, stamina, or other abilities that may enable or disable access depending on the individual and their circumstances. Similarly, the opportunity to use or develop one's opportunities may be limited or otherwise shaped by power differentials, hierarchies, social disadvantages, and other structural inequities, which may limit access to or participation in a profession. This line of reasoning is not simply about what we have in terms of ability and opportunity, but what we might become if we could change or manipulate our capabilities.

Changing capabilities

We have few intrinsic capabilities when we are born, but, as we grow, our abilities (physical and cognitive) develop and grow, in part due to genetics and organic human development, and in part due to the advantages and disadvantages (i.e., opportunities) conferred by our social, technical, and cultural contexts. Clearly, not everyone develops the same abilities, not everyone is afforded the same opportunities to develop their abilities, and not everyone wants the same abilities or opportunities. It is important to note that abilities and opportunities do not only grow, they can also be diminished or lost, for instance through injury, disease, or neglect, or through changing social circumstances. Where choice is possible, then we may consider what choices individuals make regarding changing their capabilities. Where there is little or no choice, then we may consider the implications for individuals whose capabilities are imposed on them (either through forced change or through preventing change). Clearly, capabilities can change, they often do, and when they do (or do not), then there can be many implications to consider.

As an example, a capabilities approach might focus on the ways in which Paralympians use prostheses to be able to perform at the highest athletic levels. However, as important, if not more so, are the cognitive means that all athletes employ to overcome the limitations they encounter. These include coaching that attends to challenges and failures in supportive ways (Powell and Myers 2017) and the use of biofeedback and neurofeedback to train and focus on performance (Edmonds and Tenenbaum 2011). Metacognition is central to these cases, not least because they clearly illustrate some of the entanglements of metacognition with metacapability. However, while the application of metacognition and metacapability may be implicitly a part of clinical and communication skills simulations, this theoretical framing has yet to be explored in medical education.

How then can we advance theoretical understanding of capability change? My own work has explored augmentation as a theoretical lens based on the premise that changing capabilities involves augmentation. Although augmentation in a lay sense is typically about extending or expanding capability, given that extending certain capabilities (either by changing abilities, opportunities, or both) can limit other capabilities (and vice versa), augmentation can be more productively thought of as changes to a person's overall capability state, acknowledging that such changes may involve both expansions and contractions in various abilities and opportunities. Again, there is a metacapability dimension in terms of an individual's capability to change their capabilities. This can include both the ability to change certain abilities and opportunities, and the opportunity to change certain abilities and opportunities. Some capabilities can be changed easily, while other abilities and opportunities are harder to change. Some abilities and opportunities can change quickly while others change only very slowly. Some capability changes can be reversed, while other changes are permanent. Some capabilities can only be changed by changing other capabilities, and so on. As an example of this latter point, consider how the embodied experience of cadaveric dissection or other approaches can change a learner's understanding of their own bodies as well as those of their patients. Consider how 'seeing' a body can be reframed using point-of-care ultrasound, laparoscopic cameras or even the humble microscope. Consider too how psychiatry residents are taught to 'listen through' what their patients are saying to seek an understanding of their mental conditions (Balon et al. 2020).

What are the metacognitive implications of the points I have made? One is the need to better understand ourselves (and everyone around us) by acknowledging that we have all been augmented from birth, both by the support and nurture (or absence thereof) of our parents or carers and by the means afforded by medicine, schooling, and social order. As a result, none of us is ever in a truly natural state; we are a product of our capabilities and the augmentations that shaped them, whether we will or not. In the context of medicine and medical education, this has implications for understanding patient presentations and the aetiologies of wellness, harm, and suffering. This also has implications for our understanding of others and ourselves as health professionals. After all, to be a health professional, you need to undertake or subject yourself to many augmentations, some of which you seek out (like continuing professional development) and some that simply 'come with the territory' (such as privilege as a professional). You may not be able to do much about the capabilities you already have, but you do have some agency in what you do with these capabilities. You can also consider and perhaps even change the means through which you (and others like you) came by these capabilities.

Medicine and medical education are intrinsically augmentative undertakings in that they are about changing patients' and learners' capabilities, respectively. A physician can come to see practice more holistically and more humanistically by focusing on what of their patients' abilities and opportunities they can change, both directly (for instance, prescribing pain killers to change an individual's ability to deal with pain) and indirectly (for instance, improving a patient's mobility that changes their opportunities to participate in social activities). In medical education, if instructors shift their understanding of their role from one based on imparting information to one based on augmenting their learners' abilities and opportunities, then many different perspectives on what learning and teaching might mean become possible. After all, an instructor cannot make their learners learn; they can only create the conditions and opportunities for them to do so. Our attention might be better focused on our learners' capabilities to turn knowledge into wisdom and expertise.

It is also important to understand that augmentation can be disruptive as much as it can be assistive. It can certainly be disruptive to the augmentee if one capability change disables or shifts other capabilities in unexpected and unwanted ways. Augmentation can also be disruptive to others if it contravenes the rules or conventions of the systems they work in. For instance, augmentation in one person can cause resentment, discomfort, and even revulsion in others or it may confer unfair, proscribed, or even illegal advantages. Whether it be tattooing, body piercing, the use of performance-altering drugs, or cheating in exams, or in other contexts, these uses of augmentations are often proscribed and even punished. Ask yourself, how do you feel about people who augment themselves in these ways? How do you feel about using such augmentations for yourself? How do you feel about those who object to such things? You might consider learners' use of coffee or caffeinated soft drinks acceptable but be concerned at their use of psychostimulants (such as amphetamines) or tranquilisers (such as barbiturates) to aid study (Emanuel et al. 2013). Another example, and one that is still very new at the time of writing, is medical student's use of artificial intelligence (AI) tools to enhance their performance. There is an emerging dialectic here between the opportunities afforded by AI to help to improve human capabilities and concerns that AI will be used to misrepresent human capabilities or allow them to atrophy.

The issues I have raised are not just about personal choice or bodily autonomy. Think for instance about medical learners who feel cheated when their teacher puts all their time into helping struggling learners. What about the diverging capabilities of learners who collaborate in homophilic groups to study or complete coursework compared to those who struggle to do so based in limited ability or opportunity (Keren et al. 2020)? Given the competitive nature of medical education, such comparisons and their resulting resentments are unfortunately commonplace. An augmentation lens may not solve this problem, but it can certainly make it more apparent.

If we bring together the concepts of metacognition and augmentation, we can consider ways in which metacognition might be augmented as well as ways in which metacognition might focus on augmentation and its consequences. We can augment our cognitive capabilities both by targeting our abilities directly (for instance using stimulants) and indirectly (for instance through using information technologies (Clark 2004)), and we can augment our cognitive capabilities by targeting our opportunities both directly (for instance by engaging in educational activities) and indirectly (for instance by avoiding things that distract or disturb us).

At its core, metacognition involves thinking-about-thinking, something we can consider in terms of self-awareness, intentionality, and control. Expanding on this, Baker and Brown (1984) described metacognition in terms of self-controlling, planning, evaluating, and monitoring thought processes, while Wellman (1985) described metacognition as something that involves multiple thought processes, some of which direct or control while others are directed or controlled. Alan Bleakley in Chapter 2 of this volume goes further to suggest that metacognition also includes creativity, complexity, reflective practice, dialectical reasoning, and abduction. Rather than painting myself into a corner by coming up with some canonical definition of what metacognition is or is not, I will, for the sake of argument, simply say that all these characteristics may play a part in metacognition, and all are either subject to or can be mediated by human augmentation.

As an example, by writing this chapter, I have provided you with various opportunities for metacognitive augmentation. Whether you take any of these opportunities though is up to you. If the ideas I have presented are already known to you or if you have no real interest in metacognitive development (for instance, if you are grudgingly reading this as an assignment), then reading this chapter will be unlikely to lead to metacognitive change. If, on the other hand, you are reading this in the context of an established mindfulness practice or you are looking for ideas to weave into your own teaching or clinical practices, then you are more likely to take the opportunities this chapter affords for metacognitive development. The point is that such development is contextual, relational, and complex. Not surprisingly then, although learning medicine and becoming a physician afford many opportunities for metacognitive development, whether these opportunities are recognised or taken up, and if they are taken up then to what ends, cannot be easily predicted. Indeed, it may be that the best we can do, generically speaking at least, is to be mindful of our abilities and opportunities, to be mindful of how they are woven together to create capabilities, to be mindful of how these capabilities can change and how they can change us, and to be mindful of how our cognitive landscape shifts and changes accordingly. I would also remind readers of the many less desirable aspects of augmentation and capability change such that a metacognitive perspective on metacapability should also be mindful of the many ways in which capability change can have negative outcomes, to be mindful of the many ways in which such change is resisted, protested, resented, and stigmatised, and to be mindful of the sociocultural mores that underpin such contestation and mixed feelings.

Capability, augmentation, and metahumanism

Earlier, I suggested that a capability perspective can be used to consider a much broader landscape of possibility than that afforded by traditional medical humanities approaches and I hope I have demonstrated that point. However, I do not mean to suggest that a medical humanities approach based in the arts or humanities has no value, only that it is not the only approach we might employ to develop our metahumanistic thinking. Indeed, there is much in popular culture generally that we might use to reflect and explore capabilities and capability change, both positive and negative. Capability and augmentation have long fascinated us and ancient stories and myths are full of transformations and becomings. For example, Ovid's *Metamorphoses* is replete with people being turned into different beings, and the various consequences and implications of these changes. This fascination has persisted such that contemporary culture is full of augmentative possibilities and horrors of capability changes including those associated with vampires, zombies, and mad scientists. We see augmentation as a thread that connects Kafka's *Metamorphosis* with Wells' *The Invisible Man*, and Stevenson's Mr Hyde with Verne's Dr Moreau. This thread connects the stories of Aladdin, Sinbad, the Little Mermaid, Beauty and the Beast, and other folk tales. We can see augmentation as the central theme in movies such as *The Fly*, *Limitless*, and *Lucy*, as well as the endless run of movies that have featured superheroes and supervillains. Not only can such representations of augmentation paint life-expansion as exciting or frightening, but also these stories deal with serious moral issues such as hubris, audacity, pretension, vanity, conceitedness, contemptuousness, disdain, insolence, pomposity, presumption, and pretentiousness. Rather than being a superficial or rare occurrence, augmentation would seem to be able to articulate much, if not all, of the human condition.

Given this heady mix of fascination with and bias against people trying to become more than they are (something we also see associated with crossing boundaries set out by class, caste, religion, or racialised systems), we might use these as metacognitive (and metaphorical) starting points for reflection on whether or when seeking to become a doctor is a display of hubris, a reflection of manifest destiny, or an expression of augmentative autonomy.

Conclusions

By linking a capability approach to augmentation, I have outlined a rich theoretical space that shines new and unexpected lights on medicine and medical education. It also allows us to think differently about advantage and disadvantage, surfeits and deficits, and abilities and disabilities. I would note that the human capabilities approach has primarily been used as a deficit model to understand ways in which capability has been diminished, blocked, or denied. Augmentation theory on the other hand, while relatively new and ill-formed, is less deficit-focused and more about the strangeness and otherness of augmentation, and the perception of augmentation in others. Augmentation is also a key battleground between those seeking to reject societal norms, wishing to impose their own will and wishes on their bodies and minds; and those who are repelled by the thought, let alone reality, of this. What it is to be human is at stake (Cabrera 2017), and as such, this is a compelling and generative space to engage future doctors.

From a metacognitive perspective, the synthetic construct of capabilities and augmentation affords a novel way to reflect on and understand our own abilities and opportunities and those of others; how they have been shaped, and continue to be shaped, by our various advantages and disadvantages; and how capabilities and the ways in which they change can in turn change our senses of identity and purpose. A capabilities-augmentation perspective can also afford rich insights into metacognition and metahumanity, where it can afford diagnostic and therapeutic perspectives; and it can afford a critical perspective on the social constructions of professions, services, responsibilities, and obligations.

Note

1 Note that in Chapter 13, as part of our manifesto for metacognition in medical education, we draw on John Heron's set of core human capabilities (as 'foundational human needs') that predates Nussbaum: 'to understand and be understood, love and be loved, and to be self-directing and freely engaged with the directions of a greater whole'.

References

Albanese MA, Snow MH, Skochelak SE, Huggett KN, Farrell PM. 2003. Assessing personal qualities in medical school admissions. *Academic Medicine*. 78: 313–21.

Baker L, Brown AL. 1984. Metacognitive skills and reading. In: Douglas J, Dunlosky J, Graesser A (eds). *Handbook of Metacognition in Education*. New York, NY: Routledge, 7–25.

Balon R, Beresin EV, Guerrero APS, et al. 2020. Clinical Skills Verification: a Problematic Examination. *Academic Psychiatry*. 44: 255–9.

Cabrera LY. 2017. Reframing human enhancement: a population health perspective. *Frontiers in Sociology*. 2: 4.

Clark A. 2004. *Natural-Born Cyborgs: Minds, Technologies, and the Future of Human Intelligence*. Oxford: Oxford University Press.

Clarke QK. 2023. Reimagining disability accommodations in medical education. *Postgraduate Medical Journal*. 99: 238–9.

Edmonds WA, Tenenbaum G (eds.) 2011. *Case Studies in Applied Psychophysiology: Neurofeedback and Biofeedback Treatments for Advances in Human Performance*. Chichester: Wiley Blackwell.

Ellaway RH, Malhi R, Woloshuk W, et al. 2019. An axiological case study of a medical school's admissions values. *Academic Medicine*. 94: 1229–36.

Emanuel RM, Frellsen SL, Kashima KJ, et al. 2013. Cognitive enhancement drug use among future physicians: findings from a multi-institutional census of medical students. *Journal of General and Internal Medicine*. 28: 1028–34.

Frank JR, Snell L, Sherbino J (eds.) 2015. *CanMEDS 2015 Physician Competency Framework*. Ottawa, ON: Royal College of Physicians and Surgeons of Canada.

Katz JT. 2014. Applied medical humanities: addressing vexing deficits, promoting enduring skills. *AMA Journal of Ethics - Virtual Mentor*. 16: 610–3.

Keren D, Lockyer J, Kelly M, et al. 2020. In our own time: medical students' informal social studying and learning. *Teaching and Learning in Medicine*. 32: 353–61.

Leo RJ. 1999. Competency and the Capacity to Make Treatment Decisions: A Primer for Primary Care Physicians. *Prim Care Companion J Clin Psychiatry*. 1: 131–41.

Nussbaum M. 2011. *Creating Capabilities: The Human Development Approach*. Cambridge, MA: Harvard University Press.

Powell AJ, Myers TD. 2017. Developing Mental Toughness: Lessons from Paralympians. *Frontiers in Psychology*. 8: 1270.

Robeyns I. 2017. *Wellbeing, Freedom and Social Justice: The Capability Approach Re-Examined*. Cambridge: Open Book Publishers.

Ruger JP. 2004. Ethics of the social determinants of health. *Lancet*. 364: 1092–7.

Sen A. 1992. *Inequality Reexamined*. Oxford: Oxford University Press.

Teunissen PW, Watling CJ, Schrewe B, et al. 2021. Contextual Competence: How residents develop competent performance in new settings. *Medical Education*. 55: 1100–9.

Thomas BR, Dockter N. 2019. Affirmative action and holistic review in medical school admissions: where we have been and where we are going? *Academic Medicine*. 94: 473–6.

Wellman HM. 1985. Origins of metacognition. In: Pressley D, McKinnon G, Waller T (eds). *Metacognition, Cognition, and Human Performance*. Orlando, FL: Academic Press.

Zazove P, Case B, Moreland C, et al. 2016. U.S. Medical Schools' Compliance with the Americans With Disabilities Act: Findings From a National Study. *Academic Medicine*. 91: 979–86.

10 Realising the extended mind

Quentin Eichbaum

Introduction

Our aim throughout this book has been to map innovations in this complex field onto the field of medical education. We see this in many respects as swimming against the tide, where medical education has been reduced to a narrow focus: linear, instrumental, competency-led training based on problem-solving and grounded in intolerance of ambiguity. This has been characterised by Yrjö Engeström (2018) as a 'will-to-stability' rather than the taking of necessary risk for expansion of activity (breaking new ground), the latter characterised by 'spearheads' of innovation. Here, the frame for cognition and affect embraces complexity, risk, and tolerance of ambiguity. Our chosen media for realising such innovation within medical education are the humanities (including the arts and qualitative social sciences, but also embracing aesthetic approaches to biomedical sciences). This follows a long tradition of employing the medical humanities to expand value concerns from the objective instrumental or functional to the more subjective and humanising (ethical, aesthetic, political, and transcendental concerns) (Bleakley and Neilson 2023). As the potential of the humanities is realised in this pedagogical move, so we mobilise metahumanities – humanities that (i) avoid disciplinary restrictions but operate in inter-, trans-, and circum-disciplinary manners (Bleakley 2014); and (ii) avoid epistemological frames grounded in oppositional thinking (such as science vs arts) (Beranek 2021). The pedagogical move of the humanities into the 'extended mind' (beyond the bounds of 'skin and skull') towards metahumanities provides the necessary lift to transcend such disciplinary restrictions and restrictive epistemological frames of oppositional thinking. In this chapter, I will discuss core principles for realising the extended mind and how these principles may be applied to both medical education and metahumanities.

The extended mind

The notion of an 'extended mind' might be traced back to Palaeolithic hunter-gatherers and the origins of art in cave paintings. First, small bands of hunter-gatherers would have division of labour, and in such division, a communal (or extended) mind is born. Such extension is grounded in a shared

DOI: 10.4324/9781032687339-13

language – spoken, written, sung, dramatised, and as iconography such as cave paintings of hunted animals and imprints of human hands. Along with division of labour (probably gender and age based) must have emerged agreed rules of conduct for the group – a code of morality. Cave paintings also suggest a mind extended into nature (animals killed in the hunt are considered sacred) and the transcendental (the animal must be revived for the next season's hunt and is considered sacred; perhaps there is a sense of awe in the face of natural events such as thunderstorms).

In modern times, following the invention of writing and then the printing press to disseminate writing, the concept of the extended mind gained traction as technological devices (for cognitive offloading) such as personal computers, mobile phones, and artificial intelligence (AI) were realised. Advances in neurobiology and in understanding the brain, the development of artificial and natural spaces that impacted mind and health, and the threat of climate change also point to a nuanced interaction between the environment, brain-bound cognition, and cognition outside the brain.

When Clark and Chalmers (1998) posited 'a different kind of externalism: an *active externalism*, based on the active role of the environment in driving cognition' they were drawing a distinction between their 'active' view of the extended mind and the more passive views of extended cognition (at the time) of situated, embodied, and distributed cognition. In other words, cognition is fundamentally *intentional* rather than passive. Situativity theory (see Chapter 6) in clinical education also has shades of an active externalism (Durning and Artino 2011, Torre et al. 2020), but how to operationalise the extended mind – and in particular how it pertains to the arts and humanities within a medical pedagogical frame – has received less attention.

Annie Paul (2023) suggests nine 'principles of brain extension'. Here, I elaborate on each principle to suggest how they are entwined with metahumanities.

Offloading

Wherever possible, we should *offload information* and move it out of our minds into the world. This disburdens us from having to keep details in our heads, freeing mental resources for other demanding tasks. Such offloading may entail the simple act of putting thoughts down on paper. This freeing up of cognitive load was accelerated exponentially first by the invention of the printing press and second by the development of the computer and World Wide Web. Offloading can be continuous or partial (and periodic). *Continuous* offloading demands making fresh observations in the world and keeping journals to synthesise ideas the way that poets and writers habitually do. Here, one is reminded of the speed 'stream of consciousness' writing that teachers like Julia Cameron (1999) and Natalie Goldberg (2005) developed, in which students are asked to write at speed for 20 minutes in cursive without stopping. This is a form of extended mind offloading: the mind engages with the physical objects (pen and paper) in the environment and offloads thoughts into the paper without interruption. This by-passes issues of memory for issues of attention (see Chapter 5).

Part-offloading entails designing a task such that one part is offloaded while another part receives full attention. For instance, in writing a book (or a chapter), first getting down the outline frees attention to focus on specific content without stressfully draining attention about the entire content and direction of the book. Offloading also produces a 'detachment gain' through which we can 'inspect with our senses, and often perceive anew, an image or idea that once existed only in imagination'. I would counter that from an arts perspective we would also be able to 'perceive anew' items that still linger in imagination. In creative gestures, the artist offloads not only from the moving carriages of the train (a trail of memory and anticipation), but also from the metaphorical train crashes and derailments (spontaneous irruption of ideas, utilising 'mistakes' as serendipitous innovations).

Offloading can also be *embodied* through *gestures* – such as a hand gesture – that allow the speaker to 'hold' a thought somatically they would otherwise have to hold cognitively. Gesture is key in the performing arts such as theatre, ballet, improvisation, and mime where it encapsulates items of the mind. Clinical practice has been characterised as theatre, with set roles and scripts. Lastly, offloading may occur in interpersonal contexts where we externalise our thinking processes for friends and teammates – not only to unburden our minds, but also to facilitate social interaction and collaboration.

Where we are habituated into considering intelligence as fast analytical thinking, Howard Gardner (2008) proposed a more complex model of eight kinds of intelligence, including kinesthetic (evinced by ballet dancers and sportsmen) and intra- and inter-personal intelligence displayed by people using embodied cognition to read a room and effectively offload and externalise their thoughts and feelings to facilitate social interaction.

Metahumanities might afford media to not only further explore these forms of cognitive offloading, but also explore how they align with and augment different kinds of intelligence rather than just analytical intelligence. In medical education, continuous offloading can be achieved through regular reflective writing (as done in some medical school programmes) or by requesting that students keep a journal of their clinical experiences for a specified period. This can be seen as a form of narrative-based medicine, where the student's qualitative narrative (best produced collaboratively with patients) acts as a 'parallel chart' for the standard bedside quantitative record. Also, the relevance of embodied offloading could be communicated to students making them aware of how patients from different cultures communicate differently through gestures or how a patient (e.g., a refugee) who does not speak the language used in a clinical setting is made sense of through a translator.

Making it real

Paul's second principle suggests that wherever possible we 'should endeavor to transform information into an artifact, to make data into something real – and then proceed to interact with it … '. Further, 'Humans evolved to handle the concrete, not to contemplate the abstract'. Turning abstract symbols and data to more tangible objects and sensory experiences can require the kinds of creativity promoted by the arts.

This principle is, however, contestable. While rendering the abstract 'real' and 'tangible' is one avenue for realising the extended mind, I find it hard to fully agree with Paul's assertion that we evolved 'to handle the concrete, not to contemplate the abstract' ('Making it real'). A distinguishing feature of the human brain (as it rapidly increased in size during evolution) was its increased capacity for abstraction that allowed it to learn from current 'tangible' situations and objects and to abstract to make predictions (Clark 2013) for future survival. Ultimately, this capacity also fed into the sociobiological development of religion and ethics (Wilson 1988), and to philosophy, metaphysics, and science (Wilson 2014). Unfocused abstraction (dreams, daydreaming, musing, and imagination) is also key to creativity (e.g., as serendipity).

Intellectual deliberations (of the head brain) can, with close attention, become embodied by connecting to the gut brain through interoception (a perceptive mode other than humans' default audiovisual mode). These alternate under-recognised perceptuomotor sensory modes that make the extended mind 'real' are part of what we call meta-sensory and meta-affective realms (see Chapter 1). Here again, the arts and humanities play a role by emphasising the importance of paying attention and close noticing not only to the environment and the world, but also to ourselves and our bodies. For example, in clinical education, situativity theory suggests that embodied cognition links perception and cognition to action and that perceptuomotor capacities can be channelled into action in clinical contexts through technology-enhanced simulation as well as virtual reality and AI simulations (Torre et al. 2020).

Altering our mental states

Paul's third principle suggests that we need to 'productively alter *our own state* when engaging in mental labor'. This entails inducing a state of body and/or mind suited to the task at hand. The way we think about knowledge and process information are affected by the mental states we are in. Thus, we might engage in exercise, go for a walk, meditate, stand up and stretch, plan a trip – whatever we know might work for more effective mental labour. Given how accustomed we are to commanding the brain to do our bidding, taking time to induce appropriate mental states for tasks at hand may seem odd. The brain is neither a 'machine' nor 'computer' but a context-sensitive, malleable, and fallible biological organ. Importantly, the human bodymind is an open, adaptive, complex, and dynamic system working against inevitable entropy. Computers function as closed systems, a form of 'procedural' training (discussed in Chapter 6) as 'input–output–done' that has severe limitations. Understanding that the brain evolved to navigate the body through adaptive environments while interacting with, and relating to, other members of our species should help us to see that it is not a linear-function computer. As a complex system at the edge of chaos (without generally falling into such chaos), the brain can transform spontaneously to work at higher levels of complexity.

We are ‘perturb-able’ and ‘intrinsically loopy creatures’ as Andy Clark reportedly liked to say (Paul 2023), contributing to our creative capacity for storytelling and the arts. More, we have the metacapability (metacreativity) to use the arts to critique, parody, and deconstruct the arts themselves. This is like Clark’s (2013) posited feedback loop from brain to environment, where the brain acts as predictor, and the environmental cues adjust such predictions in a future-facing feedback loop. We can change our mental status to suit the task at hand either deliberately or by interacting with the world around us, and to run processes in reverse, such as bringing abstractions back into corporeal, social, and spatial forms. The arts and humanities thrive on these loopy pathways, augmenting and altering our mental states. In part, this is the enjoyment we derive from the arts – their unpredictability, improvisation that can perturb and lead to puzzlement and surprise. The function of the arts and humanities (as well as qualitative science) is surely not as decoration but as disruption, to create the conditions for not just thinking outside the box, but without the box as ‘freefall’ cognition.

Re-embody

Wherever possible, we should take measures to *re-embody* the information we think about.

Individualist cultures maintain that thinking in the pursuit of knowledge is localised strictly within the head-brain, as if disengaged from the body. Embodied cognition calls on us to reengage the head-brain with the heart-and-gut brain, to draw the body back into the thinking process, to consider interoceptive signals, intuitions, and body gut feelings, to attend to the gestures of ourselves and others in our thinking processes. Medical education retains its intense focus on brain-bound cognition with barrages of tests and licensing exams and with little to make students aware of the connection between their body and cognition (except through occasional extracurricular opportunities). Bringing the head, heart, and gut brain into better synchrony could potentially alleviate anxiety and some of the deleterious impacts of the ‘hidden curriculum’.

The connection between interoceptive signals and brain cognition is evident, according to Antonio Damasio (1999), in people with damage to their interoceptive networks who had impaired decision-making. Neuroscientist Lisa Barrett (2017) posits that

> From your brain’s perspective, your body is just another source of sensory input … . Every thought, memory, emotion, or perception that you construct in your life includes something about the state of your body … . Every prediction you make, and every categorization your brain completes, is always in relation to the activity of your heart and lungs, your metabolism, your immune function, and the other systems that contribute to your body budget.

But such whole-body cognition is necessarily situated – how we move through space, negotiate objects, and so forth. As we place emphasis here upon flesh, so we recognise that the body is an *open* system, adaptive to the environment. We assimilate cues as we accommodate to them. Rather than regarding the body as the 'lesser animal part of our natures', we might embrace the body. Artists do not shy away from 'the state of the body' but rather attend to it as it provides the gateways for artistic perceptions. The body can become a canvas through performance or for modification. In contemporary art, this can be radical, taking the body to its limits.

Barrett provides further examples of how the senses of the body 'read the world' and construct our emotions, a concept that has implications for embodied cognition, metacognitive regulation of thoughts and emotions, and metahumanities. Barrett (2017) writes that,

> A sound, therefore is not an event that is detected in the world. It is an experience constructed when the world interacts with the body that detects changes in air pressure, and the brain that can make those changes meaningful.

Here, 'the social and the physical are intimately linked via your body and your brain, and your ability to move effectively between social and physical depends on a set of skills that you can learn'. Such warnings about whole embodiment are welcome particularly in medicine and medical education, where patients are often reduced to isolated body parts related to symptoms. We must not only resist such objectification (as disembodiment), but also recognise the multiple ways that patients 'perform' their bodies, especially through symptom, illness, and pain. In Barrett's view, effective communication and the co-construction of emotion depend on the accuracy and synchrony of our predictions (which in turn are shaped by the words we use):

> You and I communicate emotions, in the face of huge variability, by way of the brain's predictive machinery. Your emotions are guided by your predictions. And as I observe you, the emotions I perceive are guided by my predictions. Emotional communication happens, therefore, when you and I predict and categorize *in synchrony*.... Your choice of words has a huge impact on this process, as those words shape other people's predictions.

Barrett seems to echo Clark's 'predictive processing', where cognition is effectively reduced to anticipation and then a series of co-ordinated re-adjustments around the realisation (or not) of anticipations. Sociologists in the school of dramaturgy developed from Erving Goffman's (2006) work have long described such anticipation in the extended social rather than restricted personal world. Thus, as you spot a stranger or a friend from a distance, you prepare yourself socially for contact in anticipation: a mixture of defensive readiness and curiosity for the stranger, while eager anticipation and openness for the friend. This work of anticipation is, for Goffman, a work of dramatic imagination.

Barrett does not refer to this work of imagination that allows us, for example, to engage other bodies without direct knowledge of that person's experience. Imagination occupies an intangible space between psyche and soma. Barrett (2017) describes 'The co construction of experience (that) allows us to regulate each other 's body budgets' as 'one of the great benefits that we get from living in groups'. While

> All members of a social species regulate each other 's body budgets … we are the only species who can do so by teaching each other purely mental concepts and then using them in synchrony … . The social and the physical are intimately linked by your body and your brain, and your ability to move effectively between social and physical.

But *how* do we negotiate between the social and physical? Clearly, we have the power of prediction through imagination, but just where might 'imagination' be located?

Re-spatialise

Wherever possible, we should 'take measures to re-spatialize the information we think about,' says Barrett (2017). Neuroscience suggests that our brains process information in the form of spatial mental maps, but our school curricula and workplaces make insufficient application of such mental maps. Whatever we teach in a linear (procedural) flow of information acquisition, we should consider *re-spatialising* to allow us to think about topics in the sciences in medicine in more advanced ways, including spatial language map-making, sketching, gestures, charts tables, and diagrams. Medical education increasingly offers computer applications for mapping and re-spatialising knowledge to suite a range of learner needs (e.g., *Evernote™*, *Mindmeister™*, *Coggle™*, and *Roam Research™*). Here the arts and humanities also come into play, with emphasis on artistic interactional design and a willingness to enter spaces of uncertainty.

Re-socialise

Instead of keeping knowledge and information stuck in our head as a 'kind of internalized conversation' (Paul 2023), we should re-socialise it into social encounters and interactions. Research (Teixeira et al. 2022) has shown that the brain processes the same information differently, and in many ways more effectively, when other human beings participate and are brought into our trains of thought. Bringing our thoughts out into the social domain can augment them. In any case, from Socratic method to Hegelian dialectic, social augmentation patently enriches discourse. Likewise, the arts benefit from being socialised into the community space, advertised by storytelling and group singing and dancing in indigenous cultures. In medical education, we see positive trends towards collaborative and re-socialised learning in team-based learning (TBL) and case-based learning, as well as in humanities discussion groups (such as Vanderbilt University's College Colloquium described in Chapter 5) (Eichbaum 2014). A wealth of evidence, meanwhile, shows that better functioning clinical teams advertising democratic habits afford better patient care and safety and job satisfaction, while preventing burnout (Anderson et al. 2021, Jarvis and Samuel 2023).

Generate cognitive loops

Andy Clark (1998; Clark and Chalmers 1998) points to the fallacy of the mind as a model of a linear computer (input–output–done). As 'intrinsically loopy creatures', our biological intelligence benefits from being looped between external and internal modes of thinking and passed between the brain, body, and world. Moreover, such thinking is predictive. As Clark (2023) shows, prediction is laced with uncertainty and may rely on serendipity, but in the main it is accurate. The point of the feedback process is constant adjustment. Our thinking is not linear but takes a winding path so we should not try to keep our thoughts statically inside our heads 'unchanged by contours of the world beyond the skull' (Paul 2023). Such nonlinearity is a key aspect of dynamic, complex systems and of increasing relevance to education. Louis Menand (2010) has drawn attention to the nonlinear mode of learning of the new generation of students:

> A pressing pedagogical challenge right now is the problem of adapting a linear model for transmitting knowledge – the lecture monologue, in which a single line of thought leads to an intellectual climax after fifty minutes – to a generation of students who are accustomed to dealing with multiple information streams and short bursts.

By the same token, the arts by their nature are nonlinear whether we are talking about improvisation in jazz and theatre, intuitive (gut brain) abstract expressionism, or how poetry loops between different forms of attention (see Chapter 5). Given the increased awareness of the value of 'nonlinear' cognition in the arts, there have been renewed efforts in medical education in the United States through the Association of American Medical Colleges (AAMC) to better integrate the arts and humanities into medical school education through initiatives such as the Fundamental Role of the Art and Humanities in Medical Education (FRAHME) (Howley et al. 2020).

Create cognitively congenial situations

We are 'situationally sensitive creatures' and instead of demanding that our brains knuckle down, pay attention, and produce exactly the output that we demand of them – a linear approach – we can create situations and environments that elicit improved performance from the brain by recognising 'complexity' as a resource. This means creating appropriate spaces such as places where stories can thrive, and the three brains can work together in synchrony or even as a form of puzzlement. A positive trend in this direction can be seen in medical education in the 'green' and cognitively congenial architecture of some new medical schools that have gardens and light-filled collaborative meeting areas designed as environments for cognitive and somatic enrichment. Good architects create such zones with a view to stimulate rather than disengage. For example, medical schools may devise large lecture halls in an age in which learning mainly occurs in small groups (such as problem-based learning). Not only does this waste valuable resource space, it also encourages less motivated students to dis-engage, whereas small group learning demands engagement.

Embedding extensions

We should make ready use of extensions in the environment to assist thinking and the development of mental models. We are so 'technologised' that already you may be thinking of such extensions as software (e.g., virtual anatomy and dissection programmes). However, flesh-and-blood extensions exist in the form of colleagues learning together with us. Here, belonging and identity are key, stimulating the transactive (or 'shared') memory system that occurs in interactions with colleagues and friends over time and serves to distribute among the group the burden of attending to and remembering information. Once such human extensions are established, we may turn to technologies as augmentation. The use of such technologies should be judicious – for example, not becoming addicted to, or overly dependent upon, extensions such as technology devices and social media. Embedding means making these technologies part of our own mental processes rather than surrendering our cognition to these extensions. To improve attention and collaborative group cognition, medical schools are increasingly discouraging or not allowing students to be on the internet and social media during classes and group education sessions. The arts and humanities have a role in keeping our emotions agile and attention flexible, sustaining the meta-affective, meta-sensory, and metacognitive, rather than succumbing to the instrumental-procedural in surrendering to our extended devices.

Paul's nine principles of brain extension have provided an instructive framework through which I have argued for the value of the meta. Engaging with such a framework must itself be a metacognitive activity of critical attention and supplement, to expand that frame. We are doing medical students a disservice if we do not teach them critical inquiry of which metacognition and metahumanities are foundational components.

Metacognition for the extended mind

As cognition moves outside boundaries of skin and skull towards an *active externalism* with a dynamic, bidirectional, and participatory relationship with the environment (its artefacts and the minds of others), do we also need a *metacognition for the extended mind*? What would its core elements be? If the core elements of group/shared metacognition are *knowledge* of cognition, and *monitoring* and *regulation* of cognition (Garrison and Akyol 2015), what would be the components of a metacognition of the extended mind?

An extra layering of *regulation* may be needed as the extended mind engages with an increasingly complex environment. At the core of such regulation would be forms of *attention* (see Chapter 5). As the mind extends into the world, it may be at once augmented by the richness of the environment but is also at risk of diffusing its own attention while being subjugated to the demands of the environment. James J Gibson (1979) warned against always thinking (or imagining) *out* from person to world, instead considering: how are the person's perceptions *afforded* by the world? James Williams (2018), a former Google advertising strategist, now Oxford-trained philosopher, argues that 'the defining moral political struggle of our time (is) the liberation of human attention … in order to do anything that matters we must first be able to give attention to things that matter'.

Or, as another former Google employee, in testimony before the US Senate in 2019, put it: 'In an attention economy, there's only so much attention, and the advertising business model always wants more. So it becomes a race to the bottom of the brain' (Magsamen & Ross 2023). With AI and burgeoning technologies in the environment, the mind will increasingly work at what Singh and Sittig (2015) term the *sociotechnical interface* between society, the individual, and technology. Regarding clinical environments, the authors say: 'Within the sociotechnical context, many system-related factors could shape cognitive performance and critical thinking and make clinicians vulnerable to losing situational awareness'. What form of 'coregulation' is tenable at this interface remains to be seen.

Metahumanities for the extended mind

In the opening remarks to this chapter, I briefly discuss the essential need for and potential of metahumanities. Here, I return to that theme and expand it. Throughout, I refer to 'humanities' and 'metahumanities' to include the arts, qualitative social sciences, and aesthetic approaches to bioscience. My starting point is EO Wilson's (2017) axiom: 'Because the humanities … consist of everything that is human, all that is human comprises the humanities'. Here, I will focus the argument on the fit of metahumanities for the extended mind. The traditional humanities insulated themselves from the sciences and risked becoming self-limiting, restrictive, and intellectually incestuous. TS Eliot (2014), a foremost intellect of the 20th century with no background in science, understood this when he wrote that 'Knowledge of life obtained through fiction is only possible by another stage of self-consciousness. That is to say, it can only be a knowledge of other people's knowledge of life, not of life itself'.

To be apprised of knowledge 'of life itself', metahumanities must reach out into other disciplines, particularly the sciences. Wilson suggests the following

'Big Five bedrock disciplines' as 'gateways for interdisciplinary integration: palaeontology, anthropology (including archaeology), psychology (primarily cognitive and social), neurobiology, and evolutionary biology'. Tweaking the words of the great geneticist Theodosius Dobzhansky (1964), who said that 'nothing in biology makes sense except in the light of evolution', Wilson asserts that 'nothing in science and the humanities makes sense except in the light of evolution'.

In rejecting the infamous 1954 'Two Cultures' argument of CP Snow, EO Wilson (2017) argues that:

> Contrary to common belief, the humanities are not distinct from science. No fundamental chasm in the real world or process of the human mind separates them. Each permeates the other … . Scientific knowledge is the idiosyncratic, absolutely humanistic product for the human brain.

Metahumanities must therefore integrate or blend the humanities with the sciences. Wilson proposes one implication of such a blending, as a 'renewed role for philosophy to its previously esteemed position … this time as the center of a humanistic science and a scientific humanities'. More specifically, what may be needed is a revitalised *metaphysics* – that branch of philosophy that focuses on the nature of reality and existence, the relationship between mind and matter, structure of the universe, causation, identity, and consciousness. The failure of current-day philosophy is mostly due to its inattention to what has been emerging in science. We need more philosopher-scientists like neuroscientist/philosopher Patricia Churchland who can cross with seamless intellectual rigour between the sciences and humanities. We need a scientifically informed humanities that can unabashedly pose questions such as Churchland's: 'How is it that brains care about anything? To put it more tendentiously, how can neurons care? What does it mean for a system of neurons to care about or value something?' Such thinking is taken up by Alan Bleakley and Shane Neilson (2023) and Bleakley (2024) in challenging both narrative medicine's and the medical/ health humanities' continuing resistance to biomedical science, particularly in the latter's role as a generator of inventive metaphor. Bleakley suggests that the long-dead arts–science divide can be ditched. What is more important is whether any arts/humanities/qualitative social science or biomedical science approach is productive of valuable metaphors, or regresses to literalism. Where metaphors are generated, it is usually the case that an instrumental approach will blossom to embrace ethical, aesthetic, political, and transcendental values. The latter leads us into 'meta' territory.

The integrated metahumanities would not shy away from questions such as Churchland poses above. Questions like this, and the associated inquiries they engender, do not detract from, but rather augment, the humanities (and the sciences). But how do we encourage such questions in an education system that since the European Enlightenment continues to silo the branches of learning? The humanities are under attack in universities around the world and medical humanities are banished to the outer orbits of the curriculum (if they survive at all). Why are the humanities being short-shrifted?

To be sure, the onus for bringing together humanities and sciences lies also with the sciences. While scientists often have a deep interest in the arts (often as a 'hobby'), others are dismissive and driven by a quest for factual evidence in their hyper-specialised field, often under pressure of grant applications and publishing. Few are the public scientists – like Peter Medawar, EO Wilson, Richard Dawkins, and Stephen Hawking – who have crossed with intellectual ease between the sciences and humanities to ask the big cross-disciplinary questions. We also need to resist the notion that unless something can be measured, calculated, or quantified, it lacks merit or cannot be true. Quantity, after all, is just one form of quality, albeit a very important quality. Science is one way of looking at the world and reality, its power deriving in part from the narrowness of its approach. Science cannot fully grasp, let alone measure, the fullness of human subjective experience and consciousness although it might explain how we biologically perceive and process experiences. As Martha Nussbaum (2012) suggests, 'Citizens cannot relate well to the complex world around them by factual knowledge and logic alone'. Art and metahumanities remind us that science is incomplete, that some mysteries of the ghost will remain in the machine, and that we will always in part be such stuff as dreams are made of.

How can our education systems better blend the sciences and humanities within the curriculum? This has been a major aim of the (now dwindling) liberal arts education in the United States since the early 1800s starting with Jefferson's establishment of the University of Virginia to espouse the ideals of a public education. Despite many extolling the benefits of a liberal education (including business leaders, with three in four agreeing that a liberal education provides an essential background for effective leaders and thinkers), universities increasingly view the humanities as an expendable luxury that can be cut from the curriculum in favour of producing STEM professionals, lawyers, and businessmen. This devaluation is at once disturbing and perplexing. Edward O Wilson suggests that the secular humanities have been underfunded in the United States because they have had to 'compete with organized religion and religion-like ideologies for attention and volunteer public funding'.

Another reason to reconsider our traditional approaches to education in the second half of the 21st century is that our future working lives will become increasingly irrelevant as vast amounts of human labour become automated through AI and fewer jobs will be created along the way (Burmeister 2023). AI is the prime artefact the extended mind will encounter in the environment going forward. Predictions are that humans will have increasing amounts of time for leisure, and we will need to know how to apply the extended mind to fill that time. Burmeister (2023) argues that the best education to prepare people for this life is a liberal education as it fosters the essential traits of self-knowledge and self-regulation. Such an education aligns with Aristotle's notion of atelic activities involving freedom to engage in activities for their own sake essential for human happiness.

Willis Rudy (1980) suggests that a liberally educated person is one who is 'inwardly as well as outwardly free', and among the attributes this entails are self-knowledge and self-regulation, while Martha Nussbaum (2012) argues that 'liberal arts education strengthens the skills of imagining and independent thinking that are crucial to maintaining a successful culture of innovation'. A study by Winter (1981) pointed out that a liberal education provides not just cognitive, but also emotional, capabilities; and Louis Menand (2010) adds that

> the liberal arts and sciences ... are simply fields in which knowledge is pursued disinterestedly – that is, without regard to political economic, or practical benefit .... Almost any liberal arts field can be made non-liberal by turning it in the direction of some practical skill with which it is already associated .... But conversely, and more importantly, any practical field can be made liberal simply by teaching it historically and theoretically.

This kind of comment arises from dissatisfaction with the modernist opposition between the practical and the intellectual. This is a false distinction in the eyes of postmodernists, who prefer to think of all human functioning as 'activity', where the key issue is whether an activity expands (innovates) rather than contracting, crystallising, or expiring. In any activity, there is always an unknown (and unknowable) surplus, but it is this surplus that attracts and inspires us, out of curiosity.

Metahumanities fulfil this role of attraction to surplus by resisting the drive towards only instrumental skills, concerns, and information (rather than meaning). An education that resists absolutes and the purely practical and informational is comfortable exploring uncertainties, puzzlement, discomfort, and perturbations, and rests more comfortably with subjunctives and conditionals. The advantages of a mind attuned to conditionals can be argued down to the neurocognitive level, as done by Daniel Siegel (2007):

> When our minds lock onto something as being absolute, it enters our memory stores in a very different form from the way it would were we to be tentative about the contexts and conditions in which what we have just learned might apply... . Our efficient neural association machine creates memory systems that can take a 'fact' and create a rapidly accessible node of neural firing patterns that form a building block in the scaffold of our semantic knowledge of the world. But with a conditional statement, that neural nodal point must have far more intricately established conditions for it to meet the criteria for inclusion into the scaffold of knowledge.

As the extended mind reaches into an increasingly complex world, the uncertainties and conditionalities grow more intricate and daunting. With climate change, dwindling resources, and an environment populated with AI, sociopolitical tensions may increase and democracy itself placed at risk (as evident in the current rise of autocracies around the world). We will need both the sciences and humanities to deal with these threats. Martha Nussbaum (2012) argues that the humanities are best suited for promoting democracy, given how adept they are at deconstructing complex concepts and dealing with uncertainty. She further argues that another reason the humanities are being eroded in university education is the obsession with economic growth as a measure of a country's success. Governments need to show economic growth as an increase in Gross Domestic Product (GDP) to survive politically: 'For this reason, all over the world, programs in arts and humanities at all levels, are being cut away, in favor of cultivation of the technical'. Since the humanities do not serve this instrumental monetary purpose, they are being cut. Analogously, medical humanities are cut for not producing clinical and scientific evidence that can be monetised or for not educating students to that end. More perversely, the humanities are often perceived as a threat to economic growth, autocracies of power, and democratic values. As Nussbaum (2012) says: 'educators for economic growth will do more than ignore the arts. They will fear them'. For Nussbaum, 'economic growth' within our late capitalist system is merely producing greater inequity and inequality. More starkly, as Jean-Paul Sartre reportedly said, 'Why is it that in every revolution the poets are the first to get dragged out and shot?' The integrated metahumanities would not surrender their values-driven purposes such as challenging injustices, inequities, and autocracies of power.

Neurobiology may ultimately also explain and mitigate the inbuilt biases and other traps of cognition. In addition, the steadily growing field of neuroaesthetics will surely enrich the arts, augmenting their wonderment rather than detracting through reductionism. Instead of devaluing the arts as being 'too subjective', we begin to understand that, as with personalised medicine, the arts are also personalised and that does detract from their value. We also understand that value in art and other domains of our lives is not absolute but contingent. As Barbara Hernstein Smith (1988) argued some decades ago in her classic *Contingencies of Value*: 'all value is radically contingent, being neither a fixed attribute, and inherent quality, or an object property of things but, rather, an effect of multiple continuously changing, and continuously interacting variables'.

Magsamen and Ross (2023) insist that as the field of neuro-aesthetics expands, 'we will see a rise in personalized micro-dosing of aesthetics' in the arts. They provide numerous examples of how the arts and aesthetics are being effectively used across disciplines from business, education, and technology to healthcare, where they are being applied to improve the health and lives of patients and healthcare systems including, in the UK, the *Scaling-up Health Arts Programmes: Implementation and Effectiveness Research* (SHAPER) (Estevao et al. 2021), a research initiative aimed at examining the impact of arts interventions on healthcare outcomes; and in the work of renowned soprano Renee Fleming's (2005) global Arts and Health programmes (Edwards et al. 2023, Weigel et al. 2023). In the space of arts exhibition experiences, museums are no longer just repositories for artefacts but interactive spaces for relational engagement with art. Initiatives such as the interdisciplinary Team Lab Borderless in Tokyo and in London the 'Tate Sensorium' exhibition dissolved boundaries between the artwork and the viewer to bring the viewer's senses into participatory proximity with the art.

Metahumanities would embrace rather than be threatened by developments in neuro-aesthetics as they open multiple doors of exploration at the intersection of disciplines. For instance, we begin to understand the appeal of Jackson Pollock's drip paintings at a neuro-aesthetic level when we understand that they exhibit fractal patterns of the same midrange values (1.3–1.50) seen in forest twigs and branch patterns that have soothing impacts on the human nervous system and underlie the sensation of forest bathing (Hagerhall et al. 2004). (Fractals are patterns in which the same motif is repeated at different scales.) Do Pollock's paintings tap into humanity's ancient connection with nature, speaking to us through a neuro-visual signature of nature? Or take Cezanne's ambiguous *noninfinito* paintings (e.g., *Mount Sainte-Victoire seen from Lauves*) that are incomplete (to the fury of his early critics) and question the very essence of form while leaving the viewer's imagination to 'fill in the blanks'. Neuroscience now tells us how the prefrontal cortex 'first sees' an image before its starts adjusting inputs and creating an interpretable Gestalt we then view as 'reality'. Jonah Lehrer (2008) argues that the reason many great works of art (literature, music, and paintings) have lasted through the ages with universal appeal is likely because they tap into deep neurobiological signatures. Does the study of art through a neuroscientific lens reduce or detract from the art? I think not – it enriches or augments it. Such discourse makes a mockery of art/science divisions and oppositions.

The extended mind – participatory externalism

Pertinent to the active externalism of the extended mind is the finding of the physicist John Wheeler (a colleague of Einstein and Bohr) that we are living in a *participatory universe* – one in which we are not passive bystanders but active shapers and creators. Recent discoveries in physics reveal that every act of observation is in some way an act of creation and, more startlingly, that the laws of physics can themselves *change over time with different laws competing for effectiveness* (Smolin 2013, Mangabeira Unger and Smolin 2015). Every act of observation influences not only the future, but also the history, of the universe. We are not just passive observers of, but *active participants in*, the universe.

Clark and Chalmer's *active externalism* might be more aptly named *participatory externalism*. The mind does not just extend into the environment through shared, situated, embodied, and distributed cognition but, if the cosmology is right, *participates in, and changes, the world* and the way it operates. This clearly has implications for consciousness and the 'meaning of human existence'(Wilson 2014). Wheeler has devoted the last decades of his life to the question he phrases as: *'How come existence?'* – a core question for a humanities with a consilience of knowledge (Folger 2002, Meijer 2015).

The extended mind and the blessing and curse of neuroplasticity

The biological correlate of such a changing participatory universe is the universe inside the human skull – the trillions of neurons and synaptic connections that underlie our immense neuroplasticity and potentiate 'The Brain That Changes Itself'. This is the title of neuroscientist Norman Doidge's (2007) book in which he describes research countering a hardwired brain in favour of a brain that 'changes its very structure with each different activity it performs, perfecting its circuits so it is better suited to the task at hand'.

Neuroscientist Alvaro Pascual-Leone (in Begley 2007) puts it thus: 'The brain changes with anything you do including any thought you might have'. The brain is not just a receptacle for storage, or processor of information and input from the outside world, but an organ that can conjure up/create images and knowledge and process them in ways to change itself. The immense neuroplasticity of the brain, however, also has a darker side that explains both constrained and unconstrained aspects of our nature that contribute to both cognitive flexibility and rigidity. Doidge calls this phenomenon 'the plastic paradox' and says that it 'stirs up a hornet's nest of moral problems' in raising expectations of the perfectibility of human nature, our capacity for change, and the associated sociopolitical implications of such perspectives.

The unconstrained side of neuroplasticity poses a dilemma for human nature and metahumanities. Jaak Panksepp (1982) calls this *the curse of neuroplasticity*, where 'Everything in the brain is interconnected – and that of course in the problem'. This hyperconnectivity poses an issue for human identity – core for metahumanities. Heidi Ravven (2013) puts the dilemma as: 'Given the unimaginable vastness of neuroplasticity, how do we become distinctly who we are rather than mere harbourers of infinite possible actions, beliefs and selves? … how can we ever decide anything? Become a stable and recognizable personality?'. This claim of course is somewhat blinded by its location – deep in the flesh that is the brain. As we move out to interpersonal relations, groups, societies, and cultures, identity becomes less of a mystery.

A problem the unconstrained side of neuroplasticity poses for the extended mind is the limitless number of *interpretations* of behaviour (and the world) it exposes us to. Ravven (2013) continues:

> our human moral problem may be a matter of too much thinking, too much interpretation… . Openness confuses our prosocial capacities … humans are off the charts when it comes to the openness and flexibility of our behavior, or our interpretation of behavior.

To cope with such seemingly limitless flexibility, openness of neuroplasticity, and interpretative possibilities, we are impelled to view the world through what George Lakoff (Lakoff and Johnson 2008) calls 'interpretative frames' within a universe of metaphors (see Chapter 2): 'Cognitive framing exposes how neuroplasticity … links meanings to each other and to context and to our individual biographical selves … through interpretative frames, which in turn are modified in the process'. It thus seems that the extended mind for all its neuroplasticity and reach into the world is compelled ultimately to impose constraints on itself for cognitive coherence, and some sense of identity, where 'Without the invention of language we would have remained animals. Without metaphors we would still be savages… . The more advanced the civilization, the more elaborate its metaphors. Even the glossaries of physics and engineering are built with them' (Wilson 2017).

Both Wheeler's (in Meijer 2015) participatory universe and the neuroplastic human brain are susceptible to change and 'in turn are modified in the process' of change. These phenomena pose questions that loiter at the fringes of our current systems of knowledge and beyond the scope of this chapter, but that ultimately fall squarely within the realm of the emerging metahumanities.

Conclusions

In 2023, 25 years after David Chalmers collaborated with Andy Clark on *The Extended Mind*, he engaged in a public debate with notable scientist and philosopher Christof Koch on the nature of consciousness. The occasion was to follow up on a bet they had taken (in 1998 when *The Extended Mind* was published) about the nature of consciousness, and whether a locus of consciousness would be found within the next 25 years within the skull-bound human brain. The question of consciousness is core to our existence (and thus to metahumanities), and understanding its biological origins could shed light on the emergence of culture from animal instinct, and 'bring prehistory into alignment with history' (Wilson 2017). Despite extensive experimental neuroimaging studies, the debate has not been resolved. Of course, it suffers from the constrained view that, if you are a neuroscientist, the key to consciousness will be found in neuroscience. Then we are forever locked in the skull. I have ventured out of the skull to describe the territories of extended cognition. Just as John Wheeler said that there could be no universe until consciousness arose to perceive it (in Meijer 2015), so we find that extended cognition only arises where a metacognition extends to devise such a model.

The drive to understand the extended mind (and the metahumanities it brings with it) is not a denial of brain-bound cognition, not a call to ignore the individual mind, but rather to see the richness of its extension into the world. Even the use of this word 'extension' implies a brain-bound perspective. Daniel Siegel (2007) suggests that 'Our experience of life will be quite different if we approach rather than avoid the contents of our own mind'. The metaphor is telling – approaching our own minds from outside, gaining an 'intentional' perspective. As the vastness of our changing human brain coupled with the vastness of a changing universe and our participatory role in it become apparent, the need for intentional and integrated metahumanities to provide fresh meaning to human existence gains urgency.

References

Anderson JE, Lavelle M, Reedy G. 2021. Understanding adaptive teamwork in health care: Progress and future directions. *Journal of Health Services Research & Policy*. 26: 208–14.

Barrett LF. 2017. *How Emotions are Made: The secret life of the brain*. London: Pan Macmillan.

Begley S. 2007. The brain: How the brain rewires itself. *Time Magazine*: 1–6.

Beranek, N.B. 2021. The Metahumanities. *Deliberatio*, 1, 97–108.

Bleakley A. 2014. The Medical Humanities in Medical Education: Toward a Medical Aesthetics of Resistance. In: T Jones, D Wear, LD Friedman (eds.) *Health Humanities Reader*. New Brunswick, NJ: Rutgers University Press, 501–10.

Bleakley A. 2024. A therapeutic intervention for an ailing medical education: The values prism model as proof of concept. *Medical Teacher*. 46: 232–8.

Bleakley A, Neilson S. 2023. As 'synapses' become 'protoplasmic kisses': Symmetry across clinical reasoning and poetry. *Medical Education*. 57: 233–42.

Burmeister JK. 2023. Education for a post-work society. In: Araya D, Marber P (eds.) *Augmented Education in the Global Age: artificial intelligence and the future of learning and work*. New York, NY: Routledge.

Cameron J. 1999. *The Right to Write: An Invitation and Initiation Into the Writing Life*. Harmondsworth: Penguin.

Clark A. 1998. *Being There: Putting Brain, Body, and World Together Again*. Cambridge, MA: MIT Press.

Clark A. 2013. Whatever next? Predictive brains, situated agents, and the future of cognitive science. *Behavioral and Brain Sciences*. 36: 181–204.

Clark A. 2023. *The Experience Machine: How Our Minds Predict and Shape Reality*. London: Allen Lane.

Clark A, Chalmers D. 1998. The extended mind. *Analysis*. 58: 7–19.

Damasio AR. 1999. *The Feeling of What Happens: Body and Emotion in the Making of Consciousness*. Boston, MA: Houghton Mifflin Harcourt.

Dobzhansky T. 1964. Biology, molecular and organismic. *American Zoologist*. 4: 443–52.

Doidge N. 2007. *The Brain that Changes Itself*. New York, NY: Penguin Books.

Durning SJ, Artino AR. 2011. Situativity Theory: a perspective on how participants and the environment can interact. AMEE Guide no. 52. *Medical Teacher*. 33: 188–99.

Edwards E, St Hillaire-Clarke C, Frankowski DW, et al. 2023. NIH Music-based intervention toolkit: music-based interventions for brain disorders of aging. *Neurology*. 100: 868–78.

Eichbaum QG. 2014. Thinking about thinking and emotion: the metacognitive approach to the medical humanities that integrates the humanities with the basic and clinical sciences. *Permanente Journal*. 18: 64–75.

Eliot TS. 2014. *Essays Ancient and Modern*. Boston, MA: Houghton Mifflin Harcourt.

Engeström Y. 2018. *Expertise in Transition: Expansive Learning in Medical Work*. Cambridge: Cambridge University Press.

Estevao C, Fancourt D, Dazzan P, et al. 2021. Scaling-up Health-Arts Programmes: the largest study in the world bringing arts-based mental health interventions into a national health service. *British Journal of Psychiatry Bulletin*. 45: 32–9.

Fleming R. 2005. *The Inner Voice: The Making of a Singer*. London: Penguin.

Folger T. 2002. 'Does the Universe Exist if We're Not Looking?' *Discover-New York*. 23: 44–9.

Gardner HE. 2008. *Multiple Intelligences: New Horizons in Theory and Practice*. New York, NY: Basic Books.

Garrison DR, Akyol Z. 2015. Toward the development of a metacognition construct for communities of inquiry. *The Internet and Higher Education*. 24: 66–71.

Gibson JJ. 1979. *The Ecological Approach to Visual Perception*. New York, NY: Psychology Press.

Goffman E. 2006. *The Presentation of Self, Life as Theater: A Dramaturgical Sourcebook*. New York, NY: Doubleday Anchor.

Goldberg N. 2005. *Writing Down the Bones: Freeing the Writer Within*. Boulder, CO: Shambhala Publications.

Hagerhall CM, Purcell T, Taylor R. 2004. Fractal dimension of landscape silhouette outlines as a predictor of landscape preference. *Journal of Environmental Psychology*. 24: 247–55.

Howley L, Gaufberg E, King BE. 2020. *The Fundamental Role of the Arts and Humanities in Medical Education*. Washington, DC: Association of American Medical Colleges (AAMC).

Jarvis MS, Samuel K. 2023. Impact of the COVID-19 pandemic on anaesthesia training, recruitment, and examinations: a survey of UK trainees. *British Journal of Anaesthesia*. 131: e13–e16.

Lakoff G, Johnson M. 2008. *Metaphors We Live By*. Chicago, IL: University of Chicago Press.

Lehrer J. 2008. *Proust Was a Neuroscientist*. London: Mariner Books.

Magsamen S., Ross I. 2023. *Your Brain on Art – How the Arts Transform Us*. New York, NY: Random House.

Mangabeira Unger R, Smolin L. 2015. *The Singular Universe and the Reality of Time: A Proposal in Natural Philosophy*. Cambridge: Cambridge University Press.

Meijer DKF. 2015. The universe as a cyclic organized information system: John Wheeler's world revisited. *NeuroQuantology*. 13: 57–78.

Menand L. 2010. *The Marketplace of Ideas: Reform and Resistance in the American University*. New York, NY: WW Norton Company.

Nussbaum MC. 2012. *Not for Profit: Why Democracy Needs the Humanities*. Princeton, NJ: Princeton University Press.

Panksepp J. 1982. Archaeology of mind. *Behavioral and Brain Sciences*. 5: 449–67.

Paul AM. 2023. Extending Biological Intelligence: The Imperative of Thinking Outside Our Brains in a World of Artificial Intelligence. In: D Araya, P Marber (eds.) *Augmented Education in the Global Age*. London: Routledge, 157–71.

Ravven H. 2013. *The Self Beyond Itself: An Alternative History of Ethics, the New Brain Sciences, and the Myth of Free Will*. New York, NY: The New Press.

Rudy W. 1980. From Normal School to Multi-Purpose College. *History of Education Quarterly*. 20: 241–6.

Siegel DJ. 2007. *The Mindful Brain: Reflection and Attunement in the Cultivation of Well-Being*. New York, NY: WW Norton & Company.

Singh H, Sittig DF. 2015. Advancing the science of measurement of diagnostic errors in healthcare: the Safer Dx framework. *BMJ Quality & Safety*. 24: 103–10.

Smith BH. 1988. *Contingencies of Value: Alternative Perspectives for Critical Theory*. Cambridge, MA: Harvard University Press.

Smolin L. 2013. *Time Reborn: From the Crisis in Physics to the Future of the Universe*. Boston, MA: Houghton Mifflin Harcourt.

Teixeira GC, Araújo AMM, de Andrade MJO. 2022. Social neuroscience and mental processes: How does our brain process social information? *Innovations in Clinical Neuroscience*. 19: 33–5.

Torre D, Durning SJ, Rencic J, et al. 2020. Widening the lens on teaching and assessing clinical reasoning: from "in the head" to "out in the world". *Diagnosis*. 7: 181–90.

Weigel M, Hutchinson B, Magee WL, et al. 2023. Orchestrating a new path for multiple sclerosis: achieving physical, cognitive, and emotional rehabilitation goals through physical and music therapy. *International Journal of MS Care*. 25 (4): DOI:10.7224/1537-2073.2021-144

Williams J. 2018. *Stand Out of Our Light: Freedom and Resistance in the Attention Economy*. Cambridge: Cambridge University Press.
Wilson EO. 1988. *On Human Nature*. Boston, MA: Harvard University Press.
Wilson EO. 2014. *The Meaning of Human Existence*: New York, NY: WW Norton & Company.
Wilson EO. 2017. *The Origins of Creativity*. New York, NY: Liveright Publishing.
Winter DG. 1981. *A New Case for the Liberal Arts. Assessing Institutional Goals and Student Development*. ERIC. Available at: https://eric.ed.gov/?id=ED208764

11 Metacognition and pattern thinking

Rachel Ellaway

Introduction

A key capacity afforded by cognition is the ability to recognise, distinguish, and understand the world we encounter through perception (see Chapter 8). Quite how we do this has been, and continues to be, debated with different empirical and theoretical lenses applied to understanding this phenomenon (Green 2023). One of these theoretical perspectives, Pattern Theory, posits that memory, recall, and understanding emerge from nexuses or patterns of associated memories and thoughts. I have been working on a coherent Pattern Theory for several years (Ellaway and Bates 2015, Ellaway forthcoming) that is closely aligned with the architectural theorist Christopher Alexander's pattern languages (Alexander et al. 1977, Alexander 1999). This differs greatly from General Pattern Theory as formulated by Grenander and colleagues (Grenander 1994) that focused on isolating, modelling, and replicating putative cognitive patterns and basic aspects of pattern thinking.

My approach to Pattern Theory asserts that pattern is a purely cognitive phenomenon, albeit with the potential to shape the world beyond the mind, and one moreover that is metacognitive where it forms the basis of most of our other cognitive capabilities. Pattern Theory aligns with findings and ideas from neurobiology and cognitive psychology, as well as concepts and models from the philosophy of mind and information sciences. In this chapter, I explore how Pattern Theory can afford novel perspectives on metacognition and metahumanities in the context of medicine and medical education.

Introduction to Pattern Theory

Key to Pattern Theory is that patterns do not exist outside of our minds. It may seem that there are patterns 'out there' in the world around us but that is an artefact of mind. We may encounter form and regularity (although arguably they are also cognitive phenomena), but we typically perceive things in terms of patterns. For instance, you may encounter a rectangular structure in a wall that has a handle and that seems to move when you push, pull, or turn the handle. It is very likely that you may have seen things that have a similar

DOI: 10.4324/9781032687339-14

form even though you have never seen this instance before. This recurrence is a kind of regularity, and we can use this to recall previous experiences with things that look and behave like this current thing. However, when we name this class of things 'doors' – and remember what we can do with them, how they work, what they are for, and the meanings and consequences of things being doors – we are invoking our cognitive pattern for doors. Put another way, when we perceive a pattern in the world around us, we are interpreting sensory information in terms of our memories of past experiences, our memories of our interpretations, and our memories of associated things. To see patterns or to see things in terms of patterns is not only a product of mind (rather than an intrinsic quality of the world around us), our pattern thinking also imbues our current experiences with memories of our past experiences and our abstracted understanding of those experiences.

In making these arguments, I distinguish between patterns and pattern thinking. Patterns are nexuses of connected and (more loosely) associated memories, thoughts, and, potentially, other patterns. Pattern thinking on the other hand refers to the many ways in which our minds work with our patterns. Our pattern thinking is both aggregative and abstractive given that we are continuously building meanings, abstractions, and symbolic and categorical structures from our many layers of interconnected pattern memories. It should be noted that these connections are based on similarities and coincidences rather than on precise identities. As a result, pattern thinking collects and abstracts similar (but not necessarily identical) things, and the more abstract a pattern becomes the broader the range of things that it includes. Pattern thinking is the basis of Wittgenstein's 'family resemblance' problem in that we happily consider things as belonging to the same family even though none of them have all the same features in common. Pattern makes the complexity and fuzziness of family relationships (i.e., categories, classifications, types, idioms, and classes) tractable, and it can afford a reductive sense of familiarity and uncertainty, even as it accommodates variance and novelty. A key benefit of pattern thinking is that it allows us to organise our understanding of, and interactions with, the world. It also gives us the ability to build elaborate symbol systems such as language and mathematics, and to use them to systematise our knowledge of domains such as medicine.

Our patterns and our pattern thinking allow us to make sense of our experiences. Sometimes, we can easily match our current experiences to past experiences. When we do, we call this pattern recognition, which in turn forms the basis for much of clinical reasoning. Although we may recognise the exact same thing we encountered before, pattern recognition only needs similarity and not identity to work. Sometimes, when we cannot find a match between our pattern memories and a new encounter, we need to adapt existing patterns to make sense of these unfamiliar experiences; we call this 'pattern discovery'. Sometimes, if the experience is entirely novel or we are required to see something familiar in an unfamiliar way, we need to construct a new pattern nexus – we call this 'pattern learning'.

Although it might be convenient to consider pattern recognition, discovery, and learning as distinct modalities, much of the time we move fluidly back and forth between them. It is also important to note the role of time and adaptation in pattern thinking. For instance, we might initially be unsure what something is (perhaps because it is far away or otherwise indistinct) and our pattern perception may flitter back and forth between possible pattern matches. As (or if) the thing becomes more distinct, we might decide that it is a match for one pattern and yet be surprised when, on even closer inspection, it turns out to be something else altogether.

Because it works with similarities and differences, pattern recognition allows us to recognise something as an example of a class or category of things even though we may have never encountered the specific thing before. A category can be understood from a pattern theoretical perspective as a cognitive label or symbol for an underlying cognitive pattern of associated memories of instances of certain similar phenomena along with our abstracted thoughts about those phenomena. This is how we are able to say that this newly encountered thing is an instance of a cat or a door or a bicycle. Arguably, therefore, categories have no absolute or objective perimeters or boundaries. They are defined within each individual mind by the pattern associations that a particular mind holds at any one point in time. Every new encounter with, or reflection on, the category will alter the pattern nexus, which means that our patterns are dynamic and fluid rather than fixed.

Pattern thinking is not just about recognition, discovery, learning, categorisation, and heuristics, it is also the basis of our sense of significance and meaning. When we recognise something as an instance of a pattern, we 'pull' on the meanings and associations that are part of that pattern memory to tell us what this thing is, what it is likely to do, what value it has, how we feel about it, and how we should interact with it. Because our patterns can include memories of emotions and feelings, the understanding and meaning patterns can give us are not simply matters of fact, they can also confer a sense of significance and value; they tell us whether things might present a threat or an opportunity, they tell us what to pay attention to and what can be safely ignored. It is this added association and meaning that allows us to recognise things in the world (whether a cat or a dog or a melanoma), to understand them, to see meaning in them, and to a limited extent to anticipate or predict what they will do.

Pattern nexuses can come together at many different levels of aggregation and abstraction, they can function as elements of other patterns, and they can be elaborated and abstracted to form more general patterns. Micropatterns are small, fluid, and may be no more than ephemeral impressions. Mesopatterns are longer-lasting, larger, and more developed such that they form the basis of our perceptions. Macropatterns are developed over time as (variously) abstract, systematic, and rigorous as the basis of theories, models, and frameworks. Most of our patterns that we are aware of tend to be macropatterns, and they form the basis of our actions, techniques, philosophies, and languages; our social conventions and structures; our symbolic and analytical thought; and our creative, aesthetic, and ethical practices. A continuum from micropattern to macropattern reflects the ways in which we introduce abstraction, generalisation, formalisation and all the other characteristics of macropattern to our base pattern thinking capabilities. It is only in macropattern that science and medicine can be developed and codified – to be a physician and participate in the field of medicine is intrinsically to participate in collective macropattern thinking.

There are also downsides to pattern thinking, particularly when it leads to bias, error, and even delusion. Sometimes, this may be because the information we have is ambiguous or misleading, sometimes, it is because our pattern thinking habits become ingrained and inflexible (we see what we expect), and sometimes, it is because the affective and semantic aspects of pattern thinking influence our perception (we see what we want to see). Seeing patterns that are not there is called 'pareidolia', which can be the result of letting the mind wander, such as when we see faces in clouds or in trees, sometimes, or when we actively misinterpret what we see or fail to see something altogether. Attributing significance to patterns that are not there is called 'apophenia'. Although apophenia is a potentially delusional condition, a case could also be made that there is much that we perceive that is not there yet has particular significance, such as patterns of professionalism and competence.

Although intrinsically cognitive, patterns can be externalised in different ways. From a pattern theoretical perspective, the only way that pattern leaves our minds is through pattern expressions and pattern representations. A pattern expression is something we create, or shape, based on one or more patterns in our minds. A pattern expression is something that has regularity and form shaped by our pattern thinking but as it is out in the world it is no longer intrinsically linked to it. Pattern expressions can vary in how precisely they reflect pattern thought and how much adaptation and improvisation they embrace. For example, recalling the Krebs cycle is likely to be exact as abstract knowledge, whereas inserting a central line or performing a lumbar puncture requires a degree of contextual adaptation as a performed skill. We express patterns all the time in terms of our habits and dispositions and throughout our personal, working, and social lives. Acting as a physician, teacher, or medical student are all pattern expressions as identity constructions.

By contrast, a pattern representation is something we make to represent a pattern in our mind, and as such it captures (variably) the principles, structures, functions, and associations of the pattern. For example, a teacher may set out the steps required in performing a particular clinical task, or they may assess a learner's pattern expression of a task in terms of an idealised pattern representation in the form of a checklist. Pattern representations can take many forms, including instructions, recipes, blueprints, protocols, guidelines, and maps. It is interesting to note that in developing a pattern representation the reflection and abstraction this requires will also change the pattern it is trying to represent, not least by weaving memory of developing the pattern representation into the pattern it represents. Although we might create or engage with single pattern representations, they can be collected as a pattern system (a pattern of patterns) or a pattern language (a pattern system with grammar and syntax). Some of the key terms of Pattern Theory are set out in Table 11.1.

The ideas that I explore in this chapter are based on the assertion that pattern thinking is an essential if somewhat overlooked aspect of medicine and medical education. From this perspective, I will now consider ways of thinking about pattern thinking, where I explore deliberate and reflexive approaches to pattern thinking. I also consider pattern as the basis of method and methodology in acts of inquiry and consider some of the strengths and weaknesses of pattern thinking in medicine and medical education.

Table 11.1 Key Terms in Pattern Theory

Term	*Meaning*	*Examples*
Pattern	A nexus of related memories and thoughts in a mind.	An individual's pattern memories of doors, sutures, birds, and shoes.
Pattern fragments	Cognitive phenomena that are woven together into a pattern. They can include memories, thoughts, and other patterns or parts.	Memories of textures, images, feelings, thoughts, insights, meanings, significances, and associations.
Pattern thinking	A term covering the many ways in which our minds work with our patterns.	Pattern recognition, pattern discovery, and pattern learning.
Pattern recognition	Connecting current thoughts and experiences to pattern memories of past thoughts and experiences.	Recognising a person we know, a familiar odour, or recognising that this is a cat, a carrot, or a car.
Pattern discovery	Adapting existing patterns to make sense of unfamiliar thoughts and experiences.	Discovering that this is friend in disguise, discovering that a banana plant is a kind of herb.
Pattern learning	Creating new patterns to make sense of unfamiliar thoughts and experiences.	Learning about partial pressures in the lung, or the anatomy of the brain.
Micropattern	Small fleeting patterns that form the basis of our impressions of things.	A sense of melancholy related to a rainy or foggy day, a sense of excitement at the prospect of denouement in a film or novel.
Mesopattern	Patterns that coalesce micropatterns to form perceptions and provisional understanding.	Our ability to perceive discreet things reflects mesopatterns.

(*Continued*)

Table 11.1 (Continued)

Term	*Meaning*	*Examples*
Macropattern	Large, abstract, and aggregative patterns that develop over time as a way of gaining a deeper understanding of related phenomena.	Language, mathematics, medicine, categories, conventions, values, and theories.
Pattern expression	Something we create or perform based on one or more patterns in our minds.	The performance of a learned task such as drawing blood, the creation of something familiar such as preparing a meal.
Pattern representation	An externalised representation of a pattern that captures the principles, structures, functions, and associations of the pattern.	The instructions or principles for a particular task such as clinical guidelines, or the template for something such as a recipe for a meal.
Pattern system	A collection of pattern representations that collectively outline a broad domain of knowledge or practice.	A set of pattern representations that collectively outline aspects of medical school admissions systems.
Pattern language	A pattern system that includes grammar and syntax defining how representations are to be used together.	A set of pattern representations that collectively outline processes of how feedback works in clinical teaching.

Regularities and patterns

You are already pattern thinking. You have been doing it since birth, it was central to your education and training, you do it in all the aspects of your everyday and professional lives, and you even do it when you dream. You are doing it right now. Pattern and metacognition are inescapably linked. When you think about your own thinking, you are applying pattern thinking to itself. If we perceive habits and tendencies in our thinking, we are connecting the regularities of such thought and weaving them together with significance and meaning to build an understanding of our own minds. As an intrinsic pattern thinker, at the very least should you not be aware of what pattern and pattern thinking are, both in general and in the ways in which they are woven through your own social and professional worlds?

As an example of this, consider metacognition related to regularities and patterns. Patterns are discussed all the time in healthcare. There are patterns of pathology, disease, trauma, and disability. There are patterns of reasoning, diagnosis, and therapeutics. There are patterns of surgery, patient management, and rehabilitation. There are patterns of professions and disciplines, and there are patterns in service delivery (clinics, wards, attendings, referrals, discharges, and so forth). Except, are these not regularities rather than patterns? They are familiar because they recur, and, in that light, they are all regularities. What turns these regularities into patterns is our thinking about them in terms of previously encountered phenomena and the associated meanings, significances, values, and predictions these memories afford us. Put another way, the facts of these recurring examples are regularities, our individual experience of recognising and drawing meaning from that recognition is a product of our pattern thinking. That we may have learned the patterns we use to make sense of the regularities of medicine reflects the pattern learning we engaged in as new members of medical communities, as does our use of shared pattern thinking in using these concepts and categories as part of our participation in those communities.

From a metacognitive perspective, Pattern Theory can be used to query your own versions of these patterns as well as others'. For instance, what are the convergent and divergent pattern characteristics in your and other individuals' patterns (such as those of patients, trainees, or colleagues), and what are their implications? It may be that there are similarities in observations and facts but divergence in meanings and values, which in turn may account for very different understandings of what ostensibly are the same things. After all, medical students build their own pattern learning of how to take a patient history, how to conduct a physical examination, how to conduct or order tests and interpret their results, how to engage in diagnostic reasoning, and then how to devise and execute a therapeutic plan. Learning these patterns involves creating new memories and thoughts and linking them to existing ones, weaving them together and elaborating them with new understanding and insight over time. Not only does this reflect an explanatory constructivist perspective on how learning works, it also accounts for the variances and idiosyncrasies in what different students learn. Pattern Theory and its differentiation of regularities and patterns can also help us to reflect on how we developed or learned our versions of these patterns, how our patterns of these generalisations have changed over time, how we use these patterns, how we teach your patterns to others, how we assess pattern thinking in others, and how we identify pattern thinking that has gone awry.

Macropattern thinking

Earlier, I noted that patterns can involve different levels of aggregation and abstraction, that they can function as elements of other patterns and can include other patterns, and that they can be elaborated to create or contribute to more general patterns. I also differentiated between impressionistic micropatterns, perception mesopatterns, and abstract macropatterns. I should be clear that these are not distinct pattern types, rather our minds have patterns that map across a continuum anchored by these three prototypes. Although micropatterns and mesopatterns play important roles in medical thinking, our macropatterning habits are of particular interest in the context of medicine.

Macropatterns are developed from multiple patterns such that they tend to be increasingly aggregated the more macropatterned they become. For instance, a macropattern of the symptoms and consequences of a particular disease may include patterns of presentations and physiological interactions, while a macropattern of a medical procedure may include patterns for its steps as well as any variations on the procedure. A consequence of this aggregation is that macropatterns also tend to become more generalised as they become more aggregated. As an example, mesopatterns reflecting instances of similar clinical presentations may be aggregated and thereby generalised to a broader pattern for a disease within which the various presentations are understood as instances of that disease. Generalisation, broadly speaking, sacrifices individuality for commonality. However, aggregated patterns are not flattened in macropatterns, only categorised, and as such individuality and variance are not sacrificed, while detail and variance can still be interrogated.

Second, macropatterns also tend to be increasingly abstracted and formalised the more macropatterned they become. Although this is directly related to the tendency to generalise across instances of that macropattern, the tendency to abstraction goes further to weave perceptions of common abstract characteristics and relationships into the growing macropattern in the form of thoughts and memories related to hypotheses, theories, and models. Formalisation is not always required, but is often present as these hypotheses, theories, and/or models are rendered in writing, images, or using mathematics. Consider as examples: pressure changes in the ventricles and atria of a beating heart, the mathematical equations used to identify levels of oxygen in or the acid–base balance of blood, and the many mnemonics medical students and practitioners use in guiding their thinking and shaping memory. Abstraction and formalisation often elide specificity, but if they added to a macropattern rather than replacing parts – or all – of that pattern then there are still connections to the specifics and variances from which the abstractions were developed.

Macropatterns also tend to involve more collaboration and pattern sharing the more abstract and formalised they become. Again, this is not a necessary quality as an individual may manage well on their own. Indeed, this might be seen as the defining quality of great scientific thinkers such as Einstein or Mendel. However, as scholars and scientists and as healthcare professionals, we share our thinking, we subject ourselves to review and feedback, and we participate in communities of thought by sharing ideas and seeing where the collective might take them. This is particularly the case for pattern systems and pattern languages where they act as the foundation for that community to function. For example, the Ur-pattern language for much of science is mathematics, a language developed over millennia by many minds, for many purposes, and with many branches and genres. Similarly, pattern languages of biochemical, genetic, and neurological notation only develop out of collective effort. From this perspective, we might invoke Kuhn's concept of scientific paradigms to illustrate that there are also trends, factions, and ideologies in collaborative pattern thinking affording constructive debate and divergence, but such thinking can also afford controversy and control in what can and cannot be said or thought. Pattern thinking is not free of ideological bias or the imposition of complex value orientations, not least because these too are patterns. This in turn raises the complex issue of 'objectivity'. On the one hand, engaging more minds and their pattern thinking should help challenge and even out individual idiosyncrasies in the macropatterns they share (typically but not exclusively in the form of pattern representations). However, as paradigm theory makes clear, collaboration may also reinforce shared biases and blind spots, and it may prioritise the perspectives of one group over another.

A fourth characteristic of macropatterns is that the ways in which they reflect significance and meaning change the more macropatterned they become. At one level, this is a predictable product of the shift from individual patterns that have individual meanings related to individual memories and feelings to collectively held patterns that can have different meanings according to the minds in which they are realised. However, there is more to this shift in that macropatterns translate meaning and significance from individuals to collectives. For example, truth, integrity, professionalism, ethics, and even society and civilisation are the products of and the increasing focus of macropattern thinking, such that the significance of these patterns is refocused on the abstraction rather than the individual. One might even argue that all collective activity in medicine and medical education is intrinsically macropatterned, with all the implications that brings. Again, pattern recognition of what is 'out there' (such as symptoms in a patient or community) is shaped by cognitive patterning 'in here' (such as neural, sympathetic, and parasympathetic systems, and gut biome).

Another characteristic of macropatterns is that not only can they be formalised as pattern representations and performed as pattern expressions, there may be series or networks of pattern representations and pattern expressions where some expressions act as representations for other expressions. For instance, an architect may draw on rules and conventions (macropattern representations) in designing a building (an expression), after which their plan acts as a representation of which the constructed building is an expression. From an educational perspective, a teacher may draw on pattern representations in teaching a particular subject, but in doing so, they create an expression of the macropattern for 'giving a lecture' say, while their learners build macropatterns that they might externalise as a representation of their understanding of the subject matter, or as an expression by applying it in a clinical activity.

Indeed, we might conceptualise medical education as systemic guided discovery and learning of explicit shared macropatterns required of a medical thinker, and then the creation of representations and expressions in formative and summative assessments. What then are the significant macropatterns of anatomy, physiology, biochemistry, and other basic sciences; of different branches of medicine and different kinds of medical practice; and of lectures, seminars, textbooks, and assessments? How convergent and divergent are teacher and learner patterns, and is divergence or convergence a good thing or bad? There are many useful questions afforded from a macropattern perspective of relevance to metacognition in medicine and medical education.

Underlying this is the ability to discriminate between pattern perceptions that are important and those that are not. The reader may think that if everything is patterned then how do I differentiate or discriminate between the meanings of patterns for any given context?

Pattern significance

Patterns allow us to interpret things, to engage in meaning making, to develop understanding, and to appraise the significance of those things we recognise or discover. Understanding and meaning are essential characteristics of pattern and a fundamental way of distinguishing regularity and pattern. If you perceive the form of something without considering or needing to understand it or what it means, then that is perception of regularity. However, if (as we almost always do) we associate current experiences with past experiences, then we also draw on memories of how we felt about those experiences and cumulatively that can confer a sense of significance related to the current perception. For micropatterns, significance may be pure affect (emotions and feelings) associated with pleasure and pain, likes and dislikes. As patterns become more elaborated and abstract, the sense of significance we draw on through pattern recall can also become more abstract, for instance, in terms of right and wrong (ethical), aesthetic, or valuable. We should remember that all abstracted moral judgements can be configured at the level of metaphysical patterns, but that these are also within us and a part of us.

This illustrates another important aspect of Pattern Theory that flows from our patterns being nexuses of interconnected memories of experiences, thoughts, and feelings. If, say, in pattern recognition, we match a part of a pattern to our current perception we then pull that part of a pattern (such as its shape or context) into working memory and as we do so we also pull on all its associated parts. I like to use the metaphor of a cloth or membrane where pulling on one pattern part pulls on the rest such that we experience pattern recognition as a cascade of thoughts and feelings, some of which can denote or suggest significance and meaning. Think, for instance, of when you perceive indications of a delayed flight or a lost parcel in the mail; even as you acknowledge the fact of this you likely also feel frustration and annoyance, and perhaps you also get a sinking feeling associated with the additional work you will now need to do to overcome these challenges. From a metacognitive perspective, being mindful of how your patterns are activated and how you experience different aspects of an activated pattern can afford many insights into how you think.

Noting how we think about significance also raises the issue of how we assess probability and risk. Much of the theory of probability and risk is dominated by Bayes and interpretations of his models of reasoning, with much of the writing around Bayesian reasoning explaining how we, as a species, seem to struggle with even the most rudimentary concepts of probability and risk

(Levitin 2016). While Pattern Theory does not contradict or add much to Bayes and his many interpreters, it can help to explain our many biases and lacunae in dealing with probability and risk in terms of our affective pattern memories. Indeed, it could be argued that we invoke a model such as Bayes' when we fail to recognise a definite pattern, such as where we have a range of differential diagnoses affording initial confusion.

Because recalling a pattern activates feelings and emotions, our pattern memories are not based on facts and truths but on perceptions, experiences, and feelings, and only those moreover that we commit to memory. We may strive to reduce or control this through macropattern development, but we cannot escape it altogether. To that end, Pattern Theory can serve as a useful lens in examining all kinds of biases, errors, and irrationalities both on oneself and in others. It also points to weaknesses in pattern thinking, a topic I return to later.

Pattern fluidity

Another dimension of metacognition related to pattern thinking is the ability to deal with ambiguity, uncertainty, and plurality, which are a perennial concern of the medical humanities (Bleakley and Marshall 2013). A pattern has no fixed edges or perimeters; it is a nexus of whatever memories our minds have acquired and then bound together through association over time. Not only does this account for the constructivist principle that learning is unique to each mind, but also it suggests a tension between arbitrary and guided pattern learning. Some of our pattern learning is no more than a reflection of our attempts to understand our experiences, whatever they may be or may have been. Not only are medical students studying in Calgary, Exeter, and Nashville going to develop different patterns that reflect their varied lived contexts, but they will also develop patterns that may be like those of their peers but are unique to them as individuals. Indeed, it may be impossible to imprint an identical pattern on any mind as, even if the instructional experience were identical (which due to wandering attention and voluntarist tendencies is highly unlikely), the ground on which pattern memory is formed is unique to the individual. One important consequence of this is that teaching and learning are at best probabilistic and nonlinear undertakings, as are learners' journeys to professional practice, expertise, and self-fulfilment.

Moreover, our patterns are not fixed; they change over time, according to our individual mental lives and the circumstances we seek out or find ourselves in. Indeed, if our patterns did not change then we would not be able to develop and adapt them, we would be unable to learn anything new. Of course, the rate and kind of changes to patterns may vary significantly according to the individual and their circumstances. Some patterns may change little or change slowly, while others may change drastically or rapidly. Most of us can recall a lightbulb moment when our understanding of something shifted rapidly to a new configuration or Gestalt. We can also recall how our expertise can be honed over time with cycles of practice and feedback. One consequence of this is that our pattern thinking is always developing and changing, and as such no pattern is or can be perfected; patterns are every bit as alive as our minds are. This accounts for biases and errors, for the loss of learning as well as its development, and for the odd and yet compelling associations we are sometimes able to make. These associations and their implications might be useful in terms of developing new insights and understanding, but they can also be distracting particularly when our thoughts are pulled into less productive channels, for instance by 'mindworms' (distracting or destructive lines of thought).

Another consequence of the dynamic nature of pattern memory and its exponential connectivity and association is that changes to one pattern (as the result of new experiences or insights) can change all the patterns with which it is connected. We need therefore to consider the multitude of dependencies between patterns and the ways that changes can perfuse through our pattern memories and thinking. This means taking on a new configuration to accommodate the change in one of its parts. Some patterns may have few connections and therefore be less susceptible to dependent instabilities, while others may be highly connected and therefore more susceptible to changes in pattern networks. These changes may be focused on tuning an individual's pattern thinking to be more adept at being able to understand the complexities of kinds of situations and come up with reliable solutions. However, they may also be destructive when these kinds of changes reduce the coherence and performance of an individual's pattern thinking, for instance, when someone is the subject of abuse or bullying.

Not only does the dynamic nature of our pattern thinking allow us to accommodate new experiences, we can also anticipate or even imagine new configurations and possible instances of our patterns. The potential for new and different pattern configurations allows us to envisage or intuit things we have never encountered or thought about – things that are truly new in the world (or even beyond it). To that end, pattern thinking is central both to our own imaginative and creative capabilities, and to our ability to appreciate the imagination and creativity of others and to learn from it.

Setting aside the more typical kinds of creative discipline-based domains in the medical humanities (drama, poetry, literature, theatre, art, etc.) pattern thinking is also, arguably, central to creative problem-solving, to scientific insights, to leaps of diagnostic reasoning, and to the capacity for adaptive expertise. Much of this comes from the capabilities it affords us to predict (at least to some extent) what might happen in different scenarios, such as what different courses of action might lead to, or how a situation might develop with and without various interventions. Where would the medical imagination, so central to the art of medicine be without pattern thinking?

Pattern heuristics

Another way to use Pattern Theory to consider metacognition is to explore its heuristic properties. By linking pattern thinking to heuristics, I acknowledge I am also linking pattern thinking to the criticisms and debates regarding heuristics and their strengths and weaknesses. However, rather than saying pattern thinking and heuristic thinking are parallel phenomena or that pattern thinking is a kind of heuristic thinking, I think it is more appropriate to argue that pattern thinking serves as the substrate for heuristic thinking, as it does for much of our cognitive landscapes.

So, what do I really mean in suggesting pattern thinking is heuristic, and what are the implications of this? As described in Chapter 6, heuristics have key characteristics: they are used to solve problems, they work relatively quickly and efficiently, they are based on past experiences, they provide answers that are good enough (satisficing) rather than perfect, and we adapt our heuristic thinking based on our available heuristics and their apparent efficacy in solving a problem. Let us consider each of these characteristics in turn.

Clearly, pattern thinking is based on experience, as patterns are made up of interconnected memories. Pattern thinking is also central to our ability to solve problems. It is how we identify what something is, what it is related to, what it can and cannot do, and what it is likely to do. Pattern thinking can also solve the problems of what things mean, what their significance is, and how we should or do feel about them. Pattern thinking is also fast; we often recognise something before we are aware of ourselves doing so such that it seems we simply know things for what they are. We only tend to notice the speed and facility of pattern thinking when we struggle to work out what something is. The speed of pattern thinking is linked to our ability to trigger a pattern memory based on very little information; even a suggestion of something is, by definition, a minimal trigger for its apparent pattern. This would seem to be an evolutionary trait; survivability is enhanced by minds that tend to false positives rather than false negatives (particularly when they relate to danger). There is also efficiency in pattern thinking in that we generally do not hold multiple patterns for the same thing.

Rather, because our minds are always seeking to associate our patterns, similar patterns tend to aggregate and merge. Whether recognised, discovered, learned, or some combination of these modalities, a pattern solution need not be perfect or ideal, it only needs to be sufficient to our immediate needs, a behaviour that reflects both Simon's principle of 'satisficing' (Simon 1956) and Peirce's model of abductive reasoning (Fann 1970). That the solutions that our pattern thinking provides are often imperfect, as illustrated by our capacity to misidentify things when the information available to us is ambiguous. Pattern thinking is also adaptive as we evaluate whether our pattern perception of things is in fact correct and, if found wanting, our minds switch to try different possible pattern solutions until a satisficing solution is found or developed.

Although there are many advantages afforded by the heuristic characteristics of pattern thinking, they also have some critical weaknesses that should be carefully considered. First is the tendency to see (recognise) patterns that are not there. Think, for example, of the idle ways in which we see faces in natural forms such as clouds, rocks, and trees. Although this can be a source of entertainment, it can have serious implications too, particularly when we believe that our perceptions are real. Think for instance of the errors committed by scientists, physicians, and judges when they are convinced that they can see things that are not there. It is very easy to do so, we just need to match a fleeting impression to one part of a pattern to invoke the whole pattern (see Figure 11.1). This phenomenon also explains many of our tendencies to biased thought and perception and as such a pattern theoretical approach to understanding them can draw on much work in the medical humanities on image, illusion, and representation (Bleakley 2015, Neilson 2016).

While pareidolia is the misperception of our patterned minds, apophenia is a more serious problem in that it involves erroneous or illusory beliefs and meanings based on misperception. For instance, it would be pareidolia if you were to see your own face in a piece of toast or a misshapen piece of fruit, but it would be apophenia if you believed that this was a message being sent to you by some unknown entity (assuming of course that there was no message or entity). We are all subject to both kinds of errors although there are levels of

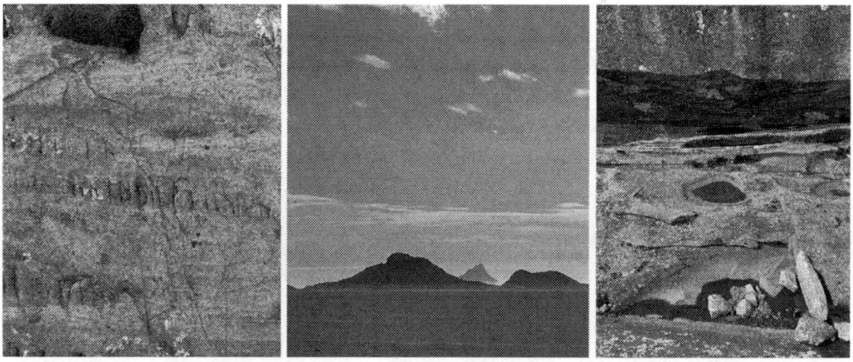

Figure 11.1 Examples of my own pareidolia. I took these images taken on a recent trip to Norway. On the left, natural intrusions in rock appeared to be some kind of runic writing; at the centre, the shape of a distant mountain looked like a giant shark was swimming by; and at the right, the random distribution of rocks and puddles looked to me like a troll's leering toothy face. While I knew these were illusions, I found them entertaining and memorable examples of pareidolic thought.

both pareidolia and apophenia where misperception and the misattribution of meaning become debilitating. It is also telling that although we can switch fluidly between possible pattern solutions, we tend to only be able to commit to one at a time. This is illustrated by the many examples of bistable images such as the drawings where you can see either a young woman or an old woman, a rabbit or a duck, but not both at the same time (Wang et al. 2013). Other pattern limitations include instances when an individual or a collective has a limited or skewed repertoire of patterns to draw on (such as those of young children or as the result of cultural genocide), or a limited capacity to form, interrogate, or adapt pattern memories (for instance because of neurological injury). To be a pattern thinker (as we all are) is not simply a matter of making the most of all it can afford us. It requires caution and critical thinking in appraising its limitations and failures as well as its strengths and affordances.

Conclusions

I do not encourage you to engage in pattern thinking. I do not need to; it is far too late to think of beginnings and introductions. We are all pattern thinkers and we always have been. If you make use of language, if you partake in societal structures and activities, if you think in any way that draws on experience, that works with associations and abstractions, then you are already a dyed-in-the-wool pattern thinker. Because we are always seeing the world through patterns, the world often seems patterned to us, but what we are really seeing are reflections of our own minds. Indeed, we often struggle to perceive our own pattern thinking, let alone that of others.

In exploring issues in metacognition and metahumanities from a pattern theoretical perspective, I have not simply suggested that it might be useful here or interesting there. I have tried to argue that pattern thinking is implied in every aspect of metacognition. I might even argue that Pattern Theory is meta-metacognitive. Similarly, pattern thinking is implied in every aspect of metahumanities, and I have only suggested some of its many possible applications and uses. Rather, I have encouraged you to think about what it means to be a pattern thinker, what its strengths and limitations are, what it means to be surrounded by other pattern thinkers, and what it is to be working and living in a society that is framed by its shared patterns at many levels, not least those of medicine and medical education.

To be human is to be a pattern thinker. To understand this is to gain perspective and agency in one's own pattern thinking and in working with the pattern thinking of others, both individually and collectively. If we are not mindful and deliberate in our pattern thinking then it can lead to harm or allow harm to flourish. However, rather than asking what pattern and pattern thinking have to do with metacognition and metahumanities in medicine, we might instead ask why have pattern and pattern thinking not been discussed or considered in these contexts before?

References

Alexander C, Ishikawa S, Silverstein M. 1977. *A Pattern Language: Towns, Buildings, Construction*. Oxford: Oxford University Press.

Alexander C. 1999. The origins of pattern theory: The future of the theory, and the generation of a living world. *IEEE Software*. 16: 71–82.

Bleakley A. 2015. *Medical Humanities and Medical Education: how the medical humanities can shape better doctors*. Abingdon: Routledge.

Bleakley A, Marshall R. 2013. Can the science of communication inform the art of the medical humanities? *Medical Education*. 47: 126–33.

Ellaway RH, Bates J. 2015. Exploring patterns and pattern languages of medical education. *Medical Education*. 49: 1189–96.

Ellaway RH. (Forthcoming). *Pattern Theory: Memory, Interpretation, Understanding, Meaning*. Abingdon, Routledge.

Fann KT. 1970. *Peirce's Theory of Abduction*. The Hague: Martinus Nijhoff.

Green EJ. 2023. The perception-cognition border: architecture or format? In: BP McLaughlin, J Cohen (eds.) *Contemporary Debates in Philosophy of Mind*, 2nd ed. London: Wiley, 469–92.

Grenander U. 1994. *General Pattern Theory*. Oxford: Oxford Science Publications.

Levitin DJ. 2016. *A Field Guide to Lies: Critical Thinking with Statistics and the Scientific Method*. New York, NY: Dutton.

Neilson S. 2016. Pain as metaphor: metaphor and medicine. *Medical Humanities*. 42: 3–10.

Simon HA. 1956. Rational Choice and the Structure of the Environment. *Psychological Review*. 63: 129–38.

Wang M, Arteaga D, He BJ. 2013. Brain mechanisms for simple perception and bistable perception. *Proceedings of the National Academy of Sciences*. 27 (110): E3350–9.

12 From empathy to compathy in medical education

Alan Bleakley

Empathy and its discontents

Three quarters of a century ago, Carl Rogers (1951) proposed the three core principles of person-centred care: congruence (genuineness), unconditional positive regard (trust), and empathy (fellow feeling). Of these, empathy has remained the unquestioned anchor for clinical-communication skills in medical education (Lloyd et al. 2018). Surely everybody in healthcare and its educational wings knows what 'empathy' is and how it operates? Seemingly not, where clarity has proved elusive. Veloski and Hojat (2006), writing on empathy, suggested that 'there is no agreed upon definition of the term', while a 2022 special edition of *The Journal of Social Psychology* on empathy argued that it remains a problematic concept:

> The concept of empathy as it is used in scholarly discourse has been challenged for over 50 years, yet the same ambiguities and controversies associated with the concept persist and, indeed, have accelerated with the accumulation of definitions, subconstructs that are included under the empathy umbrella, and measuring instruments.
>
> (Hall and Schwartz 2022)

Sulzer et al. (2016) found that 90% of the studies they reviewed lacked any definition of empathy, used the term inconsistently, and/or were over-reliant on self-assessment of a contested notion – that is, whatever 'empathy' was supposed to be. These flaws undermine the validity of the reported studies and of course the validity of the very term 'empathy' itself. Moreover, despite differences of opinion on what 'empathy' is, the notion has been instrumentalised – reduced to crude linear scales. The immeasurable has been measured, such that empathy has been transformed from an abstraction to an embodied trait – even at the level of the neuron (Iacoboni 2009a, b) – and there have been few willing to challenge this desire to instantiate (Steuber 2019).

At one level, this is like Alice in conversation with the mad Queen. If philosophers and psychologists find it impossible to agree on what empathy is, how can we (for example) locate it substantially in the brain as the work of

DOI: 10.4324/9781032687339-15

'mirror neurons' (Iacoboni 2009a, b)? Such assumption of certainty in an uncertain realm is disturbing. In arguing that: 'Empathy is a cornerstone of mental health and well-being', did Iacoboni (Iacoboni 2009a, b) mean that those suffering from mental ill-health are unable to empathise? And quite what is meant by 'well-being'? Is a soldier trying to kill the perceived enemy both unwell and incapable of empathy? When Iacoboni (Iacoboni 2009a, b) argued that 'empathy also helps us to infer and predict the internal feelings, behavior, and intentions of others' is he shifting empathy from an innate capability to a social grace? That empathy can be relational is a point to which I will return later, in recognition of the core notion of this book – the framing of the 'meta' as social or collective.

Moving from neuroscience to philosophy, the Scottish physician and medical educator Jane Macnaughton (2009) argued that empathy in clinical contexts is a short-lived experience and is in essence inauthentic, while empathy in intimate personal encounters is tangibly different, and patently authentic: 'A doctor who responds to a patient's distress with "I know how you feel" is likely, therefore, to be both resented by the patient and self-deceiving'. Arno Kumagai (2008) warned against teaching 'empathy' to medical students, suggesting that students may benefit more from learning a generalised 'perspective taking' as part of developing a wider narrative sensibility of the nature of clinical care. There is a big difference between imposing a medical narrative on a patient and engaging constructively with a patient's narrative.

Revisioning 'empathy'

We start by outlining how 'empathy' drifted from the field of early 20th-century aesthetics to become a key concept in academic and applied psychology. The etymology of the word 'empathy' in the English language paradoxically has little to do with feelings between persons, as it referred to aesthetic responses such as one's feeling states towards a painting.

Einfühlung (translated into English as 'empathy') was coined by Lotze in 1858. In 1903, Lipps used the term to refer to an aesthetic state of 'entering into' a work of art – literally 'in' (*ein*) 'feeling' (*fühlung*), often translated as 'aesthetic sympathy' – while Titchener used the term *einfühlung* to denote a metaphorical entering the being of another person, as a sympathetic state. The term was translated to English based on the Greek word *empatheia* meaning 'a state of emotion', or a passion, drawing on the root word *pathos* that means 'suffering' (hence, 'pathology') (etymonline.com).

The idea of empathy as an aesthetic response to art was reinterpreted by early 20th-century psychologists with reference to an aesthetic response in the presence of another person (such as love, affection, or friendship). This was further instrumentalised in the context of psychoanalysis by treating empathy as a technique that could be learned. This allowed empathy to be treated as an essential attribute for medical psychoanalysts and lay psychotherapists and counsellors alike. This trend culminated in the work of Carl Rogers, as we noted above, who lionised empathy. The standard professional view was that the physician-analyst, therapist, or counsellor held large empathy capital (exercised in managing the transference), acting as a substitute 'good mother' or 'good father'. The patient or client was treated as being drained of empathy as they regressed to an infantile state. We still see this reflected in instances where medical students find themselves drained of their own natural empathy through participation in training that is formulaic, generalised, and divorced from the realities of patient care (Bleakley et al. 2011).

As much as there are many examples of individualist and trait-based empathy, including art appreciation and person-centred counselling, there are other perspectives. For instance, Alfred Adler not only invented what we now call 'social work', but also, well over a century ago, developed what we now refer to as 'relational empathy' (Eichbaum et al. 2023). Here empathy is not situated in a person but is a product of familial and social relationships. Adler called such a spirit of community *Gemeinschaftsgefühl* (literally 'social feeling', 'social interest', or 'community feeling', although there is no direct English word translation).

Towards compathy, a meta-empathy

Empathy can refer to both a cognitive state of identification with another ('I know what you mean') and an affective state of identification ('I feel for you, I've been through the same myself') (Bleakley 2014, 2015; Bleakley and Marshall 2017). Building on this, Jeffrey (2016) suggested that empathy is empty without action or intervention (a behavioural dimension) and is given authenticity by held values such as concern for others (a moral dimension). A disembodied cognitive state is perhaps better termed 'sympathy' than 'empathy', while in contrast an embodied affective state admits greater identification with another's condition (such as suffering) and can be more appropriately described as 'empathy'. However, we want to push deeper, and to that end we will develop the notion of 'empathy' into both a concept and a practice of 'compathy'.

While you are likely to be familiar with the terms 'sympathy' and 'empathy', 'compathy' may be new to you, described as 'a higher level of emotional maturity, which helps in achieving better quality care' (Kalra et al. 2024). Compathy can be understood as a meta-empathy, empathy that is reflexively and critically examined and interrogated by those who express it. While 'empathy' has its roots in the ancient Greek *em* and *pathos* (as *empatheia*) – respectively, 'in' and 'suffering', 'compathy' has its roots in the Latin *com* and ancient Greek *pathos* – respectively, 'with' and 'suffering'. Again, a physician expressing compathy is not simply aware of the emotional state of others (such as the suffering of patients or the grief of relatives), she also shares some of that emotional state through identification. Compathy is a more heightened, sensitive, and attuned experience than everyday empathy. It is an attunement that could benefit physicians and other healthcare professionals, for instance, when it affords better insights into the specific affective dynamics of their patients' conditions.

However, compathy could also require more of physicians than they are initially willing or able to invest in individual patient relationships (for instance, in high acuity and high turnover contexts such as emergency rooms). We do not argue therefore that empathy is insufficient, only that there is a continuum between empathy and compathy that healthcare professionals and educators need to traverse mindfully.

Like empathy, compathy too is a contested term – even though the notion has already been instrumentalised, where measurement of compathy is mooted (Kalra et al. 2024). Such instrumentalization affords a paradox where Kalra and colleagues (Kalra et al. 2024) (translating between Urdu and English) define the difference between empathy and compathy as: 'empathy means being able to put oneself in another's shoes, while compathy is the ability to feel another's emotions as if one is in the other's heart'. My scepticism about measurement is offset by my admiration of the poetic quality of definition in these clinician-authors' paper, where compathy is articulated through metaphor, not measurement. For example, the authors echo Morse and Mitcham's (1997; Morse et al. 1998) definition of compathy from nursing culture as 'the contagion of physical distress' (Kalra and colleagues give the example of a husband feeling compathy for a pregnant woman somatically and not just psychologically).

That 'compathy' can have a cost is reflected in the ground-breaking work of Morse and Mitcham (1997) (who claim to have coined the term) in describing, as noted above, what they call 'the contagion of physical distress'. Here, a person identifies so much with another person's physical distress that she feels similar bodily symptoms, even if they have not suffered from that illness (e.g., a nurse feeling pain in a leg as she cares for somebody who has broken a leg). The authors then call compathy 'the physical equivalent to empathy' (Morse and Mitcham 1997). However, this frames compathy instrumentally, where there is no apparent qualitative dimension. Nor is there reference to ethical and political (power) issues such as how a patient might feel as the care provider may appear to 'own' the patient's suffering herself, displacing ownership. Morse and Mitcham's use of 'compathy' can be read as contradictory in that it can be both a welcome relational quality and an unwanted interruption to the rhythm of care as the care giver inadvertently takes over the wheel of the cared for.

Bleakley (Bleakley 2014) introduced compathy into medical education in 2014, first describing the term as over-identifying with another's feeling states. Over time, this view has been revised, such that compathy is now understood as *authentic identification* with another's feeling states – a deepening and completion of empathy. Where Morse and Mitcham stressed physical identification or embodiment of empathy as the defining feature of compathy, Bleakley takes a broader view, where compathy describes any kind of *holistic* (complete, overlapping) cognitive and affective identification with another's state of being as an acknowledged sharing without imperialistic overtones. This recognises not only a political shift in values (a democratising of compathy) but also an ethical shift. Compathy affords a moral stance against potential colonising of another's being.

In a recent online article on compathy, Sofia Salazar (2020) summed up the differences between sympathy, empathy, and compathy as:

> A sympathetic person says, 'I see you're sad. I'm sorry your mom passed away.' An empathic person says, 'I see you're sad. I've lost someone too. I feel FOR you.' A compathic person says, 'Your sadness is my sadness. I feel WITH you.'

The *Shorter OED* does not have an entry for compathy, but the *Collins English Dictionary* (2019) does, and it is distinctly underwhelming: 'feelings, as happiness or grief, shared with another or others'. The online *Cambridge Dictionary* has a more vibrant and rather beautiful definition:

> The sharing of another person's feelings such as happiness, sadness, or pain. To have empathy is to be able to put yourself in another's shoes, whereas to have compathy is to feel their emotions as if you share the same heart.

This offers a clear distinction between empathy and compathy. To make clear that distinction, we need a metaphor ('heart'). As an example of use, the *Cambridge Dictionary* suggests 'In holistic nursing an advanced form of empathy is demanded, namely that of compathy'. The key descriptor here is 'holistic', returning to Bleakley's definition above. So, we might conclude that compathy again can be treated as a meta-empathy.

Distributed compathy

What empathy 'is' depends on the paradigm at hand. Neuroscience studies of empathy generation provide exact impersonal brain locations. In social psychology, sociology, human geography, or anthropology empathy is a product of social relationships, occupying the nexus of exchanges between persons. Here, we might see empathy and compathy as distributed phenomena, engaging several actors contextualised in habitats, and embracing shared languages and artefacts. In the discourses set up by these social accounts, compathy becomes dispersed, shared, negotiated, and contested. Each discipline viewpoint has developed its own rhetoric.

This shift from individual to social empathy (and here, as compathy) is commonly termed 'relational empathy' and comes from the work of Broome (1991) and later De Turk (2001) as a 'possibility for alliance building'. But surely all kinds of empathy are 'relational' by definition, as empathy is always shown to another or others? (At a stretch, I suppose that self-care can be seen as an introverted form of empathy or compathy). Returning to Alfred Adler well over a century ago, we can again directly equate 'fellow feeling' with 'relational empathy'. Indeed, the latter term directly echoes 'fellow feeling'. Russell Kirkscey (2018) published an article on relational empathy in the context of shared decision-making concerning bioethical dilemmas a year before Fagiano. Monika Betzler (2019) also describes the relational value of empathy as a value stance:

> Philosophers and scholars ... have long discussed the role of empathy in our moral lives. The distinct relational value of empathy, however, has been largely overlooked. ... Empathy is both intrinsically and extrinsically valuable in virtue of the pleasant experiences we share with others, the harmony and meaning that empathy provides, the recognition, self-esteem, and self-trust it enhances, as well as trust in others, attachment, and affection it fosters. Once we better understand in what ways empathy is a uniquely relational phenomenon, we can unveil its relevance to morality, which avoids the strictures of both partiality and impartiality.

Betzler argues that relational empathy is a condition of moral calling within a particular relationship. In other words, empathy is revisioned not specifically as a cognitive or affective identification, but as a moral call to action. Thus, 'To realize empathy's relational value, we are not constantly required to empathize', because, for example, friendship already implies a constant current of empathy. Betzler's model chimes with professionalism in medicine, where physicians are required to empathise as a duty of care, but this may result in an inauthentic empathy-by-numbers that Jane Macnaughton (2009) is so concerned with. This raises important questions about differences between empathy as a 'natural' response of compassion, and as a professional duty of care. It also raises the issue of why medical students need to be 'taught' empathy at all, given that empathy is a part of the human condition (or, that lack of empathy, for example in psychopaths, sociopaths, and narcissists, raises questions about what the 'human condition' means). The perceived need for such 'training' in empathy implies that there is a special kind of professional empathy exercised in medicine that must be learned – a rather dubious notion.

The same dynamics advertised by the three extracts above apply equally to compathy. Below, I further expand the meaning and practice (or activity) of compathy as it is displaced from individuals to become dispersed among social groupings or collectives as a political gesture – one involving power relationships. I emphasise the political nature of such situating of compathy as a problem of translation across cultures in healthcare settings shaped by power. Empathy and compathy afford capital – produced by emotional and cognitive labour – both used and abused through exchange and trade. For example, empathy is regularly commodified through communication skills training courses.

Empathy and compathy as affective capital

In common with other forms of labour-producing capital, Western/Northern hemisphere/high-income cultures have tended to act in imperialist ways in colonising low-income cultures' home-grown empathic and compathic labour. We call for a paradigm shift not just in our understanding of empathy and compathy, but also in our cross-cultural applications through medical and healthcare pedagogies. We inquire into issues of both translation and transaction between actors in cross-compathy exchanges. While these transactions are foregrounded in neo-colonial encounters between high-income and low-income countries, they happen too at a micro-level – for example within multi-disciplinary clinical teams, where, typically, medical professionals act as the coloniser while healthcare professionals such as nurses identify as the colonised (and often oppressed). This reflects not just in professional status, but also in income.

The dangers of exporting individualistic models to collectivist cultures

Despite the legacy of Alfred Adler's championing of 'fellow feeling' or 'social feeling', Western/global Northern psychology side-lines this model where individualism prevailed. The values complex behind individualism is Protestant-Capitalism – the two ideologies were tied by the sociologist Max Weber (1905) in *The Protestant Ethic and the Spirit of Capitalism*. This complex was fused with a masculine-heroic 'frontiersman' set of virtues that culminated in the birth of 'self-help' movements in the late 19th and early 20th centuries (Bleakley 2020). Protestant virtue demanded that individuals take responsibility for their own actions, where capitalism saw personality as a market commodity (hence, the birth of the 'snake oil' slick salesman and the development of the cult of personality in show business). The movement culminates in the 1980s UK Prime Minister Margaret Thatcher claiming that 'there is no such thing as society' (or there are only individuals in competition with one another).

A counter movement was developed in psychoanalysis in response to excessive individualism, based around bonding and attachment to the mother figure as the key factor in personality development (e.g., the work of Anna Freud, René Spitz, John Bowlby, and Donald Winnicott). As Alfred Adler (1929) said a century ago: 'it is also the mother who interests the infant in other people and enlarges its social circle'. This, however, was overshadowed by masculinist ego psychology that shaped personality theory after the Second World War and to this day infects medical cultures worldwide. Such a masculinist virtue ideology has also dominated post-war medical education. Despite the need for collaborative teamwork in healthcare, heroic masculine and strenuously individualist medicine has up to recently resisted interest in the mother (and feminism in general). For example, militaristic masculinist metaphors (conflict, and strife) – such as the 'war on cancer' – have dominated modern medicine, as opposed to feminine metaphors of inscribing patients through tender and nourishing care such as Hélène Cixous' (1976) 'writing in white ink', referring to a metaphorical 'writing' with mother's milk.

Because of this dominance of the individualist masculine-heroic value complex, empathy has been framed as personal capital, rather than a consequence of quality of interaction between persons and then shared capital. Empathy also became part of the capital of medicine (in the emergent arenas of 'communication skills' and 'patient-centred' practices) in the wake of Carl Rogers' work as noted earlier. However, a new era of medical education calls for a new paradigm of 'empathy'. This is signalled by two major shifts: first, from an autocratic medicine based on historical hierarchies (multi-professionalism) to democratic team process (inter-professionalism); and second, in the challenge to high-income Western/Northern hemisphere imperialism in the emergence of 'cultural crossings of care' (Kristeva et al. 2018) as a resistance movement.

As the transition from empathy to a more complex compathy demands reflexivity, so we note paradoxes engaging the political, such as exercise of empathy as an instrument of sovereign power. Seeing through, or reflecting on, such power issues in a collaborative setting gives birth to a reflexive and embracing compathy to displace a potentially manipulative empathy (e.g., showing care for others only to inflate one's own ego, or to gain advantage). Kristeva (personal communication 2018) notes how productive translations between caregivers and newly arrived immigrants in French psychiatric settings are impossible without reflexive political stances drawing on compathy. Here, potentially oppressive sovereign power is displaced by potentially productive capillary power in the employment of reflexive micro-mechanisms that sensitively adjust conversations, non-verbal communications, and allied semiotics in support of another.

The Western individualist model of empathy is not applicable to collectivist cultures and, where exported, offers a form of imperialism or neo-colonialism. This can lead to empathic 'dissonance' if not 'disjunction' (Eichbaum et al. 2023) and a lack of 'empathic accuracy' that can negatively impact patient care. Indeed, the tables can be turned on the neo-colonist where relational empathy is exported from low-income to high-income countries that have become increasingly multicultural. Here, the indigenous individualism of high-income countries may be tempered by a new-found subscription to collectivism and collaboration. Our template is clinical teamwork, found to be more effective in terms of quality of patient care, generation of patient safety, and increase in work satisfaction where democratic (collaborative or authentically inter-professional) practices are adopted (Bleakley 2014).

While a relational empathy can suggest a passive arrangement of mutual understanding and respect, this can be progressed where transactions and translations occur that expand activities or innovate. In this case, we can describe a 'translational' and 'transactional' compathy as noted above. We can also think of this again as a meta-empathy. Not only is empathy exercised at the higher level of compathy or distributed emotional identification – rather than cognitive empathy as understanding without identification – but it also has wider ramifications across cultural barriers.

Let us give an illustrative example. A young West African Islamic woman refugee suffering from persistent earache is initially assigned to a male doctor in a Paris clinic. She speaks little French and is wearing a headscarf. A male doctor arrives and makes signs for her to remove her headscarf and is irritated when she shows concern and refuses to do so. A West African female nurse happens to be working in the clinic and comes upon the scenario by chance. Sensing the young woman's frustration, she asks the increasingly irritated and exasperated doctor if she can help. He shows no concern for the patient and is focused only on the technical aspects of the investigation: it is after all just a simple examination of the ear. The nurse talks with the patient to reassure her and turns to the now irritated doctor to explain the cultural barrier. The doctor leaves, and a woman Islamic doctor is found who shows compathy, echoing the nurse. A translational and transactional cultural crossing is achieved, so that the activity of care can be expanded to include the patient's wishes. Nobody is compromised because nobody adopts 'sides', as compathy capital is distributed equally. The locus for compathy drifts from the individuals to the quality of their interactions, as a generative process and not a fixed quantity (as personal capital). Sovereign power transmutes into capillary power. This process has also been amply demonstrated in Cultural-Historical Activity Theory (CHAT) research, as expansive learning through 'boundary crossings' in cross-cultural settings (Kerosuo and Engeström 2003).

The male doctor failed to show professional empathy, never mind basic human concern beyond treating symptom. No context was then generated for promoting boundary crossings. As women collaborating, the nurse, woman doctor, and patient achieve insights into each other's worlds, and a supportive examination of the ear follows with a ready diagnosis and treatment – in this case, just a simple earwax removal. Importantly, the young woman is assured that she will not be culturally embarrassed in future visits and the patient assures the nurse and doctor that she now feels confident to trust public health services. Boundary crossings occurred, expanding the object of the activity system (as safe and caring treatment of the patient).

Educating for compathy in complex settings

Empathy – and then compathy – are best learned in medical education through work-based placements that offer exhaustive and reflexive collaborative debriefing. This can be called 'learning refractive practice' (Bleakley 1999). As noted in the Preface, where reflective practice describes consideration of one's actions either during or after events, reflexive practice describes gaining enduring insights from reflection, particularly concerning values that shape activities. Refractive practice takes reflective and reflexive activity from location in the individual to a product of social interaction. The 'refraction' occurs as each participant engaging in a social field finds that actions and values must be constantly refracted through a commonly agreed value complex such as 'democracy' or 'patient safety' in collaborative teamwork. Just as a stick plunged into water appears to bend, so individual contributions plunged into common activities will adapt to the democratic key. Key to engaging in (and with) refractive practice is compathy.

If we decide that we can teach and learn both cognitive and affective empathy, as clinical-communication skills courses in medical education routinely assume (McNally et al. 2023), we should be able to provide evidence for the outcomes of such learning. For example, evidence is routinely published for 'empathy decline' amongst medical students as they progress through an undergraduate course (McNally et al. 2023). But, again, such claims are made based on the measurement of a notion that we have already seen is complex, multifaceted, and slippery (even contradictory), where the measurement reifies the concept (again, empathy is what empathy scales measure). Can ostensibly validated instruments for measuring empathy – such as the Jefferson Scale of Empathy (JSE) (Hojat et al. 2001, Hojat et al. 2018) – be reliably applied to determine whether teaching and learning empathy has increased empathic capacity where the reliability and cross-cultural validity of the JSE has been questioned (Williams and Beovich 2020)? And how might we progress such measurement to 'compathy', as noted earlier? If empathy decline is indeed pervasive, what hope is there for compathy gain?

To address these dilemmas, we need a paradigm shift in how we both conceptualise and actualise patient care. We must shift from linear to complex models. A linear medicine is based on problem-solving and closure, where a complex medicine is based on problem-stating (or problematising) and tolerance of ambiguity. Here, compathy is a complex, open-ended state of being that is context sensitive. Compathy then embodies what Jacques Derrida (1974) describes as 'surplus' – where closure (such as definitive models) is impossible because both the concept and the experience of compathy are not just complex but dynamic. For example, as the dynamic system operates at the edge of chaos, it is in danger of falling into chaos, but also, it can spontaneously re-organise at higher levels of complexity.

Compathy acts as a strange, nonchaotic attractor for a variety of cognitive and affective phenomena. An analogous system would be the overall economy of a country determined by several interacting factors such as unemployment rates, level of inflation, and costs of borrowing. The ideal is to move to a stable condition, but the reality is that stability is relative, again as maximum complexity of the system at the edge of chaos. Compathy capital, as noted, is subject to lingering hierarchical systems in healthcare including the larger picture of neo-imperialism by high-income countries within a global market. We illustrate this below with an example of how 'obesity' is framed as an illness by medicine in high-income countries, riding rough-shod over competing views of obesity from low-income countries.

As a strange, nonchaotic attractor, compathy might re-organise at a higher level of complexity through, for example, radical democratisation of healthcare activity, including authentic patient-centredness. Such democratisation refuses imperialisms as it operates with a capillary or distributed power principle rather than a hierarchical sovereign power structure. Quality of compathy might both expand and intensify across a complex system, for example a healthcare team, due to alignment of several disparate practices such as briefing, debriefing, dialogue rather than monologue (e.g., asking questions rather than making statements), democratic division of labour, clarification of roles, and emergence of situational awareness (Allard et al. 2007, Bleakley et al. 2013). Compathy acts here as an inter-professional heuristic, where 'solutions' can be fluid, bootstrapped, and temporary, leading again to re-organisation of the system at a higher level of complexity. Problem stating is not overshadowed by problem-solving. Rather than 'teams' as complex interpersonal objects, we can think of 'teeming' as a process – here, effective communication is achieved through 'negotiated knotworking' and 'spearheads of innovation' (Engeström 2018).

Neologisms are important here because they introduce new concepts and innovative directions of thought and action. To again rehearse the model, compathy is conceptualised as a strange, nonchaotic attractor in an open, non-linear, dynamic, complex system that is constantly evolving or expanding, able to re-order at higher levels of complexity. The attractor is a state towards which the complex system tends to evolve that may or may not remain stable. The purpose of compathy is to maintain stability across relationships while generating the conditions for innovation towards horizons of possibility. These are horizons that, again, Derrida would describe as 'surplus' – a goal towards which a phenomenon is impelled as an ideal, but one necessarily without closure, or a finishing point. To draw on a hackneyed saying, the goal is not the destination but rather the journey itself. 'Democracy' is such a goal: an ideal, as a work always in progress. 'Compathy', as argued here, is another such phenomenon.

As an illustrative example of how complex translational compathy may work, we will draw on Emily Yates-Doerr's (2018) account of translating the notion of 'obesity' across cultures. Yates-Doerr highlights the dangers of medical neo-colonialism and the value of anthropological relativism and situated ethics as counters to such imperialistic gestures. Western/Northern hemisphere medicine is all too eager to export its model (and treatments) of 'obesity' as an illness globally. Such an approach to obesity is linear – there is a problem, let's find a solution (and then export it).

The commonly adopted pedagogical technique of problem-based learning (PBL) – first proposed in 1974 by Howard Barrows at Canada's McMaster University, but just a variation of John Dewey's methods from the early 1900s – has been commodified and marketed globally. But PBL is inappropriate, for example for Japanese medical students who are culturally conditioned to learn passively by formal instruction and are reluctant to study in collaboration with unfamiliar peers (Lin-Aung et al. 2022). Asian students in general appear to prefer passive, lecture-driven learning to active, small group work requiring high levels of participation (Khoo 2003).

Returning to Yates-Doerr's study, she adopts an anthropological approach that also (while she does not explicitly describe this) embraces complexity. For 'obesity' is a complex, culturally relative notion demanding culturally sensitive understandings and interventions. Western/Northern hemisphere medicalising of body shapes and eating habits – leading to standard 'treatments' – can be countered by cross-cultural insights that remain complex and dynamic, resisting 'one size fits all' problem-solving (in this case, literally, as overweight bodies are stigmatised). Rather, the notion of 'obesity' itself is problematised: for example, obesity as a symptom produced by cultural norms, food manufacturers, the advertising industry, and relatively low-income lifestyles (and then not a 'choice').

Yates-Doerr is not ignoring some very real somatic problems caused by over-eating and lack of exercise. Rather, as noted, she extends compathy to those who may suffer from poor diet because of structural inequities (such as poverty) for example. She gives an example from the 1970s in Amsterdam where Surinamese immigrants showed higher rates of obesity than other groups. A campaign was started to get these people to walk or cycle around the city centre in Amsterdam. However, most of the Surinamese had settled in a district on the outskirts of the city, 11 kilometres from the centre. It was thus unreasonable to suggest to this group that they should walk for exercise with a view to engaging with the civic life of the city centre.

Where anthropologists claim a more reflexive position on global health issues than physicians, medical education has listened, adopting the term 'translational competency' to describe the kinds of cross-cultural conundrums that Yates-Doerr describes. But she suggests that courses on translational competency in medical schools tend to pay lip-service to the notion of authentic cross-cultural empathies. Indeed, the unreflexive use of the term 'competence' advertises such inauthenticity. Just as empathy is superseded by the deeper form of compathy, so competence is superseded by 'capability' (see Chapter 9). 'Competence' literally means 'good enough', where capability implies a reaching for new horizons, or 'spearheads of innovation' (Engeström 2018).

While, considering the previous remarks, we would question her use of 'competency' here (rather than 'capability'), Yates-Doerr (2018) explains that:

> A premise of translational competency is that, because interactions are dynamic, it is simply not possible to communicate without transforming meanings. To be competent in translation is to maintain awareness of the necessary equivocation that happens in interactions, where people speak using terms that will not mean the same thing between speakers, and which do not, in fact, have fixed meanings at all.

Again, social compathy understood as both cognitive and affective *negotiated reality* in complex settings. As shifts from the linear to the complex and the individual to the collective are now well underway, so we encourage medical educators to engage with a paradigm shift from empathy to meta-empathy or compathy.

References

Adler A. 1929/1964. *Problems of Neurosis: A Book of Case Histories*. New York, NY: Harper & Row.

Allard J, Bleakley A, Hobbs A, Vinnell T. 2007. 'Who's on the team today?': The status of briefing amongst operating theatre practitioners in one UK hospital. *Journal of Interprofessional Care*. 21: 189–206.

Betzler M. 2019. The relational value of empathy. *International Journal of Philosophical Studies*. 27: 1–26.
Bleakley A. 1999. From reflective practice to holistic reflexivity. *Studies in Higher Education*. 24: 315–30.
Bleakley A. 2014. *Patient-Centred Medicine in Transition: The Heart of the Matter*. Dordrecht: Springer.
Bleakley A. 2015. *Medical Humanities and Medical Education: How the Medical Humanities Can Shape Better Doctors*. Abingdon: Routledge.
Bleakley A. 2020 *Medical Education, Politics, and Social Justice: The Contradiction Cure*. Abingdon: Routledge.
Bleakley A, Allard J, Hobbs A. 2013. 'Achieving ensemble': Communication in orthopaedic surgical teams and the development of situation awareness – An observational study using live videotaped examples. *Advances in Health Sciences Education*. 18: 33–56.
Bleakley A, Bligh J, Browne J. 2011. *Medical Education for the Future: Identity, Power and Location*. Dordrecht: Springer.
Bleakley A, Marshall R. 2017. *Re-juvenating Medical Education: Seeking Help from Homer*. Newcastle-Upon-Tyne: Cambridge Scholars Press.
Broome, B.J. 1991. Building shared meaning: Implications of a relational approach to empathy for teaching intercultural communication. *Communication Education*, 40, 235–49.
Cixous H. 1976. *The Laugh of the Medusa*. Chicago, IL: University of Chicago Press.
Derrida J. 1974. *Of Grammatology*. Baltimore, MD: Johns Hopkins University Press.
De Turk S. 2001. Intercultural empathy: Myth, competency, or possibility for alliance building? *Communication Education*. 50: 374–84.
Eichbaum Q, Barbeau-Meunier CA, White M, et al. 2023. Empathy across cultures– one size does not fit all: From the ego-logical to the eco-logical of relational empathy. *Advances in Health Sciences Education*. 28: 643–57.
Engeström Y. 2018. *Expertise in Transition: Expansive Learning in Medical Work*. Cambridge: Cambridge University Press.
Hall JA, Schwartz R. 2022. Empathy, an important but problematic concept. *Journal of Social Psychology*. 162: 1–6.
Hojat M, Mangione S, Nasca TJ, et al. 2001. The Jefferson scale of physician empathy: Development and preliminary psychometric data. *Educational and Psychological Measurement*. 61: 349–65.
Hojat M, DeSantis J, Shannon SC, et al. 2018. The Jefferson Scale of Empathy: A nationwide study of measurement properties, underlying components, latent variable structure, and national norms in medical students. *Advances in Health Sciences Education*. 23: 899–920.
Iacoboni M. 2009a. Imitation, empathy, and mirror neurons. *Annual Review of Psychology*. 60: 663–70.
Iacoboni M. 2009b. *Mirroring People: The Science of Empathy and How We Connect with Others*. New York, NY: Picador.
Jeffrey D. 2016. Empathy, sympathy and compassion in healthcare: Is there a problem? Is there a difference? Does it matter? *Journal of the Royal Society of Medicine*. 109: 446–52.
Kalra S, Selvan C, Rathore SK. 2024. Communicative compathy and chronic care. *Journal of the Pakistan Medical Association*. 74: 178–9.
Kerosuo H, Engeström Y. 2003. Boundary crossing and learning in creation of new work practice. *Journal of Workplace Learning*. 15: 345–51.
Khoo HE. 2003. Implementation of problem-based learning in Asian Medical schools and student's perceptions of their experience. *Medical Education*. 37: 401–4.
Kirkscey R. 2018. Bioethical communication: Shared decision-making and relational empathy. *Journal of Communication in Healthcare: Strategies, Media and Engagement in Global Health*. 11: 164–74.

Kristeva J, Moro M-R, Odemark J, Engebretsen E. 2018. Cultural crossings of care: An appeal to the medical humanities. *Medical Humanities*. 44: 55–8.

Kumagai AK. 2008. A conceptual framework for the use of illness narratives in medical education. *Academic Medicine*. 83: 653–8.

Lin-Aung H, Masumoto D, Linn Z, et al. 2022. Students' perception of problem-based learning at a Japanese medical school: An exploratory sequential mixed method. *International Journal of Medical Education*. 13: 322–34.

Lloyd M, Bor R, Noble LM. 2018. *Clinical Communication Skills for Medicine*. London: Elsevier.

McNally G, Haque E, Sharp S, Thampy H. 2023. Teaching empathy to medical students. *Clinical Teacher*. 20: e13557.

Macnaughton J. 2009. The dangerous practice of empathy. *Lancet*. 373: 1940–1.

Morse JM, Mitcham C. 1997. Compathy: The contagion of physical distress. *Journal of Advanced Nursing*. 26: 649–57.

Morse JM, Mitcham C, van der Steen WJ. 1998. Compathy or physical empathy: Implications for the caregiver relationship. *Journal of Medical Humanities* 19: 51–65.

Rogers C. 1951. *Client-centered therapy: Its current practice, implications and theory*. Boston, MA: Houghton-Mifflin.

Salazar S. 2020. There's Sympathy and Empathy, but Have You Heard of Compathy? Dec 26, 2020. Available at: https://medium.com/@sofia.salazar_55503/theres-sympathy-and-empathy-but-have-you-heard-of-compathy-d747981c3f3a. Last accessed: 09/11/2023.

Steuber K. 2019. Measuring empathy. *The Stanford Encyclopedia of Philosophy*.

Sulzer SH, Feinstein NW, Wendland CL. 2016. Assessing empathy development in medical education: A systematic review. *Medical Education*. 50: 300–10.

Veloski J, Hojat M 2006. Measuring specific elements of professionalism: Empathy, teamwork, and lifelong learning. In: D Stren (ed.) *Measuring Medical Professionalism*. New York, NY: Oxford University Press, Chap. 7.

Weber M. 1905/1930. *The Protestant Ethic and the Spirit of Capitalism*. London & Boston: Unwin Hyman.

Williams B, Beovich B. 2020. A systematic review of psychometric assessment of the Jefferson Scale of Empathy using the COSMIN Risk of Bias checklist. *Journal of Evaluation in Clinical Practice*. 26: 1302–15.

Yates-Doerr E. 2018. Translational competency: On the role of culture in obesity interventions. *Medicine Anthropology Theory*. 5: 106–17.

Part III

13 Metahumanities in medical education

A manifesto

Rachel Ellaway, Quentin Eichbaum, and Alan Bleakley

Metahumanities in medical education

What metahumanities are in the context of medical education has not previously been clearly articulated and here we collectively seek to address that gap in the literature. Throughout this book, we call for a shift in register in medical education – from a reductive instrumental frame to an expressive complex that embraces morality (ethics); qualities, beauty, and form (aesthetics); power (politics); and meaning (the transcendental). We argue that this transition to a meta-education involves the curriculum medium of the medical humanities. Our vision of the medical humanities also requires a shift in register, where metahumanities provide the pervasive media through which medical pedagogies are both refined and expanded for innovative gain.

'Metahumanism' is introduced in the opening chapter of this book. First mooted by Jaime del Val in 2002 and later refined in collaboration with Stefan Lorenz Sorgner (Del Val 2024a, b), 'metahumanism' refers to a philosophical stance that rejects the modernist and pervasive mind–body dualism of humanism and, as noted in Chapter 1, sits between the concepts of transhumanism (extending humans through technologies) and posthumanism (rejecting the authority and values of a traditional humanism – developed from the Renaissance through to High Modernity – that can privilege the human over other species).

As much as our thinking aligns with approaches to the humanities that seek to challenge and deconstruct hegemony and structural violence (Bleakley 2019, 2021), we do not see this as the only or the inevitable positioning of humanism. Indeed, we see a difference between ideological schemes to improve human nature and relativistic educational or pedagogic formulations that can raise the quality of life, such as Lev Vygotsky's concept of 'second stimulation'. For example, if we were worried about forgetting something, we might tie a knot as an aide-memoire. Another example is the alarm clock that provides a second stimulus for waking on time. These simple examples can be raised in value and complexity. An elaborate and complex second stimulus is the 'meta' process of critical reflection on any topic or issue, of which there are many illustrative examples throughout this book, to begin to see that topic or issue

DOI: 10.4324/9781032687339-17

differently, or 'slant'. If we tell you that seeing things 'slant' is derived – slantwise – from a term coined by the poet Emily Dickinson ('tell all the truth but tell it slant'), then Dickinson's poems themselves can become a second stimulus for the act of reflection. Poetry itself, as the medium *par excellence* for innovation and application of metaphor, reminds us of metaphors that by their very essence act as second stimuli (Bleakley 2017).

The medical metahumanities offer, and must embrace, a naturalistic perspective (humans as we are) rather than, solely, a normalistic perspective (humans as we should be), as both Sorgner and de Val have proposed. Not only must medical metahumanities be inclusive of difference, but also we must strive for realisation of potential – humans as they could be if certain chronic social, familial, and cultural conditions were addressed. For instance, John Heron (1977) provided a typology of such vulnerabilities, grounded in emotional life, that offers a catalogue of pedagogic formulations to improve human life: the need to love and be loved; the need to understand and be understood; and the need to be self-directing and to be freely engaged with the directions of a greater whole. This is ground zero for medical metahumanities.

Our everyday life involves frustrations, distortions, and perversions of these natural human impulses, largely grounded in systemic inequities and inequalities, but also bound with upbringing and education. A medical metahumanities can address these distortions as part of the overarching aim of medicine to address suffering while doing no harm, knowing also that physicians cannot wish away or deny the diseases, traumas, and suffering of their patients. Medical humanism must embrace the fact that medicine is an impossible task, aiming to maintain health in the face of inevitable suffering and mortality. Indeed, we would argue that medicine has hampered its primary task by adopting an apolitical stance in the face of inequity and injustice that contributes to ill-health. While Sorgner and del Val rejected traditional humanism as irredeemably flawed and therefore to be rejected, medicine cannot do this. The 'meta' in medical metahumanities is not above the human condition.

The work of metahumanities in medical education is not just expansive but is largely – like the work of psychoanalysis – one of lifting repression to realise a potential. An instrumental initial medical education can be seen to progressively de-sensitise students to create emotional insulation, loss of empathy, and creeping cynicism. It attempts to defuse resistance and the production of identities of resistance through conformist subscription to a professional code – an ideological interpellation into mainstream medical culture. It resists both democratisation (through maintenance of hierarchy) and feminising (through continuing masculine domination). It refuses to educate for psychotherapeutic capability that could improve communication potential with both patients and colleagues while improving self-care in the face of an epidemic of burnout. In this respect, students do not learn adequate tolerance of ambiguity (or negative capability). A primary medical metahumanities curriculum intervention aims to correct such a systematic miseducation to reveal a more potent pedagogy.

There are other ideas that we can draw on in the work of both Sorgner and del Val. For instance, Sorgner (2015) argued that 'genetic enhancement by modification and education are structurally analogous processes' mirroring arguments that Rachel Ellaway made in her chapter 9 on augmentation. However, Sorgner (2015) was particularly interested in how 'the categorical distinction between genetic and environmental influences will dissolve' and how posthumanist and transhumanist perspectives will be integrated into curricula. This suggestion is, we think, well-aligned with medical metahumanities in that it seeks to understand the many ways in which humans can be changed or change themselves, and from the expanding varieties and identities of the individuals and populations for which medicine is responsible. Indeed, we may need new ways to think about wellness, harm, and healing from such a perspective.

Del Val (2024b) argued that metahumanism has two main principles. One is to 'stop being the planet's pandemic' whose radical version would include stopping human reproduction, embracing 'radical veganism', care of self, and ambient resistance. The other was to 'mutate reinventing our movement' that embraces neurodiversity and non-rational thinking. To some extent, his manifestos reflect a particularly European, radical antagonistic relationship with power and society, but his work does nevertheless illustrate the deliberate expansion and variance in human experience, and to an extent it parallels the ancient principle of *primum non nocere* as well as more contemporary pushes towards the inclusion of planetary health in medical education programmes (Bleakley 2021, Luo et al. 2022).

Essentially, medicine (and therefore medical humanities and metahumanities) cannot reject old and conventional humanisms. However, medicine and medical humanities can engage with the shifting ground of humanism, which has moved from a Renaissance interest in selfhood as an aesthetic project towards a Protestant-Capitalist sense of selfhood as private – indeed private property – properly challenged by models of democratic collaboration. This modernist project has in turn been challenged by the postmodern notion that self is made in the image of the Other. The culmination of this thinking is that the Other is environmental destruction created by humanity and so self must be re-made in the mirror of this realisation. As we have noted, the fallout of this within medical education is to shift the axis of interest from downstream hospital-based care to upstream community and primary care with a focus on prevention and management of chronic illness.

Medicine and medical education find themselves in the paradoxical position of both supporting and rejecting traditional humanisms. While person-centred care is grounded in classical humanism, medicine also provides many of the mechanisms that afford the pursuit of posthuman and transhuman goals and identities. These include the promise of immortality (realistically, life extension), invulnerability (such as that afforded by vaccines and the survivability of erstwhile fatal conditions such as aneurisms and cancers), and the multitude of medical augmentations (such as drugs, prostheses, transplants, and relational care). This, together with a response to the health fallout from climate disaster and mass migrations.

We can learn from interactions with philosophical concepts of metahumanities without subscribing to the ideology or its more radical agendas. We also acknowledge that it would be easy to get lost in Wittgensteinian word games with all these conflicting meanings and intents of 'human' and 'humanism' and of meta and its implications, so let us be clear what we do mean. First, we note the tension between humanism and the humanities. Humanism is a Western European concept that emerged in the Renaissance (Italian *umanista*) as a reaction to scholastic domination of society and an assertion of principles of human rights and the integrity of self-determination. In doing so, the focus of authority shifted from the Bible to ancient Greek and Roman scholars, and it retained and was often used to champion white, male, and cis-het supremacies and the pursuit of aggressive capitalism and European empire building, while allowing slavery, economic and military oppression, and many other ills to continue and even flourish. The humanism project was completed by Immanuel Kant's (1784) essay 'An Answer to the Question: What is the Enlightenment?' in which the philosopher asked humans to grasp the opportunity to release themselves from the dogmatic authority of both Church and State to form an identity of resistance that signals the birth of the modern 'self' (Schmidt 1996).

As much as traditional humanism diffused in the face of the withering critiques of deconstructive postmodernism thought (reconstructive postmodernism however retained interest in humanism [e.g., Jencks 1996]), contemporary humanism is still positioned in opposition to theist philosophies and aligned with the broad (and vague) pursuits of human rights. Whatever its moral authority, the centring of responsibility in the individual reflects broader Nietzschean existential concerns of liberalism and scepticism to orthodoxy and established authority. It is difficult therefore to assert a humanistic position without invoking and aligning with its historical implications. But metahumanism for contemporary medical education must critically address the historical project of humanism. We have done this throughout this book and will summarise our efforts by providing a manifesto for metahumanities in medical education.

Metahumanities in medical education: a manifesto

How then does medical metahumanities differ from medical humanities? As noted throughout this book, Bleakley (2023) suggests a shift in register from a dominant instrumentalist perspective (the medical humanities as means-end) to embrace a range of values: ethical, aesthetic, political, and transcendental (meaning). This shift constitutes the 'meta'. It directly mirrors TS Eliot's notion of a progression from 'Information' through 'Knowledge' to 'Wisdom'. 'Wisdom' is a loaded word however, and we prefer 'Meaning'.

We have discussed many 'meta' issues in this book, including (but not limited to) metaphor, metacognition, metaphysics, metacapability, meta-heuristics, and meta-affect. As a prefix in ancient Greek 'meta' referred to above, after, and beyond. But, as Bleakley argues in Chapter 2, 'meta is not just higher, but deeper and wider'. Moreover, these are spatial concepts and 'meta' can just as readily refer to time, as transcending ordinary perceptions of time. We see this illustrated throughout the book with reference to Andy Clark's (2023) notion of cognition as predictive – living just ahead of ourselves in time or 'surfing uncertainty' to use Clark's metaphor. Contemporary meanings situate 'meta' as a prefix referring to that which it sits 'above' – metalinguistics is the linguistics of linguistics. There is a sense of a recursion, of abstraction, and of logical and conceptual testing of the integrity of something by applying its methods to itself. As an example, in medical education, Ritz and colleagues (2014) critiqued the pursuit of social accountability on the basis that its espoused values were not applied in its development, effectively an act of meta-social accountability. Meta can also be used as an adjective; to say that something is 'meta' is to suggest it is self-referential and abstracting in doing so. To be meta is to consider underlying principles and commonalities, to reflect on the nature of something and how it is understood.

'Meta' might be applied differently by considering 'metamedical' humanities. This would involve applying the tenets of medicine to itself, which could include the nature of health (human, other species, and collectively as planetary health), the diagnosis and healing of the ills of medicine and medical education, and the examination of the profession's understandings and applications of ethics, professionalism, and autonomy. Better that we apply the tenets of pedagogy to contemporary medical education where we find a host of symptoms shaped by linear instrumentalism as noted throughout this book. To rehearse the key symptoms again: medicine promises to educate for sensibility but produces insensibility; linearity is preferred to complexity and certainty to tolerance of uncertainty, even though clinical practice is patently complex and ambiguous; syllabus (as content) is mistaken for curriculum (as process); downstream (hospital based) work experience is privileged over upstream (community based) work experience; there is failure to educate for psychotherapeutic acumen and self-care and for authentic inter-professional teamwork grounded in democratic habits.

In terms of the scope of medical metahumanities, as we have set out through this volume, this is much wider, inclusive, and holistic than an understanding of the humanities as equivalent to the 'liberal arts'. Medical metahumanities would reintegrate topics that are part of a wider reading of the humanities such as those of philosophy, law, the study of faith and religion, and the philosophy of science. We also argue for medical metahumanities to be inclusive of politics and economics – professions that have stood aside from such matters to remain 'clean' of the taints of being involved have simply subjected themselves to being dominated by local and national political and economic philosophies.

We do not exclude science and technology from medical metahumanities. Indeed, we have appealed to neurological and psychological sources as often as to literary and philosophical ones in this volume. We note several key reasons why medical metahumanities must include the sciences. First is the ongoing relationship between medicine and science and the deep (but neither uniform nor exclusive) immersion of medicine in the cultures of biomedical and post-positivist philosophies of science. If these are not a part of medical metahumanities, then how can the very basis of much that constitutes contemporary medicine be examined and how can it be integrated with all the other concerns medical metahumanities embrace?

Second, medical metahumanities need to encompass the ways that scientific medicine changes and diversifies the identities and pursuits of humanity. For example, the transhumanist and posthumanist movements we described earlier are dependent on medical and scientific advances. Third is that medical metahumanities need to make a meaningful contribution to medicine and medical education and as such must legitimately participate in the spaces in which medicine and medical education are conceptualised and enacted.

The title of our book – *Metacognition, Metahumanities, and Medical Education: Thinking Without the Box* – brings focus on our manifesto for medical metahumanities. We have been particularly concerned with how trends in metacognition and metahumanities progress medical education (and not 'medicine' per se). Our focus is therefore primarily pedagogical. Below, we set out 10 organising principles of metahumanities in medical education, as manifesto:

1 To respect foundational human needs: to understand and be understood, love and be loved, and to be self-directing and freely engaged with the directions of a greater whole (metahumanities are thus inclusive of human experience, and respectful towards the individual and the variant as well as the collective and normative)
2 To raise value concerns from the reductive instrumental and economic to embrace the ethical, aesthetic, political, and transcendental
3 To engage science and technology in consilient, translational and participatory conversation with arts, humanities, and qualitative social sciences
4 To be curriculum-focused (as process) rather than syllabus-focused (as content), where curricula are treated as differing texts – such as the historical, political, aesthetic, ethical, and so forth
5 To facilitate learning-to-learn that goes beyond brain-cognition towards the extended mind and the application of cognitive extensions through artefacts.
6 To promote learning across cognitive, affective, intuitive, and psychomotor domains
7 To note that curriculum shapes identities and these may be identities of resistance
8 To promote curricula that promise integration and holism, uniting mind, body, social, technical, and existential experience and knowledge
9 To cherish innovation, where curricula are transformative, adaptive and expansive, encompassing the many ways of being human and as such encompassing the possibilities as well as the limitations of the human condition
10 To place critical reflexivity at the core of learning

These ten points can collectively form a foundation for the development of a new wave of values-based medical humanities in medical education that is patient-centred and humane but does not subscribe to outdated models of humanism-as-personalism where the individual is lionised and humans are seen as the crown of creation. We envisage new democratic structures for medical humanities in medical education in which ontologies of humans and artefacts are not arranged hierarchically, but horizontally and collaboratively. Here, objects have (or should have) voices, as detailed in Actor-Network Theory (ANT) (Latour 1996) and Object-Oriented Ontology (OOO) (Harman 2018). In an era in which the voice of persons has been reduced to one of linearity and the functional or instrumental in medical education, we see metahumanities restoring human potential through proliferation of values perspectives as these apply to medical pedagogies.

Specifically, we see a future for such enriched medical pedagogies as expressions of curricula as texts (ethical, political, aesthetic, and transcendental) as detailed in the body of work that is the 'curriculum reconceptualisation' movement (Pinar 2019). We do not explore that horizon in this book. What we have done here is to remind readers of the enormous potential of humanity, especially in collaborative work and utilising extensions of cognition through artefacts. This potential can be released without a shift from a carbon-based to a silicon-based lifeform largely because humans – while relatively restricted cognitively in relation to the potential for artificial intelligence, have enormous potential to develop their overall body–mind through three channels: emotional life (affect), intuitive life (and the imagination), and registers of language (particularly metaphor). Let's go to work!

References

Bleakley A. 2017. *Thinking With Metaphors in Medicine: The State of the Art*. Abingdon: Routledge.

Bleakley A. 2019. Invoking the Medical Humanities to Develop a #MedicineWeCanTrust. *Academic Medicine*. 94: 1422–4.

Bleakley A. 2021. *Medical Education, Politics and Social Justice: The Contradiction Cure*. Abingdon: Routledge.

Bleakley A, 2023. *Medical Humanities: Ethics, Aesthetics, Politics*. London: Routledge.

Clark A. 2023. *The Experience Machine: How Our Minds Predict and Shape Reality*. London: Allen Lane.

Del Val J. 2024a. Metahumanist Manifesto: its genealogy, evolution and relevance 10 years after. Author's website: https://metabody.eu/metahumanist-manifesto-10-years-after/. Last accessed: 5 Feb 2024.

Del Val J. 2024b. Metahumanism. Author's website: https://metabody.eu/metahumanism/ Last accessed: 5 Feb 2024.

Harman G. 2018. *Object-Oriented Ontology: A New Theory of Everything*. London: Pelican.

Heron J. 1977. *Catharsis in Human Development*. Guilford: University of Surrey.

Jencks C. 1996. *What Is Post-Modernism?* (4th ed.). London: John Wiley.

Latour B. 1996. On actor-network theory: A few clarifications. *Soziale Welt*. 47: 369–81.

Luo OD, Wang H, Velauthapillai K, Walker C. 2022. An approach to implementing planetary health teaching in medical curricula. *Canadian Medical Education Journal*. 13: 98–100.

Pinar W. 2019. *What is Curriculum Theory?* (3rd ed.). London: Routledge.

Ritz SA, Beatty K, Ellaway RH. 2014. Accounting for social accountability: Developing critiques of social accountability within medical education. *Education for Health*. 27: 152–7.

Schmidt J. (ed.) 1996. *What is Enlightenment? Eighteenth-Century Answers and Twentieth-Century Questions*. Berkeley, CA: University of California Press.

Sorgner SL. 2015. The future of education: genetic enhancement and metahumanities. *Journal of Evolution and Technology*. 25: 31–48.

Index

Pages in *italics* refer to figures and pages in **bold** refer to tables.

Made in the USA
Las Vegas, NV
19 September 2026

272f8235-ae89-47bd-a1cf-60f6e5c4f06eR02